'In this book Professor Jelinek details the path for recovery from Multiple Sclerosis and in doing so provides the blueprint for managing modern chronic illness.'
DR SAM GARTLAND, MB ChB BSc (Hons) MRCP (UK) FRACGP, Australia

'If you are a skeptic, read this book with an open mind, and you might just discover that overcoming multiple sclerosis is possible. If you are already a believer in lifestyle disease management, then get ready to be inspired.'
JANINE STASIOR, Ph.D., M.S., ABPdN, Board Certified Pediatric Neuropsychologist, Child Development Network Inc., Lexington MA, USA

'For people living with MS, or their families, this is the book you need to read. Through reading it you will take hope—a lot of hope—not just from inspiring stories of recovery, but from a mountain of research all pointing in the same direction. There is much you can do to change for the better the course of MS and your life by following Professor Jelinek's OMS program. These 7 steps are the essential management of MS although it may take the wider medical profession another generation or two to catch up to that fact.'
ASSOCIATE PROFESSOR CRAIG HASSED, Department of General Practice, Monash University, Australia

'This book has proved a life line. When I was first diagnosed with multiple sclerosis it made such a difference to have a template to live. Now 22 years on after my first MS episode I have remained relatively unscathed and here is the revised edition to provide me with the inspiration to maintain my cognition and an opportunity to confront the risks that come with a MS in the long term. Through *Overcoming Multiple Sclerosis* I have been given back a rich and blessed life that felt so close to being torn away. Thank you.'
DR HEATHER KING, general practitioner, New Zealand

'George Jelinek's book is the Science, Art and Heart of Multiple Sclerosis. It provides a mountain of evidence showing his 7 step "total change of life, for life" program gives people with MS real hope of leading a normal, healthy life.'
PROFESSOR ROB MOODIE, AM, Professor of Public Health, Melbourne School of Population and Global Health, Australia

'We once believed the earth was flat and it took a brilliant mind and a very long time before the world understood this was not the case. My one hope is that the world of Neurology and Medicine is much quicker to catch on to the brilliance of the many minds whose research has been summarised here in simple terms by Prof Jelinek for everyone to understand.'
DR JOANNE SAMER, MB. BS, Post Grad Dip Health Sciences, GAICD, Australia. Living well with MS since 1991.

'This is the book everyone diagnosed with MS should read! As a clinical psychologist and as a person diagnosed with MS, I cannot recommend it highly enough.'
DR RACHAEL HUNTER, BA (Hons), MSc, DClin Psychol, UK

'I am a super sceptical medical doctor with MS and I had the great good fortune to be given George Jelinek's *Taking Control of MS* 15 years ago. It was the best gift ever and the concepts and recommendations were a revelation to me. The information was all based on sound scientific evidence and that made it easy to accept and embrace the recommended lifestyle factors. The only side effects were better health. The new edition is extensively updated and we need to disseminate the enclosed valuable the information widely to our fellow MSers and educate our medical colleagues that there is hope of recovery.'
DR VIRGINIA BILLSON, pathologist, Melbourne, Australia

'Professor George Jelinek distils years of experience as a clinician-researcher to provide people with MS with a tool to navigate the vast array of information in the scientific and lay press to make informed decisions about their health. He does not profess to have all the answers but his approach offers measured hope and optimism for people with MS.'
DR PETER VAN WIJNGAARDEN, Principal Investigator, Centre for Eye Research Australia

2 433689 21

'A lot of people glibly refer to patient-empowerment and self-management as if it was easy for everyone with multiple sclerosis to do and know how to do. *Overcoming Multiple Sclerosis* is a self-help guide that will not only empower people living with MS, but act as a manual on how they should manage their disease and their life, written by a person with medical knowledge and a personal story to tell makes the book more authentic. I would have no hesitation in recommending it to my patients, but also to my friends and colleagues. This book is not just about living with a disease, but it sets out a philosophy of how to live your life, be an active participant in decisions about your health and it makes you think very deeply about wellness. Being self-disciplined is clearly one of George Jelinek's strengths and not everyone will have his self-discipline nor the desire to follow all of his recommendations. But the inspiration you will get from reading this book is that you, yes you, could also set-out on a journey of empowerment and change the way you live for the better. Tomorrow, today will be yesterday; there is no time like now to start living differently.'

PROFESSOR GAVIN GIOVANNONI, MBBCh, PhD, FCP (S.A., Neurol.), FRCP, FRCPath, Chair of Neurology, Blizard Institute, Barts and The London School of Medicine and Dentistry

'George Jelinek's *Overcoming Multiple Sclerosis* is a remarkable and unique book. Born of his harsh personal experience of multiple sclerosis, it offers sound scientific evidence-based advice to optimise the chances of people with MS leading a normal healthy life. *Overcoming Multiple Sclerosis* combines hard scientific evidence with practical advice and compassion. It will be of benefit to nearly everybody affected by MS and I heartily recommend it.'

DR PETER FISHER, FRCP, Physician to Her Majesty Queen Elizabeth II, and Director of Research, Royal London Hospital for Integrated Medicine

'Fifty years ago my wife was diagnosed with MS and I was told by her neurologist what her future would be. At first I lied to her, in order not to take her hope away, until I realized lying would not solve her problem. It was at that time that I began exploring the field of holistic medicine and learning from physicians like George. She is still by my side today. Yes, she has some effects of the disease but has also far exceeded the predictions made decades ago. So take the challenge and understand it is not about failing but about participating in one's life, exceeding expectations and taking responsibility for your own health and well-being.'
BERNIE SIEGEL, MD, author of *The Art of Healing* and *Love, Medicine & Miracles*, USA

'As a Pediatrician who has been controlling his MS for 21 years, I wholeheartedly recommend this book for all people with MS. Diet and lifestyle changes offer enormous potential in facilitating recovery from this illness.'
JOHN HOVIOUS, MD, USA

'Professor Jelinek is inspirational in his approach to empower patients to take control of their multiple sclerosis and responsibility for the management of their disease. His holistic approach encouraging patients to consider more than just a pharmaceutical approach to the disease has proven itself as the modern approach to the management of multiple sclerosis. This is a book that all patients with multiple sclerosis should read and use as a platform for discussion with their neurologist.'
DR PETER L SILBERT, MBBS (Hons) FRACP, Neurologist, Perth Neurophysiology, Australia

'I cannot recommend this book highly enough whether you are diagnosed with MS, a support person or a medical professional. Through his work and research George Jelinek changes the paradigm of managing MS. Based on scientific evidence and a deep understanding of the mind body connection this book provides the tools to take your health and wellbeing back into your own hands.'
DR. MED. MIRIAM NEATBY, Berlin, Germany

'This book, written by a professor of medicine, himself a person with MS, gives a lot of information on dietary treatment and supplementation with vitamin D, to prevent an unfavourable course of this extremely multi-facetted disease. The work is actually a scientific one which is written, however, in a non-specialist language. The book should be on the shelf of anyone with MS, and others interested in this subject.'

KLAUS LAUER, MD, Assistant Professor, Department of Neurology, Klinikum Darmstadt, Germany

'A must read for people diagnosed with multiple sclerosis, their doctors, and family members. Professor Jelinek provides a comprehensive summary of the evidence supporting a lifestyle approach to living well with multiple sclerosis and gives clear guidelines about what people with multiple sclerosis can do to optimise their health.'

PROFESSOR ANNE KAVANAGH, University of Melbourne, Australia

'Every person with MS should have access to this information and the support of their family, doctors, and all health care providers to implement it.'

DR ANNETTE CARRUTHERS, general practitioner, NSW, Australia

'Many people with MS are made to feel like their illness is a mystery and not much can be done. This book provides the evidence based proof that taking that view is not only wrong, it's also misleading. Professor George Jelinek's thoroughly researched program not only demonstrates that recovery from MS is possible, it's actually pretty straight forward.'

SHANNON HARVEY, director and producer, *The Connection* documentary, Australia

2ND EDITION

PROFESSOR GEORGE JELINEK MD

OVERCOMING MULTIPLE SCLEROSIS

The evidence-based 7 step recovery program

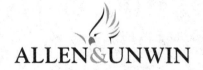

ALLEN&UNWIN

First published in Great Britain in 2016 by Allen & Unwin

First published in Australia in 2016 by Allen & Unwin

Allen & Unwin
c/o Atlantic Books
Ormond House
26–27 Boswell Street
London WC1N 3JZ
Phone: 020 7269 1610
Fax: 020 7430 0916
Email: UK@allenandunwin.com
Web: www.allenandunwin.co.uk

A CIP catalogue record for this book is available from the British Library.

Trade Paperback ISBN 978 1 76029 319 2
E-Book ISBN 978 1 95253 374 7

Internal design by Midland Typesetters
Internal illustrations by Tor Ercleve
Index by Puddingburn
Set in 11/14 pt Berkeley by Midland Typesetters, Australia
Printed in Great Britain by Bell & Bain Ltd, Glasgow.

10 9 8 7 6 5

For Eva Jelinek
1923–1981

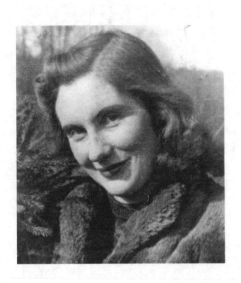

CONTENTS

LIST OF TABLES
AND FIGURES

TABLES

FIGURES

ACRONYMS AND ABBREVIATIONS

ACNEM	Australasian College of Nutritional and Environmental Medicine
ALA	alpha-linolenic acid
ARMS	Action for Research into Multiple Sclerosis
BBB	blood–brain barrier
BDNF	brain-derived neurotrophic factor
BMI	body-mass index
CAMS	Cannabinoids in MS (study)
CIS	Clinically Isolated Syndrome
CNS	central nervous system
CoQ10	Coenzyme Q10
CSEP	Canadian Society for Exercise Physiology
CSF	cerebrospinal fluid
CT	computerised tomography
CV	curriculum vitae
DHA	docosahexanoic acid
DHQ	Diet Habits Questionnaire
DMD	disease-modifying drug

DRI	dietary reference intake
EAE	experimental auto-immune encephalomyelitis
EBV	Epstein-Barr Virus
ECTRIMS	European Committee for Treatment Research in Multiple Sclerosis
ED	emergency department
EDSS	Expanded Disability Status Scale
EPA	eicosapentanoic acid
GDP	gross domestic product
HHV-6	human herpes virus 6
HOLISM	Health Outcomes and Lifestyle Interventions in a Sample of people with Multiple Sclerosis (Study)
HSCT	Haematopoietic stem cell transplantation
IFN	interferon
Igs	immunoglobulins
IL	interleukin
IOM	Institute of Medicine (US)
IPAQ	International Physical Activity Questionnaire
IRIS	immune reconstitution inflammatory syndrome
IV	intravenous
IVIgs	Intravenous immunoglobulins
JCV	John Cunningham Virus (or JC Virus)
M-G	mitoxantrone followed by glatiramer
MBP	myelin base protein
MBSR	mindfulness-based stress reduction
MitoQ	Mitoquinone
MP	methylprednisolone
MRI	magnetic resonance imaging
MS	multiple sclerosis
MSQOL-54	MS Quality of Life-54 (questionnaire)
NARCOMS	North American Research Committee on Multiple Sclerosis
NGF	nerve growth factor
NHMRC	National Health and Medical Research Council (Australian)
NICE	National Institute for Health and Care Excellence (UK)
OCT	optical coherence tomography

OMS	Overcoming Multiple Sclerosis
PML	progressive multifocal leukoencephalopathy
PMR	progressive muscle relaxation
PPMS	primary progressive MS
PRT	progressive resistance training
PSA	prostate-specific antigen
PwMS	people with MS
RA	rheumatoid arthritis
RDA	recommended daily (or dietary) allowance
REP	Rest–Exercise Program
RIS	radiologically isolated syndrome
REM	rapid eye movement
SLE	systemic lupus erythematosus
SPMS	secondary progressive multiple sclerosis
STOP-MS	STudying Outcomes of People attending MS retreats
T1D	type 1 diabetes
T2D	type 2 diabetes
TNF	tumour necrosis factor
TRIGR	Trial to Reduce IDDM in the Genetically at Risk
UL	upper level (or upper intake level)
VZV	varicella-zoster virus

PREFACE

I leant over and kissed her on the cheek. She was already cold. Strangely, I couldn't feel sad—only overwhelming relief. Relief that the suffering had finally stopped. Relief that Mum wouldn't have to fight any more.

So this is how it ends, I thought. The insidious tentacles of multiple sclerosis (MS) had taken sixteen years to pull her down, but they couldn't beat her in the end. Mum had chosen to take her own life rather than get any worse, rather than be completely degraded.

She looked so peaceful. I had kissed her goodnight the previous night, not knowing it would be the last time I would see her alive. What must she have been going through? To have been so brave right to the end, to have not let on as she said goodnight to the most precious parts of her life for the last time. I felt my eyes misting, but no tears would come. We had all known this was coming for a long time. Most of us had already grieved while she was alive. But now it was real. The image of me sitting there alone on her bed will stay with me forever.

How could I know that, eighteen years later, I would be sitting in a neurologist's office some 7 kilometres away, listening but not listening as he was trying to tell me I had MS? I would not let myself hear what he was saying. When it did hit me, all the memories of Mum came flooding back. I relived the gradual deterioration, the descent into paralysis, the indignity of urinary catheters and bedpans, the loneliness and frustration. And it was going to happen again. To me.

I don't know when I resolved that it wouldn't. Things just seemed to lead me down a path where answers kept turning up—real answers. Now, approaching two decades of good health, relapse-free, I am confident about my future, and also about the possibilities for others diagnosed with this illness.

How old was Mum when she got MS? I don't know. Perhaps 42 or 43. One night Mum was on her way to a night shift when she had a car crash that landed her in the Intensive Care Unit at Royal Perth Hospital. That's when it started. A few months later, Mum started dropping things. Soon there were doctors' appointments and tests, but the real significance of what was happening still didn't sink in. Until she began to deteriorate.

At first it was just the occasional stumble. I can't remember when she went into a wheelchair. Modifications started appearing around the house: shower rails, showering chair, ramp up the front stairs. The car was modified too. More and more, as time went on, when I'd come home for the night I would catch Mum looking at me from her wheelchair with a tear in her eye. You knew, when she had that look, that the big things in life were going through her mind: loss, separation, death, the burden she felt she was. This was her recurring theme: she was adamant she wouldn't be a burden to anyone. It was also one of my first thoughts when I was told I had MS.

I could see the neurologist's lips moving, but I couldn't hear anything. It was a beautiful late Sunday afternoon in Perth. The light was coming through the leaves from a low angle, firing them up with late autumn colour. In an instant, my whole world had changed. I was not to know it, but I would never feel the same way about life again, and my orderly, seemingly successful life would soon fall apart.

'It's not the worst thing I could be telling you right now,' I heard as if in some sort of dream. It certainly felt like the worst. We were suddenly talking about me having a magnetic resonance imaging (MRI) scan that night at the hospital. He was ringing the radiologist. All I could think of was my family. My daughter was only seven. All the plans I had, all the aspirations. Suddenly a big hand had reached into my life and taken away my future. And inexorably altered that of my family.

On the outside, I was calm and grateful that he had taken up so much of his valuable Sunday afternoon to see me and make the diagnosis. Inside, I was numb. Why hadn't I realised that I had MS? I now know that it is many times more common in family members, but somehow I had just assumed that lightning wouldn't strike twice. Not me!

One morning at work, I noticed that the shoelace on my left shoe kept falling down into my shoe. But every time I looked for it, it was no longer there. As the day wore on, the feeling of something being there became more and more marked. By the next day, it was a feeling of numbness—like having been to the dentist—over all the toes of my foot. By now I was starting to remark on how odd it was. By the next day, it had spread up the outside of my lower leg. I was getting nervous. Being an emergency physician, I am not prone to panicking. I started thinking about all the possibilities. A slipped disk? I had had back problems for years, but swimming regularly had fixed that. Some unusual peripheral neuropathy? I let it go for another day, but by the Thursday I knew I was in trouble. The numbness was progressing pretty rapidly all the way up the leg, and around my backside. I hardly slept that night. The next morning I had a colleague from the emergency department (ED) look at me. I spent an anxious hour or two waiting in x-ray while another friend tried to squeeze me into the burgeoning Friday queue for the MRI.

To my surprise, there was nothing there. But what you find depends on where you look, and they looked for a slipped disk and missed the MS lesion two levels higher. I found this really puzzling. On the Sunday, I asked a neurologist with whom I worked to look me over. The MRI gave me the answers I did not want.

The first few days were awful. Should the kids be told? Should I tell anybody? What about the financial implications of not being able to work? The boys had only just started at an expensive private school. There were just no answers. But I realised I had to face this. My initial reaction of not telling anyone just wouldn't work. How could I deal with this illness without acknowledging to the world that I had it? Keeping it a secret was impossible. I realised I had to start somewhere. Over the course of the day, I resolved to tell my brother and sisters. First, though, I had an appointment at the hospital to get my first dose of high-dose intravenous steroids. I wasn't prepared for how difficult that would be:

there was just no way to avoid the diagnosis. I could feel the pity in the eyes of the staff. I had nothing to hang on to. I felt like a man sentenced to a merciless, gradual destruction from which there was no escape.

That evening, it was hard to organise telling my brother and sisters all together, but I did the best I could, and we cried together all night. Driving home from my sister's place, I was feeling really empty but surprisingly calm. I now realise how important this immediate expression of grief was, and how it so quickly led me to start finding answers in myself and to gain some feeling of control over the disease. Feeling so calm allowed me to start thinking logically and without fear. I began thinking and wondering, as I was driving down the freeway, why this illness had happened to me just when it did. Why did I have MS? What emotional needs was it serving for me to get ill just then? Was my subconscious knocking on the door of my seemingly well-ordered life, trying to tell me something was wrong? I was beginning to tackle MS.

So I arranged a meeting with my old mentor from intern days, Dr Ian Hislop. In his calm and measured way, he led me through the feelings I was experiencing. Every time I mentioned Mum, I found it almost impossible to speak without becoming tearful. It was clear that I was seeing my own illness and future through the filter of Mum's disease and history. Until I could separate myself from those feelings a little, I would not get anywhere.

Ian listened quietly, occasionally interjecting with something to prompt me. Finally he gave me some assessment of what he thought I could do. First and foremost, he said, put yourself first. He suggested I take a long time off work in order to start doing some work on myself. This was great advice, but really difficult for me. Just the day before, I had told my colleagues I would be back in two weeks. For such a great challenge to one's life, two weeks simply doesn't do it justice. Ian was suggesting that perhaps I may not want to go back to work at all—that I should consider all possibilities. I knew he was right. I was at a crossroads, and anything was possible.

I wasn't to know it, but the simple process of trying to put myself first was to start a chain reaction of events that led my outwardly appearing 'perfect' life to simply fall apart, to head in directions I had never anticipated, to cause seismic shocks in the lives of my immediate family and many of my friends. Continuing to trust in this process of having faith in myself and my feelings, and going where they led me, has been extremely difficult at times—both for me, and for many of those I love and have loved. But my life has now finally reached a point of stability.

Finally, Ian asked a question that was to start me on a greater journey than confronting MS. He wanted to know whether I had ever thought much about my spirit. I searched for an answer. I soon realised that this was an extremely important part of me, one of which I was aware but that I had put to one side because of the demands of the rest of my life. It was a simple question, yet I didn't even have the vocabulary to answer it. Within the question lay the beginnings of a whole new journey for me.

Saturday morning arrived and I had finished my steroids. Now I was doing what the neurologist had termed 'doing nothing', and waiting. He had said that if I was still okay in six months we should repeat the MRI to see whether there were any new 'silent' lesions. I wasn't sure I liked this idea. If there were new lesions, surely finding out about them would just knock my optimism and confidence. The steroids had done their job. I still had numbness and pins and needles but in a smaller area, and I still had a bit of trouble telling where my leg was in space unless I was looking at it.

I was following Ian's advice and had let everyone at work know that I would not be back and that my leave was indefinite. I refused to say how long. I needed to marshal every resource I had to start this process. On Ian Hislop's advice, I had bought a copy of Carolyn Myss's wonderful book *Anatomy of the Spirit* and was starting to explore my own spirit.

The thing that started my search was a small, insignificant email from my brother, about Tuesday. I haven't kept it, because I didn't realise its significance at the time. It said something like, 'A friend's wife reckons you ought to try gamma-linolenic acid. She's taken it for ten years and hasn't had a relapse. There was something in the medical journals about it a few years ago.' A message like that tends to wake you up when you feel there's no hope.

I fired up MEDLINE and plugged in the key words 'gamma-linolenic acid', then cross-referenced it with multiple sclerosis. A few abstracts of papers came up from the 1980s. I was a bit surprised to see that, yes, there did seem to be a small benefit for patients with MS who took gamma-linolenic acid. In one of the papers, there was a bit about linoleic acid deficiency in MS, and it referred to another paper on patients getting better with linoleic acid supplements.

My search had begun in earnest. What I discovered in the literature shocked me. It rapidly became clear that with a preventive medicine approach, there was a real possibility that people with MS (PwMS) could slow or stop the otherwise relentless progression of MS into disability. Paper after paper reinforced this view, until I simply had to make the information public—and, of course, I immediately adopted it myself. Within months, I had collated all the evidence that went into the first book I wrote, *Taking Control of Multiple Sclerosis*, which later became *Overcoming Multiple Sclerosis* as I continued to build the evidence base.

From there, I began running live-in retreats for PwMS in early 2002, started a website with a community forum in 2008 and became a frequent user of social media so as to better disseminate my important message. As the number of PwMS who were doing well following this approach grew, I found I had more and more willing volunteers to help spread the news. Overcoming Multiple Sclerosis, or OMS, the community-based charity and support for PwMS grew from this process in 2012, through the passion and enthusiasm of Linda Bloom, a participant who had been to one of my early retreats and had recovered.

But spreading the message about the research findings of all the scientists in the world who had looked into this illness in detail was one thing. It was quite another to find credibility among my medical peers by undertaking my own research in the area. So began not only my research into the outcomes of people who had attended our retreats, but also a novel project recruiting PwMS from social media sites, where I had garnered quite a following, to try to find more evidence of the potential effect of lifestyle factors on the progression of and outcomes from MS.

This book represents a distillation of the evidence I have accumulated over nearly two decades since my diagnosis, as well as the experience I have gained of overcoming MS and watching countless others recover. I hope it helps on the journeys of many people diagnosed with this illness as they do the same.

ACKNOWLEDGEMENTS

There are many, many people to thank. First, I thank my wife, Sandra. Our lives have been inextricably linked since early in this millennium. Whenever I am confronted with doubt or fear, I instinctively reach for her and she is always there. Thank you, sweetheart, for never wavering. I thank my children, Sean, Michael, Pia, Ruby and John, for the love, support and humour they bring to my life, and for just being who they are. I am also grateful for the unfailing support of my siblings and extended family. Special thanks to a wonderful neurologist and good friend, Dr Peter Silbert, for his constant support and the very constructive suggestions made to the manuscript. I cherish the close connections I share with the OMS team, an international group of wonderful people that continues to grow, and particularly thank Emily Hadgkiss for her help with the figures, Dr Keryn Taylor for all that she does for people with MS, Dr Claudia Marck for the drive she brings to our research, and Linda Bloom and Gary McMahon for the enormous passion they have for the important work of OMS. Thanks also to my emergency physician colleague and friend, Dr Tor Ercleve, whose drawings have added significantly to the book. And to the colleagues, friends, and MS community with whom I have shared my life, I offer my continuing gratitude for your support and wisdom.

PART I

BACKGROUND

CHAPTER 1

ABOUT MS

Multiple sclerosis (MS) is a highly variable, unpredictable disease and one of the most life-altering diagnoses a person can receive.

Nancy Holland and Michele Madonna

WHAT IS MS?

Multiple sclerosis is a disease of the brain and spinal cord, usually resulting in progressive disability. It is the most common disabling neurological disorder in young adults, and has a very uneven distribution geographically, being common in so-called Western industrialised countries but also progressively more common further away from the equator. MS is a disease of affluence,[1] as are other auto-immune diseases;[2] research clearly shows that it is generally more common in countries with greater gross domestic product (GDP)—that is, with greater spending power.

MS is usually a progressively disabling disorder more common in affluent countries further from the equator.

3

MS is described as an inflammatory demyelinating condition. This means that parts of the brain and spinal cord (together called the central nervous system, or CNS) become inflamed, resulting in loss of the fatty coating—called the myelin sheath—around the connections between nerves. At a microscopic level, the immune system sends its first line of defence—white blood cells—to the area. These cells secrete messenger chemicals that cause the inflammation, and destroy part of the myelin around some nerves.

The brain and spinal cord are mainly made of fat; the type of fat depends on what we eat. The membranes of cells—their outer envelopes—are made of a double layer of fat. After changing to a diet consisting of different types of fats, there are quite marked changes in the make-up of these cell membranes.[3] This is because our bodies are not static, unchanging structures; we are literally what we eat. Deepak Chopra says, 'Just one year ago, 98 per cent of the atoms in our bodies were not there. It's as if we live inside buildings whose bricks are being systematically taken out and replaced.'[4]

Importantly, because of the different melting points of the various different types of fats we eat, the cell membranes of people who consume mainly unsaturated fats are more fluid and pliable than those of people who consume saturated fats. For people who eat mainly saturated fats, cell membranes are more rigid and inflexible, and more prone to degenerative changes.[3]

Typically, inflammation of a portion of the myelin sheath of a nerve in the brain or spinal cord is followed by loss of some of the myelin. This forms the so-called lesions of MS. In these inflammatory lesions, white cells of the immune system gain access to the myelin sheath, which they usually can't do because of what is called the 'blood–brain barrier' (BBB), a tight junction between the blood vessels around the brain and the brain itself. Further white cells are probably attracted by some of the chemical messengers released by these initial white cells. The demyelination strips the insulating coating on the connections or axons between nerves; this is followed by some repair and scarring, as with any episode of inflammation. The result is that nerve impulses don't travel along the nerve as well as they did before.

SYMPTOMS OF MS

The symptoms of MS depend entirely on which particular parts of the brain or spinal cord are affected, which is why symptoms vary so much from person to person. If a nerve axon in the spinal cord bringing sensory messages up from the legs to the brain is affected, then the person might notice tingling or numbness. If it is carrying motor messages down from the brain to the leg muscles, there may be some weakness. If they are nerves inside the brain responsible for, say, the sense of balance, the person may become very unsteady. Because inflammation causes swelling, there is some pressure on surrounding axons, causing them to work less well. As this swelling subsides, these surrounding nerve cells start to work again. So there is some recovery for this reason alone, but there is also some repair of the damaged nerve cells (a process called remyelination)—particularly early in the disease—so the symptoms settle further. This remyelination is a process whereby certain cells in the nervous system start to wrap themselves around the axons again. It occurs throughout the disease, and is more prominent than previously thought.[5]

 Symptoms of MS vary markedly from person to person.

Thus the area of numbness or tingling may become smaller, or the weakness may improve gradually, as the lesion heals and scars. Recovery is often incomplete, though, and people are left with persistent symptoms—although less severe than when the attack was at its peak—in the same part of the body. These residual symptoms typically wax and wane depending on numerous factors. Heat makes nerves conduct less well, and so makes these residual symptoms worse for most people. But it doesn't actually damage the nerves. So exercising that heats the body up is fine, even if it makes the symptoms temporarily worse. Some people find the reverse is true: that cold makes their symptoms worse.

As the disease progresses, these lesions grown in number, and more and more pathways are knocked out. Hence the person notices a gradual decline in function. Some of these lesions occur in 'silent' parts of the brain and are not noticed. Those we really notice occur in the spinal cord or in the nerves leading to the eye. Virtually all of these nerve fibres in the spinal cord are essential for things like sensation, power, balance and vision. Even a small lesion here is therefore usually noticed.

The nervous system has an amazing capacity to regenerate, so that impulses can now 'detour' around the damaged lesion.[6] The brain changes as well, recruiting new nerve cells and pathways to compensate for what is missing, in a process of 're-wiring' called neuroplasticity. This is well described in Norman Doidge's book *The Brain that Changes Itself*.[7] When there are only a few lesions, the brain is really good at this regeneration and compensation process, even if there isn't much remyelination. If the damage continues, these processes become overwhelmed and progressive disability occurs. That is why it is so important to stabilise the illness and prevent further damage as quickly as possible.

Optic neuritis

The first attack of MS quite often affects an eye. This is called optic neuritis, where the optic nerve—the major nerve carrying visual information from the retinas behind the eyes to the brain—becomes inflamed. Optic neuritis is a common cause of relatively sudden loss of vision in one eye in young people.[8] People who develop optic neuritis have a 40–50 per cent chance of developing MS in the next fifteen years.[9] The best predictor of the risk of going on to develop MS for someone who develops optic neuritis is whether they have other lesions in the brain on MRI at the time of the attack.[10] About 25 per cent of people with no lesions at the time of the attack go on to get MS, but if there is one lesion or more, the risk is about 75 per cent. Women are also more likely than men to go on to develop MS after an attack. If there are spinal cord lesions at the time of the initial attack, that increases the risk of ultimately being disabled.[11]

Optic neuritis is the first sign of MS for about 15–20 per cent of people with MS (PwMS).[12] Between one-third and one-half of all PwMS develop optic neuritis at some point in the illness. Even for those people, the long-term outlook for vision after an attack of optic neuritis is good, with 72 per cent having normal vision in at least one eye and two-thirds having normal vision in both at fifteen years.[13]

Many neurologists argue that people developing optic neuritis who have MRI changes that suggest a greater likelihood of developing MS should start on one of the disease-modifying medications immediately.[14] Such therapy has been shown to delay or prevent the onset of MS considerably.[15] This book makes the case that the OMS approach of an ultra-healthy diet, exercise, vitamin D and stress reduction should be started as early as possible after such an attack, whether or not one opts to take a medication. This should provide optimal protection against the development of MS.

The role of steroids in optic neuritis is not clear. Intravenous steroids are commonly prescribed to speed up recovery, but they don't seem to affect the long-term outcome for vision.[16]

Cognitive function

Cognitive function describes higher level functions of the brain, such as reasoning, judgement, abstract thought, awareness, perception, the ability to learn and remember details, and so on. If nothing is done about stabilising MS, cognitive function is generally progressively impaired, often quite subtly. The impairment seems to relate quite closely to the loss of nerve cells that accompanies MS progression in people who are not proactive about the illness. MRI scans reveal a gradual shrinking or atrophy of the brain.

A decline in cognitive function is common in MS—even in those people with so-called benign MS.

Some doctors have been inclined to put complaints by PwMS about mild cognitive problems down to depression or other mental health issues, but studies have shown that such complaints are mostly due to genuine cognitive impairment and need to be taken seriously.[17] Studies show that between half and three-quarters of PwMS have some degree of impairment of cognitive function, and many others probably have more subtle cognitive issues.[18, 19, 20] Cognitive decline becomes progressively worse the longer people have had the disease, the worse the damage in the brain has become, and the more disabled people are—although more recent research shows that it occurs even very early in the disease and has an effect on quality of life.[19, 21] Even people with so-called benign MS, such as those who have only had one episode of optic neuritis and otherwise appear to be well, have been shown to have significant cognitive decline many years later.[22]

Researchers have suggested that PwMS be tested for any decline in cognitive function, as this is the most sensitive index of disease progression, and can even be used to measure whether disease-modifying therapies are working,[23] although most neurologists would not be keen to pursue this strategy, as it is very confronting for the individual with MS. One important aspect of cognitive decline is that it can affect the ability to make decisions, and this can have a profound effect on daily life for PwMS, and also contribute to disability.[24]

HOW COMMON IS MS?

As a rule of thumb, MS occurs in about one in 1000 people. But that proportion varies a lot between and within countries. In the United Kingdom, it occurs in approximately one in 800 people, affecting around 90,000 people in total, and in Northern Europe it affects approximately one in 1000. In Australia, there are around 23,000 people with the illness, and there is a marked increase in how common it is with distance away from the equator. In Australia, for instance, the disease affects about twelve people per 100,000 in Far North Queensland, rising to about 36 per 100,000 in New South Wales and peaking at around 76 people per 100,000 in Tasmania. This effect of MS being more common the further one gets from the equator applies from country to country as well as within countries. In the United States, there are generally said to be between 250,000 and 350,000 PwMS, although a 2013 study put this much higher at around 570,000.[25] There are said to be about 2.5 million PwMS worldwide, although this is almost certainly an under-estimate.

MS is becoming more common, probably because of less healthy lifestyle choices.

The disease is becoming more common. A 1922 review from the United States showed that the incidence had increased over the preceding twenty years.[26] A 1952 report indicated that the incidence of MS doubled in Europe early in the twentieth century, and other data from Montreal show a 50 per cent increase from 1935 to 1958.[27] A 2005 study from Sardinia, a high-risk area for MS, showed that the incidence of the disease on the island had increased more than five-fold over the 30 years to 1999.[28] There are now data from several countries, including Japan, Canada and Ireland, showing that the incidence of MS is increasing.[29, 30, 31] A US study showed that MS had become 50 per cent more prevalent there over the 25 years to 2007.[32] Similar increases are being noticed everywhere.

Researchers in Tasmania have provided important data over many years on how common MS is. They have showed that the number of new cases per year per capita roughly doubled from the 1950s to the 2000s, and the number of people with the illness tripled from 1961 to 2009, going from about one in 3000 people to about one in 1000 people in Hobart.[33] An editorial by Dr George Ebers from Oxford suggested that this was unlikely to be just due to detecting more cases because of MRI, because most of the change happened before MRI was available.[34] More cases were being diagnosed in the elderly, and the increased longevity of the population may partly explain the increase, as more people now live long enough to get the disease, and the age of the study population had increased. However, the death rate from MS over the period had halved.

MS is a 'modern' disease. The first cases were described in the mid-1800s. By the turn of the twentieth century, the disease was commonly recognised. As environmental influences are the most important risk for developing MS, it is very likely that environmental factors have changed in a way that increases the risk of getting MS. These factors are the common environmental triggers for MS, such as sun avoidance, low levels of vitamin D, a diet high in saturated fat, omega-3 deficiency, lack of exercise and so on. There is little doubt that these risk factors are much more common today in developed countries than they were in the past, and are responsible for the explosion of chronic disease faced by our communities. Like heart disease, type 2 diabetes, high blood pressure and cancer, MS is becoming increasingly more common. It is interesting to note the interplay between these diseases, because having MS is no guarantee that we won't get another of these diseases related to our lifestyles.

MS and other diseases

While the research has been patchy in this area,[35] it seems that, quite apart from MS, PwMS are sicker than other people in the population. They have more mental illness, with around half having depression at some stage during the illness and a third anxiety.[36] But they also have considerably more physical illness, with high cholesterol and a poor fat profile in their blood (we will see later that this is no coincidence), high blood pressure, heart and blood vessel disease, and chronic lung disease. Having these additional diseases accelerates the progression of MS to disability, and results in worse quality of life.[36-39] Heart disease is more common in PwMS than the rest of the population,[40, 41] and heart and blood vessel disease occurring at any time during the illness has the effect of making progression to disability more rapid.[42] Canadian researchers looked at 8983 PwMS enrolled in the North American Research Committee on Multiple Sclerosis (NARCOMS) Registry, and analysed them according to whether they had vascular conditions such as heart disease, high blood pressure and diabetes.[42] They found that having a vascular condition at the onset of MS, or developing one later, resulted in around a 50 per cent increased risk of having difficulty walking. The risk increased the more vascular conditions a person had. Whereas it took about nineteen years for a person with MS who did not have any vascular conditions to need assistance with walking, it took only thirteen years for someone with a vascular condition.

Sex and age distribution

MS mainly affects people in their twenties or thirties, but no age group is immune. It is the most common disabling neurological illness in young adults. MS has now been found in very young children and in the elderly; as many as 20,000 children in the United States may have the disease but are not yet diagnosed. Children have been diagnosed with MS at as young as eighteen months old. Women have always been affected more commonly than men, in a ratio of around 3:2, but the ratio is changing towards 3:1. This changing sex ratio shows that environmental factors play a major part in the risk of getting the disease, and therefore that many cases are preventable by changing these factors.

GENETICS OF MS

MS is more common in family members of PwMS. Many are unaware of this, and so are some doctors. If one has a first-degree relative with MS, like a brother or mother, the risk is 20–40 times greater that of the general population. Identical twins have 300 times the risk of other people of getting MS if the other twin has the disease. For 100 pairs of identical twins in which one of each pair gets MS, 24 of the other twins will get the disease—that is, a 24 per cent risk. For non-identical twins, the risk is 3 per cent.[43]

 MS is a disease that runs in families.

The Canadian Collaborative Study Group has published a number of important papers on various aspects of the family risks of getting MS. Initial studies showed that the increased risk of MS in a family was due to genetic factors—that is, factors passed from parent to child—not factors in the shared family environment. The group has shown that adopted family members and step-siblings have no higher risk than the general population of getting MS; one has to be related to have the increased risk.[44, 45] The risk to a sibling of someone with MS is three to four times higher if a parent also has or had MS, if the disease occurred at an earlier age in the sibling (five times higher if the brother or sister got MS at age twenty years or less), and if the person in question is female. Thus, for sisters of someone with MS where a parent has had it as well, the risk is as high as 8 per cent, and even higher if that person got MS under the age of twenty.[46] If environmental risk factors are present—for example, if the person smokes cigarettes—the risk is higher again: up to one in five.

There has been contradictory research on whether the majority of the risk comes from the mother or the father having MS; they probably confer equivalent risk.[47, 48, 49] MS is not inherited as a result of a single gene, like cystic fibrosis or muscular dystrophy, but as a result of the interaction of several genes—probably over 100 of them, each with small effects.[50, 51, 52] Hence predicting the occurrence of MS in one's children is not possible at present, so genetic counselling is not particularly helpful. But it is important to remember that our children are at significantly increased risk, and that there are ways to reduce that risk by modifying the environmental influences on children.

Important research has shown that only around 2 per cent of the population has the genetic predisposition to MS.[53] While men are slightly more likely to have this genetic background, women are much more likely to get the disease because they are more influenced by environmental factors. In this study, the environmental risk factors for getting MS were noted to be vitamin D level both prior to birth during the mother's pregnancy and in childhood, and infection with the Epstein-Barr Virus (EBV), the glandular fever virus.

Genetics plays an important part in risk of developing MS. Interestingly, for someone in the 2 per cent of people with the genetic make-up to develop MS, one of the factors that reduces the risk is childhood exposure to a wide range of infectious diseases.[54] It is felt that this exposure makes the immune system more tolerant of challenges to it later in life. This is often referred to as the hygiene hypothesis.

Environment

So around a quarter of the risk of getting MS is genetic, and only about one in 50 people has this genetic make-up. What, then, makes that risk of MS turn into an actual diagnosis of the disease? We now know that the majority of the risk of developing MS—the other three-quarters—is environmental. There are many risk factors in the environment that act in concert with the genetic risk to cause MS to develop. This book is really about going into those in great detail, because the majority of these factors are modifiable—that is, one can do something about them to reduce the risk, not only of developing the disease but also of it progressing. Later, we will see that while the environment is responsible for most (75 per cent) of the risk of actually getting MS, it is completely responsible for the risk of progression of the disease, although some of these environmental factors are not necessarily modifiable. The book will go into those risk factors that are able to be modified in great detail, from diet—especially the role of the balance between healthy and unhealthy fats—to sun exposure and vitamin D, smoking, and stress, in addition to certain viral infections—most of which we cannot currently control.

So environment is around three times more important than genetics in the risk of developing MS in the first place. But in terms of the disease progressing once someone is diagnosed, it is vital that everyone is aware of the ground-breaking research of the International Multiple Sclerosis Genetics Consortium, published in *Nature*, one of the world's most important and influential journals. This group has mapped and compared the genome (all or most of the genes of a person) of 9772 PwMS of European descent with that of 17,376 other people without the disease.[55] This massive study was done to assess how genetic variations are associated with the development and progression of MS. First, they confirmed that many genes interact to create the risk of getting MS, and the stronger that genetic background risk, the earlier in life one is likely to get the illness.

But—and here is the key reason secondary prevention is an essential part of MS management—they found that genes and genetic predisposition did not account *at all* for the clinical course or severity of disease. To quote directly from the paper, 'We found no evidence for genetic associations with clinical course, severity of disease or month of birth . . .' This means that environmental factors, rather than genes, influence the course of MS once a person has the disease; while some of these factors are out of our control—like previous viral infections—most of these environmental influences can be controlled. Many authorities are now recognising this role of the environment in determining outcome from MS; however, questions still remain about which particular factors are responsible and to what extent.

Genetics contributes about 25 per cent of the risk of developing MS, but has no role in progression of the disease.

TYPES OF MS

MS occurs in several forms, but it has still not been established whether the underlying disease process is different in these or whether there are more distinct types. Up to 20 per cent of PwMS are said to have benign MS, but most authorities put this figure at around 6 per cent. This means that they suffer one or two attacks, but either that is all or they have only very occasional further episodes and remain active. Often these are people whose first attack was of visual disturbance, or other sensory symptoms. Researchers have suggested, however, that we probably over-estimate the number of people who have benign disease because we don't account for subtle problems like cognitive disturbance, fatigue, and social and psychological disturbances.[56] It is becoming apparent that benign MS may in fact not be benign at all. Most definitions say that benign MS is where the patient remains fully functional fifteen years after the onset of the disease. However, recent findings show that although there may be no physical sign of classic MS symptoms, around 45 per cent of people diagnosed with so-called benign MS have problems with cognitive function.[57, 58] In some studies, the presence of cognitive dysfunction was also associated with higher handicap scale scores, suggestive of considerable disease-related psycho-social problems.

We now know that the brain is not fixed, but constantly changing, with the theory of neuroplasticity explaining how new neurons are born and new connections are formed, based on life experiences. This new understanding of how flexible the brain is goes some way towards explaining why people with benign MS retain function.

It has been suggested that people who do well on the OMS Recovery Program probably do so because they have benign MS, but this is very unlikely. The aim of the program is to reduce the risk factors responsible for disease progression, and therefore limit the amount of nervous system damage through a program based on immune modulation, coupled with the prevention of degeneration, so that people actually stay quite well and do not deteriorate, either physically or mentally. This is quite different from so-called benign MS. If people are told they have benign MS after being on this program for some years, it is because healthcare workers find it hard to believe that it is possible to stay well after a diagnosis of MS, and conveniently apply that label.

At the other end of the spectrum is primary progressive MS. This is said to occur in about 10 to 15 per cent of cases. In this form of MS, disability progresses steadily from the first attack, usually without obvious attacks or remissions.[59] Around 65 per cent of PwMS begin with typical relapsing-remitting MS. This means that they have an attack, followed by some recovery—partial or sometimes total—then a period in which they have no further attacks. This period may be called a remission, because the symptoms remit. Remission is a bad term, though, because it implies that the disease is not active during this period. We know that it usually is, and can often see continuing nervous system damage on MRI scans. This period is then followed by another attack, or a relapse.

After some years of relapsing-remitting disease, most of these people end up progressing to secondary progressive MS. This is the typical later stage of relapsing-remitting MS, where disability again progresses steadily—presumably due to continued accumulation of lesion upon lesion. Evidence is coming to light now that, because damage continues to occur to the CNS even during periods of so-called remission, there may be progressive loss of brain tissue. This may become evident in subtle ways, such as the development of memory problems. The obvious attacks are only the tip of the iceberg, and this is one reason it is so important to get started with therapies to slow down or stop the disease as early as possible.

 Relapsing-remitting MS is a poor term, as damage commonly still occurs during periods of remission.

More recently, doctors have begun to recognise a form of the disease that is progressive but still involves relapses. This is termed relapsing-progressive MS. It is important to remember that classifying MS in a particular individual is not an exact science. Essentially, the doctor looks at how the illness has gone over time, whether there are relapses and whether disability is progressing, and then chooses the most appropriate category. If things change—such as the person making major lifestyle changes and modifying risk factors—it is quite possible, and frequently happens, that the disease changes and a different label has to be applied. People on the OMS Program, for example, have been told they have benign MS after initial diagnosis of primary progressive MS, or relapsing-remitting MS after being called secondary progressive MS. This is a good sign that the course of the illness is changing as risk factors are modified, indicating that risk factor modification is actually influencing the underlying disease process.

IMMUNITY AND AUTO-IMMUNE DISEASE

The immune system is a set of structures and functions within the body without which we could not survive, as it protects us against a range of things that cause disease. When a bacterium or virus invades the body and starts to multiply, the immune system recognises the bug as foreign, and either sends cells to the site to try to eliminate it, or instructs particular cells to secrete antibodies to try to neutralise it. The cells performing these tasks are white blood cells called lymphocytes. Lymphocytes are classified as either T or B lymphocytes, both derived from bone marrow. To simplify very complex processes, T cells help to get rid of the invader or toxin essentially by recognising them as foreign, going to the area and destroying them, whereas B cells secrete antibodies, which are complex proteins specially and individually designed to recognise the foreign material, bind to it and neutralise it.

When the immune response is activated like this, it leads to inflammation. Inflammation can best be thought of by picturing how angry a wound gets when it becomes infected. It may help to recall a cut or abrasion that has become infected. Typically, the wound gets hot, red, swollen and painful, and the area experiences a loss of function. So the inflamed part stops working as well. These are the typical features of inflammation. At a microscopic level, the immune system sends white blood cells to the area. These cells secrete messenger chemicals that cause the inflammatory reaction, and they dispose of bacteria, debris and foreign substances in the wound.

Naturally, the immune system needs to have a balance between switching on this immune response that causes inflammation in the body as the lymphocytes secrete their inflammatory chemicals, and switching it off. It would make no sense to have a permanently activated immune response to each foreign chemical or organism with which we make contact. Our bodies would be in a constant state of inflammation. Life would be miserable, with hot, swollen, painful body parts that refused to work properly. So the immune system, like all other bodily systems, has an off switch. In simple terms, the on switch is called the Th1 response and the off switch the Th2 response. We need the ability to switch on the immune response and the associated inflammation to deal with external threats, but we also need the ability to switch it off. Without the Th1 response, we would not recover from the most trivial infections; without the Th2 response, inflammation would be present all the time, and we would never return to normal.

 The immune system is in balance between switching on inflammation (Th1 response) and switching it off (Th2 response).

MS is well-known to be a Th1-predominant inflammatory condition. That is, PwMS have an exaggerated Th1 response, with a tendency towards inflammation. That needs to be balanced by a stronger Th2 response. Interestingly, a variety of environmental and other risk factors increase the Th1 response, including a predominantly high in saturated fat, Western diet, excess omega-6 fatty acids, obesity, stress, smoking, lack of exercise and depression; the Th2 response, in contrast, is increased by exercise, meditation, omega-3 fatty acids and vitamin D. This is one of the reasons these risk factors, discussed in much greater detail later, influence MS progression.

The immune system is a highly advanced, complex system that develops a detailed memory of every foreign agent or toxin it fights, so the next time it encounters the same agent, it can rapidly use that memory to begin a precise response tailored to that particular agent. This, of course, is the basis of vaccination. A non-toxic sample of whatever virus or bacterium one is vaccinating against is introduced to the body by injection or by mouth. The immune system develops this response and remembers the agent. If the agent is ever encountered again, the immune system remembers immediately, and cells and chemicals respond rapidly to neutralise the threat.

This is where the concept of molecular mimicry comes in. In the case of MS, it is widely thought that exposure to a particular protein in cow's milk at a young age in certain people leads to the immune system recognising this as foreign. For this to happen, the individual has to have some disturbance of the lining of the intestine ('leaky gut') that allows whole pieces of the protein to get into the bloodstream. Normally, proteins from cow's milk are broken down by enzymes in the intestine and absorbed into the blood as the individual amino acids that make up the protein. With leaky gut, fragments of the protein are absorbed whole without being broken down, and the immune system recognises them as foreign and mounts an immune response. Naturally, it would be counter-productive for the immune system to recognise amino acids—the building blocks of proteins—as foreign, as we have amino acids floating around in our bloodstream much of the time.

The issue in MS is that parts of cow's milk protein are identical to the protein in myelin. This has been elegantly shown in experiments from the Max Planck Institute.[60] In line with Poser's theory of MS causation being a cascade of environmental impacts on a genetically susceptible individual[61], people with leaky gut, exposed to cow's milk from an early age, with a genetic susceptibility to MS, develop this immune system recognition of cow's milk protein as foreign. Something disrupts the blood-brain barrier at some point (like EBV infection or trauma) and the lymphocytes that carry this memory get access to the brain, which they normally can't access. When they encounter myelin protein, their memory of it as being foreign—because it looks just like cow's milk protein—is triggered. This may result in some local immune response, with inflammation and formation of a lesion or two. Later—perhaps many years later—an environmental event like a death of a loved one or a trough in vitamin D levels, through their Th1 stimulating effect on the immune system, triggers full-blown MS.

DEGENERATIVE DISEASE

But MS is not just about the immune system.[62] It is now well established that degeneration is also a key mechanism in MS right from the beginning of the illness,[63] and particularly in the later, progressive phases. Degenerative disease is where the function or structure of tissues or organs progressively worsens over time, due to normal body wear and tear or lifestyle choices such as exercise or diet. So lifestyle choices can and do result in degeneration, and in Western countries, poor lifestyle choices are the commonest cause of degenerative diseases like heart disease, diabetes, high blood pressure, cancer, Alzheimer's disease and osteoarthritis.

There is now solid MRI evidence that the process of degeneration of nerve cells begins very early in the course of MS.[64, 65] Even early on, when there may be only a few lesions on an MRI scan, damage to the CNS is very widespread in MS and is not just confined to these lesions. It is important to remember that the MRI is only a picture, a visual representation of what is going on in the brain and spinal cord. MRI can only 'see' abnormal tissue down to a certain size or resolution; smaller than that, and damage is essentially invisible to MRI, even though it is widespread. The concept of MS as a focal, demyelinating disease really does need to be re-examined: we should regard it as a diffuse disease of the brain and spinal cord with a major degenerative component.[66, 67] Increasing loss of nervous tissue over time seems to be what ultimately leads the disease to become progressive.

But while the disease has a degenerative component throughout its course, it appears to be largely immune-mediated early on (although perhaps not in primary progressive MS), and later mainly degenerative once secondary progressive disease has occurred—although some would argue that the distinction between immune and degenerative diseases of the nervous system is blurred, and that both processes probably contribute.[68]

The immune system drives the MS disease process early in the disease; later, degeneration is more important, but both processes are present throughout.

It is useful to keep in mind that both of these components—immunity and degeneration—contribute to the development and course of MS, as this helps when looking for lifestyle interventions that can affect the course of the disease. For instance, polyunsaturated fats have been shown to be useful in degenerative diseases of the nervous system, such as Huntington's disease,[69] Parkinson's disease[70] and the memory loss and deterioration in mental function that accompany ageing,[71, 72, 73] as well as degenerative disease in general.[74] One of the omega-3 fatty acids in fish oil, DHA, has been shown to be powerfully neuroprotective, and to prevent degeneration in a rat model of brain injury.[75, 76] Being overweight predisposes one to many degenerative diseases, including heart disease, diabetes and arthritis. Eating fewer calories—even every second day—can dramatically improve health and longevity.[77, 78] Fasting causes a shift to a Th2 cytokine pattern in animals with the animal model of MS (experimental auto-immune encephalomyelitis, or EAE) and delays the onset of the disease, with milder clinical symptoms observed.[79]

Many other lifestyle modifications affect the ageing process and associated degeneration. For example, daily walking prevents age-related dementia[80] and a plant-based wholefood diet dramatically improves heart disease.[81]

CAUSES OF MS

Genetics

MS is often described by MS societies and fund-raising bodies as a mystery disease. This is rather surprising, because a great deal is known about what causes MS, and subsequently what influences the rate of progression. MS develops because of an interplay between genetic predisposition to the disease and environmental factors, many of them related to lifestyle. Without the particular genetic background towards developing MS carried by about 2 per cent per cent of the population, no matter how many adverse lifestyle and environmental factors there may be, one cannot develop the illness. Of course, other illnesses may develop—such as heart disease and diabetes—but not MS. That doesn't mean that someone has to have a relative with MS to develop MS; our DNA comes half from our mothers and half from our fathers, so that each of them may contribute some susceptibility to MS, but it is only when it comes together that there is enough susceptibility for the person to be at risk of developing the disease.

Blood–brain barrier

This genetic predisposition represents around a quarter of the risk of getting MS; the remainder is due to the effect of environmental and lifestyle factors in these people who are susceptible. A challenge to the immune system of such a genetically susceptible person then occurs, and it is likely that this challenge involves some kind of disruption to the blood–brain barrier. The BBB is really the interface between the blood circulating around and through the brain and the brain substance itself. This is a very tight interface, specially developed so that cell membranes of these blood vessels really tightly wrap around all the brain tissue, allowing very little of what is in the blood into the actual brain substance. Immune cells themselves normally cannot get through this barrier. It is only after it has been damaged that the immune cells (Th1 cells) at the heart of MS inflammation can get into the brain and spinal cord to start the disease process. Often this immune challenge that damages the BBB is a viral infection such as Epstein-Barr Virus (EBV), or one of the other viruses known to be associated with the development of MS. EBV has now been shown to cause damage to this sensitive BBB.[82]

Apart from viral infections like EBV, other insults can damage the BBB. Some research has suggested that trauma may damage this barrier. Researchers from Taiwan have found, in a very large case-control study involving nearly 300,000 people, that traumatic brain injury nearly doubles the risk of developing MS over the subsequent six years.[83] Using insurance databases, they examined the records of 72,765 people with traumatic brain injury and their risk of developing MS over the next six years, and compared this with the incidence of MS in a matched group of 218,295 people from the database who had not had such an injury. The risk of developing MS over the subsequent six years was nearly double for those with a head injury. On average, in this study, MS developed around eighteen months after the injury.

A more recent study, also from Taiwan, looked at nearly 12,000 people who had sustained traumatic injuries to their spinal cords, comparing them with nearly 60,000 people without such injuries, to see whether those with the spinal cord injuries had a higher incidence of MS.[84] In fact, their incidence was around eight times higher. This confirms the belief of many PwMS that significant injury to the CNS can predispose one to MS. There are a number of mechanisms through which this association may operate, including disruption of the BBB, vascular disruption and possibly the stress of the event.

More recently, Dr Raymond Damadian, the original inventor of the MRI, discovered something along similar lines. He scanned eight PwMS in a newly invented upright MRI machine, showing that a number of the MS lesions in these people communicated with the cerebrospinal fluid (CSF) in the ventricles (cavities) within the brain, around which most MS lesions usually form.[85] The researchers suggested that CSF leaking into the brain surrounding the ventricles, possibly due to blockages related to old trauma to the neck, might be involved in the causation of MS, tying in with the Taiwanese study about previous head trauma increasing the risk of MS.

Damage to the blood–brain barrier is an important step in the development of MS.

Evolution of the clinical disease

Whatever the cause, the challenge to the BBB doesn't actually cause damage to the nervous system and may never evolve into full-blown MS, but leaves the person with what Poser calls the 'multiple sclerosis trait'.[61] This means a person with this particular genetic predisposition and subsequent immune challenge is now primed to develop MS, even without any symptoms or any illness. Typically, susceptibility is now increased by a number of adverse background lifestyle factors, particularly lack of sun exposure and vitamin D, a diet high in saturated fats and low in omega-3 fatty acids, cigarette smoking (active or passive) and chronic stress. If a certain environmental trigger event then occurs, it can turn the trait into actual clinical MS. The trigger event precipitates the immune system to be activated in a Th1 response to form a lesion or lesions with the typical clinical features of MS, such as loss of sensation, power, balance or vision. This trigger event could be any of the lifestyle factors that have been linked in long-standing research studies to MS risk, but for many people it is a particularly stressful life event. The person may then remain symptom-free, with perhaps only a lesion or two in non-critical areas of the brain on MRI, and no noticeable effects, or go on to develop symptoms.

Conversely, a person in this situation who may be closely related to someone with MS, increasing their risk, and who also has a number of adverse lifestyle risks, like having had glandular fever, having major stresses in life or living where there is little available sunlight, can do much to prevent the development of MS by modifying lifestyle factors so that the immune system is tipped towards a Th2 or suppressant response. Taking vitamin D, getting more sun exposure, meditating, quitting smoking, eating more fish, exercising more and so on may well prevent MS from ever developing for a significant proportion of those who are genetically susceptible.

The appearance of just a lesion or two in the brain or spinal cord without noticeable symptoms is often now called a radiologically isolated syndrome (RIS). If the lesion or lesions cause one episode of clinical symptoms or signs, like loss of sensation or power, that is usually called a Clinically Isolated Syndrome (CIS). If the lesion or lesions cause more than one attack, then that satisfies the definition of *multiple* sclerosis. It is quite apparent, though, that this process has been going on for quite a while for most people—often well before the actual diagnosis of MS—and that these convenient clinical distinctions between RIS, CIS and MS are really just part of a continuum. For most people, if the underlying environmental and lifestyle predisposing factors don't change, they will move on to the typical course of the disease, with progression to disability.

A large Italian study demonstrated this particularly clearly. Researchers chose PwMS from families where there was no recorded MS (sporadic cases) and where there was a history of MS (familial cases). They performed MRI scans on 296 first-degree relatives of these PwMS and also people without MS.[86] All people in the study had no symptoms of MS and had not been diagnosed with MS. They found that 10 per cent of relatives of familial cases had MRI brain lesions that looked identical to MS lesions. In relatives of sporadic cases, 4 per cent of people had these lesions. In people unrelated to someone with MS, there were no lesions. So it is clear that these people with genetic backgrounds in common with PwMS were some way along the path to developing MS, probably having had appropriate immune challenges and adverse lifestyle factors, and with the right trigger, might go on to develop actual MS. That is, they had the MS trait, but not the disease yet.

Auto-immunity

The initial immune event primes the immune system into ultimately attacking its own nervous tissue. The immune system recognises some component of the myelin sheath around nerve channels as foreign, and tries to get rid of it by attacking it. This is called auto-immunity, and is the basis for most of the theories about MS causation. There is now compelling evidence from a range of genetic studies examining the actual genetic make-up of PwMS that multiple genes associated with the immune system are involved in the development of MS.[87, 88] As we have seen, part of this is the process of molecular mimicry. The immune system recognises particular proteins that have a strong resemblance to myelin as foreign, mounts an immune response to them, and is later tricked into doing the same against myelin, also seeing it as foreign. A number of different molecules have been suggested as mimicking myelin, including dairy protein[60, 89] and gut bacteria.[90]

Fat metabolism

Consistent with all of this background, a new all-encompassing theory from a forensic anthropologist outside medicine has tied these threads together. Dr Angelique Corthals argues that MS is a disorder of fat metabolism (metabolism refers to the chemical reactions within cells) that in many respects parallels cardiovascular disease, but occurs in people with genetic susceptibility to MS.[91] Noting that the formation of plaque on the walls of arteries (atherosclerosis or hardening of the arteries) in heart disease is remarkably similar to the formation of plaque in the CNS in PwMS, Corthals suggests that MS happens predominantly to women who have disordered fat metabolism and atherosclerosis happens mainly to men—although neither is excluded from getting the other disease, and must be susceptible to it first.

This explains why the risk factors for MS progression are so remarkably similar to the risk factors for heart disease—that is, a high saturated fat and processed food diet, lack of omega-3, smoking, lack of exercise, low vitamin D, stress and so on. Similarly, it ties in with the research showing more cardiovascular disease in people who have MS.[92] One extraordinary paper showed that the common Framingham Risk Score, used to score the risk factors for people developing heart disease, and shown in elegant studies to accurately predict that risk, also accurately predicts the level of disability and disease severity for PwMS.[93] Similarly, as with heart disease, recent work shows that increased body weight increases the risk of progression of MS.[94]

 One compelling theory is that MS is a disease of fat metabolism related to diet and lifestyle choices.

Gut bacteria

There are other theories about why a high saturated fat and processed food Western diet predisposes us to MS. These concern the effect of such a diet on the bacteria that live in our intestines. This research area is expanding rapidly. The number of bacteria living in our gut is around ten times the number of cells in our bodies, numbering in the trillions. We live in a kind of symbiosis with this enormous number of organisms, and our health is affected profoundly by the particular type and number of different organisms we harbour. The effects are particularly noticeable on our immune system and the chemical processes in our bodies.

Put simply, the different types of foods we eat are preferred by different types of organisms in our gut, and in turn overgrowth of certain organisms changes the immune system balance. Diet is just one of the lifestyle factors that influences the types of organisms that grow in our gut, others include stress, the influence of different medications particularly antibiotics, age, exercise, and others. But diet is critically important. A high-calorie, processed, low-fibre, high-saturated fat and refined-sugar diet—that is, the common Western diet—results in an overgrowth of certain bacteria (such as *Firmicutes*), while low-calorie, high-fibre diets rich in complex carbohydrates and low in fat favour other bacteria (such as *Bacteroidetes*).[95] This is because these particular bacteria thrive on these different dietary components. The typical Western diet also leads to a reduction in the biodiversity of the bacteria in the gut.

These changes induced by the Western diet change the settings of the immune system towards a Th1 profile—that is, towards inflammation.[96] Interestingly, they also change the way the gut lining works, allowing more and bigger pieces of protein into the body's circulation, which has great relevance for the way cow's milk triggers auto-immunity. The potential for dietary changes to trigger MS lesions has been shown very elegantly in the animal model of MS.[97] Based on analysis of these and other factors affecting the bacteria in the gut, Italian scientists have suggested that the key dietary factors to avoid to control inflammation for PwMS are saturated fats, trans fats, red meat, sweetened drinks, high-calorie diets rich in refined carbohydrates, salt and cow's milk proteins.[98] It is interesting to see how closely this aligns with the OMS Recovery Program diet.

Another compelling paper from German researchers published in the eminent journal *Immunology* in 2015 provides some key insights into how dietary factors interact with gut bacteria to cause central nervous system inflammation.[99] In the animal model of MS, they showed that long-chain saturated fatty acids in the diet consistently made the disease worse by increasing the Th1 and Th17 cell lines of bacteria in the gut; this effect was not seen with shorter-chain unsaturated fats, which improved the disease and reduced the loss of axons.

Viruses

Viruses almost certainly play a role in causing MS. The evidence for this is largely epidemiological. The very uneven worldwide distribution of

MS is related to diet and exposure to sunlight, but probably also to viral infections. People who migrate to other countries change their risk of getting MS,[100] but the age at which they migrate seems to be very important, raising the possibility that something happens to them before that age—possibly infection with a certain virus.

In other words, a child under the age of fifteen years going from a country of high incidence—say, Denmark—to one of low incidence—say, Singapore—acquires the risk of the new area; that is, the chance of getting MS goes down substantially. But an adult doing the same keeps the same risk they would have had if they had stayed in Denmark. This strongly suggests some environmental agent—possibly a virus—affects the individual around the age of fifteen. Potentially, this provides the right 'soil' for the later development of MS, precipitated by dietary fats and perhaps a lack of sunlight. Australian epidemiological data, however, has disputed these observations about age at migration being important,[101] and it seems that the way we live in terms of lifestyle choices is more important than whatever early exposures we may have had as children.

Several viruses, particularly the glandular fever and herpes viruses, contribute to developing MS.

Other epidemiological studies have shown a correlation between the incidence of varicella (chickenpox, shingles or herpes zoster) infection and MS.[102] Compared with other viruses, this virus—the varicella-zoster virus (VZV)—is very commonly (95 per cent) present in immune cells of PwMS having relapses, but not commonly present in people without MS.[103, 104] In a study using electron microscopy—a method that highly magnifies bodily tissues and fluid so that minute particles are visible—that looked at the spinal fluid of PwMS compared with healthy volunteers, researchers found particles identical in appearance to VZV in the spinal fluid of the PwMS who were having relapses, but none in those in remission or the healthy volunteers.[103] The number of particles fell away steadily as people recovered from the relapses. None of the healthy people in another study had VZV in their immune cells, whereas

95 per cent of PwMS having a relapse had VZV, as did 17 per cent of those in remission.[104] Six of 82 consecutive patients with MS had either varicella or zoster concurrent with the development or progress of their illness in one study.[105] Another study found no healthy people with the virus, about 10 per cent of people with other neurological diseases with the virus, and over 40 per cent of those with MS with the virus,[106] suggesting that VZV has a role in the development of MS.

So VZV is likely to play a direct role in the development of MS and the initiation of relapses. As VZV is one of the herpes viruses, and is able to be prevented and treated with the cyclovir group of anti-viral drugs, this might open up the possibility of using these drugs for MS treatment. There have been regular reports of clusters of cases of MS occurring in particular geographical areas,[100] and several epidemiological studies showing that relapses occur much more frequently after viral infections.[107] It is not clear whether this is due to the particular virus triggering or causing the relapse or a general activation of the immune system.

A lot of work has gone into finding which particular viruses are involved. The most likely are the herpes virus, human herpes virus 6 or HHV-6, and the Epstein-Barr virus that causes glandular fever. Herpes viruses include herpes simplex, which causes common cold sores and genital herpes, and herpes zoster, discussed earlier. Herpes viruses are good candidates for causing CNS problems because—after an attack of cold sores, for example—they persist in the nervous system and are reactivated to again cause infection. HHV-6 causes a common condition in children called roseola. HHV-6 protein and DNA have been found in active MS lesions,[108, 109] and antibodies to HHV-6 have been found in PwMS after relapses.[110] PwMS have also been found to have higher antibody levels to HHV-6 than levels in the general population.[111]

Reactivation of HHV-6 infection is closely associated with relapses in MS.[112] The risk of relapse is much higher for patients with active HHV-6 infection than for those with inactive infection, raising the potential for suppressing MS activity by suppressing herpes infection with medication. HHV-6 is also present in post-mortem specimens from PwMS at a higher rate than in the rest of the population.[113, 114, 115] Treatment with interferon reduces the amount of HHV-6 in PwMS having relapses but not those in remission, also suggesting a role for HHV-6 in causing relapses.[116]

HHV-6 is found more often in PwMS with relapsing-remitting MS than those with secondary progressive disease.[117]

There is now quite a bit of research implicating the virus known to cause glandular fever, the Epstein-Barr virus (EBV), in the development of MS.[118, 119, 120] One study looking at blood samples collected from around three million US military personnel at their time of enlistment found that those with high antibodies to EBV on enlistment—that is, those who had had the viral infection even up to five years before the onset of MS—had a 20 to 30 times higher risk of getting the disease than those with low antibody levels.[120] Nurses enrolled in the US Nurses Health Study who developed MS were 2.5 times as likely to have had EBV in their blood when first enrolled in the study before diagnosis, compared with those who did not develop MS.[121] Others have confirmed these findings.[122, 123] A Canadian population study showed that PwMS were more than twice as likely to have had an EBV infection than their spouses.[124] These data and others were summarised in one meta-analysis of all the studies on EBV and MS, which concluded that the combined risk of MS after glandular fever from fourteen pooled studies was more than double (2.3) that of the population who had not had EBV infection.[125]

So the evidence shows that EBV infection is associated with the development of MS. Interestingly, it is also implicated in other auto-immune diseases such as rheumatoid arthritis where evidence of EBV infection has been found in affected joints.[126] Whether this will help us to determine some way of preventing or treating the disease, however, is another question. Researchers have suggested that vaccination against EBV may prevent MS developing in susceptible people,[127] although to date a vaccine has not been developed.

DIAGNOSIS

For many years, the diagnosis of MS was made largely on the basis of clinical findings—that is, assessing the course of the illness and whether it was typical of MS. So diagnosis was somewhat difficult, often delayed and sometimes not accurate. The diagnostic breakthrough came with the development of MRI scanning. MRI is an imaging method that, unlike computerised tomography (CT) scanning, doesn't use x-rays or other forms of radiation. Instead, it uses powerful magnets and sensors to detect minute magnetic fields within cells, so it can be used again and again without any radiation risk. The scans enable visualisation of tiny defects in the nervous system. The lesions of MS usually show up even if they are very small, although some don't. MRI reveals lesions in 95 per cent of people with clinically definite MS,[128] but it isn't definitive. Other diseases can produce lesions that look like MS on MRI. It needs to be used in conjunction with the doctor's clinical diagnosis—that is, assessment of features of the person's symptoms—as well as findings on clinical examination. It should be noted that a very large review has shown that MRI is not particularly accurate at diagnosing MS, and tends to lead to over-diagnosis and over-treatment.[129] Certainly, a good clinician is necessary to interpret the MRI and make the diagnosis.

For many years, people presenting with a first attack of neurological symptoms that suggested MS would be told that a diagnosis of MS could only be made once there were further attacks. Put simply, *multiple* sclerosis meant multiple attacks of neurological symptoms, separated both in time—that is, occurring at two different times at least—and separated in location—that is, occurring in two different parts of the nervous system. The first attack, or Clinically Isolated Syndrome (CIS), was often called transverse myelitis if it occurred in the spinal cord. Many people at their diagnosis of MS are convinced that they have had previous episodes of neurological symptoms that represented earlier MS attacks, but were either not investigated or dismissed as not serious. Many neurologists take this history into account when considering whether the person has MS. Canadian researchers have shown that even five years before the diagnosis of MS, PwMS were seeing doctors around 15 per cent more than others in the general population, supporting this suggestion of earlier episodes.[130]

The diagnosis of MS can now be made in many people on the first attack.

The criteria for diagnosis of MS are always changing as new diagnostic methods and techniques evolve. The McDonald Criteria are the diagnostic criteria that are most widely adopted; they have been used for many years by neurologists to diagnose MS. The 2010 McDonald Criteria contained a number of changes from previous versions, the most important being that MS can now be diagnosed on the first visit to a neurologist if there is MRI evidence of more than one attack arising from more than one location in the brain.[131] This allows the diagnosis to be made, contrary to what PwMS are often still told, in people who have experienced only one attack and had only a single MRI scan. In effect, what is needed is a minimum of two lesions on the first scan, with one of them being gadolinium (contrast) enhancing, indicating that it is recent, versus the other or others being older; this indicates at least two attacks separated in time and location in the brain.

In a recent study, Dutch researchers examined how often these 2010 criteria would allow the diagnosis of MS to be made in 178 people who had had a single neurological episode (CIS) consistent with MS. Using these criteria, the diagnosis could be made at the first presentation to a doctor in 33, or 19 per cent, of them. This is of great value, as evidence shows that secondary prevention strategies, both with lifestyle changes and medication, appear to be more effective the earlier they are started, and the earlier a definite diagnosis is made, the earlier one can start on the OMS Program. Given the evidence presented in this book, there is also a very strong case for starting the lifestyle program after a CIS and not waiting until a formal diagnosis of MS is made. This may stop MS ever being diagnosed.

One of the difficulties of using MRI for diagnosis is that both doctors and PwMS have started to place undue faith in the images produced by the MRI. There is now a lot of evidence to show that the number of lesions seen on MRI often doesn't correlate well with a person's physical condition. For instance, we may show that a particular therapy decreases the number of new lesions, yet we may not see any difference in the person clinically.[132] The power of such medical images can be profound, and the MRI can sometimes be interpreted by both doctor and patient as a 'report card'; if there is a bad report, yet the person feels well and doesn't have any worsening of the disease, it can be an extremely

negative experience for the patient—and indeed, management decisions can be made by the doctor that might not actually be sensible or
appropriate, as the patient is actually doing well. Conversely, in some
respects it is important for PwMS to know that there is often continuing damage occurring in this disease in periods of so-called remission.
If used sensibly, this information can highlight the importance of a
proactive approach, and of starting a multi-faceted prevention program
as early as possible.

Despite the relatively poor correlation of MRI lesions with a person's
physical condition, large studies correlating MRI findings with clinical
course have now shown that PwMS have significant atrophy (shrinkage)
of both white and grey matter in the brain.[133] Secondary progressive
patients have more atrophy than relapsing-remitting patients and a
higher lesion load—that is, a greater number of lesions. Lesion load and
atrophy in this study significantly predicted Expanded Disability Status
Scale (EDSS) score, and grey matter atrophy was the most significant MRI
predictor of final disability.

Being told the diagnosis

In the past, it was quite common for doctors not to tell people they had
MS after making the diagnosis, so as to spare them anxiety or worry
about the future. Even today, some doctors still avoid such disclosure.
Many wait until there are more attacks, even if the McDonald Criteria
indicate that the diagnosis is MS at the first visit. This doesn't seem a
particularly sensible approach. Until patients become aware that they
have MS, they can't begin to do anything about it. This partly stems from
the old-fashioned view that it is better not to know the diagnosis as there
is nothing much that can be done about MS anyway. Hiding the diagnosis,
though, denies the person with the illness a chance to be proactive and
take control early in the illness. The evidence strongly suggests that the
earlier people adopt a comprehensive prevention approach to MS, the
less likely it is that they will become disabled over the long term. Put
simply, the earlier treatment is started, the better the outcome.

Italian research sheds important light on this question. Researchers
enrolled 229 people with MS or CIS in the study.[134] Of these, 93 (over

40 per cent) were unaware of their diagnosis, suggesting that this practice on the part of treating doctors of not disclosing the diagnosis is still relatively common. After measuring their quality of life and psychological state, the diagnosis was then disclosed. Interestingly, 30 days after this disclosure, measures of quality of life, anxiety and depression were better than before the patients knew the diagnosis, and this improvement in quality of life and psychological well-being persisted over the following two years.

These findings fit with what many PwMS say about finding out the diagnosis. While the diagnosis of MS is 'considered one of the most life-altering diagnoses a person can receive',[135] it is important for the person to know what they are up against. As one newly diagnosed person with MS noted, 'the potential challenges of the journey ahead have to be viewed with realism, optimism, and meaning',[135] and this journey can't begin until people know what they are facing. Many people are actually relieved to finally know what is wrong, and to have an explanation for what can be baffling and not always well-understood or appreciated symptoms.

 People with MS generally want to be informed of the diagnosis.

While it is important to have this confirmation that PwMS really do need their doctors to be frank and honest with them, it is disappointing to note that, at least in this Italian clinic, over 40 per cent of PwMS in the study had not been told the diagnosis prior to the study. Anecdotal evidence from PwMS confirms that this is still common practice in many countries. It has actually long been known that PwMS wish to be told the diagnosis. A study in *The Lancet* in 1985 showed that people overwhelmingly want to be told they have MS after diagnosis. Only six out of 167 surveyed MS patients preferred not to be told.[136] More recently, a very large Greek study reported that, of 1200 PwMS, 91 per cent favoured being told immediately, yet only 44 per cent had been told.[137] For 27 per cent it took longer than three years to be told.

Likewise, previous guidelines for the management of MS issued by the UK National Health Service National Institute for Health and Care

Excellence (NICE) recommended that 'if a diagnosis of transverse myelitis is made, the individual should be informed that one of the possible causes is MS'.[138] Updated guidelines in 2014 suggested offering people suspected of having MS further review, and offering them information about support groups and national charities.[139] One qualitative study reported that all 23 people interviewed with MS reported the moment of diagnosis as powerfully evocative and unforgettable.[140] Its effect on partners should not be under-estimated either, with one study reporting feelings of helplessness and isolation.[141] Unfortunately, very poor levels of support and information were sometimes given, and this is something commonly reported by PwMS.

Telling others the diagnosis

Once diagnosed with MS, most people are faced with the very difficult issue of whom else to tell. For many, their partners may have been with them at the time of diagnosis. While there is little research about this, having your partner there can be very helpful. Being able to share the very difficult emotions that come up immediately around such a life-altering diagnosis is very important. But then the questions often start. 'Should we tell the children?' 'What about my siblings . . . parents . . . friends . . . work colleagues?' These are very difficult and individual choices. My experience of interacting with many thousands of PwMS over many years now has taught me that there is a significant cost to keeping such a secret.

In one of the early retreats I ran, one of the participants—let's call her Janet—was wheelchair bound. Janet had been diagnosed with MS for over 25 years, but had told only her husband. She had built an elaborate story for other family members, friends and colleagues as her condition worsened. By the time she came to the retreat, in a wheelchair, she was profoundly depressed and had a very poor quality of life. Later, we will see that depression makes MS worse, physically as well as mentally, and that it is very important to proactively take steps to avoid becoming depressed.

The retreat atmosphere is such that people often open up about very difficult issues, sometimes for the first time. Janet discussed her decision not to tell people and the price she had paid for this decision, both practically and emotionally. Above all, it became clear that she had denied her friends an opportunity to help her over many years. Later, in keeping in touch with the group, I was to find out that Janet had told many of her close friends and relatives about the diagnosis on returning home from the retreat. I met Janet several times over subsequent years at presentations I was giving to PwMS; the difference was amazing. Janet radiated happiness, and surprisingly good health. She remained wheelchair bound, but it was clear that an enormous burden had been lifted from her life. She reported that her long-standing depression had lifted, she was no longer on anti-depressants and her enjoyment of life had returned.

There has been some research around this area to back up the personal anecdotes I have witnessed. With respect to the work environment, many PwMS are concerned about whether to disclose the diagnosis of MS to their employers. Some see such disclosure as very risky, and fear that disclosure may have negative repercussions in terms of their employers' views of their capabilities, leading to issues with job retention and support at work. Such fears seem to be well founded in many cases, with evidence showing over three-fold higher rates of unemployment for PwMS than those in the general population[25] and others with comparable disabilities. Many who do disclose, though, maintain that employers and colleagues are actually very helpful and supportive once they become aware of the diagnosis.

Researchers from Monash University found that while level of disability certainly predicted whether someone with MS was still working, those who had disclosed their diagnosis in the workplace were more likely to still be working and for longer periods than those not disclosing, even allowing for level of disability.[142] In contrast, neither age nor gender predicted employment status. While the authors acknowledged the risk of discrimination for some people in certain organisations after disclosure of a diagnosis of MS, with about 8 per cent of the sample reporting dismissal after disclosing the diagnosis, they note that the majority of workplaces respond in a positive, supportive manner to the disclosure.

 Telling others about the diagnosis of MS can relieve the heavy burden of keeping secrets.

This is an extremely difficult issue for many PwMS, particularly early on after diagnosis. It is difficult enough to try to plan for the future when one has been confronted with such a life-altering diagnosis, but many find the issues about whether to tell family, friends, work colleagues and employers an added and difficult burden. This study should finally add some evidence that can help in making these difficult decisions in the workplace a little easier. In the right workplace circumstances, disclosure may actually help someone maintain employment, although individuals should make their own judgements about the particular culture within their workplace and whether disclosure is likely to be helpful or harmful.

COURSE OF MS

It is important to be realistic about what can happen to PwMS if they don't actively engage with the illness by adopting a program to prevent progression. MS is a progressive condition, and it is usual for PwMS to progress to disability over time. The rate at which this happens has been the subject of much conjecture and mythology, but recent studies have clarified this considerably. One large study of the natural history of the condition showed that a relapsing course is followed by chronic progression in around 80 per cent of cases within 20 years.[143] While there is considerable individual variation in the rate of progression, this process is relatively typical in most patients and the disease seems likely to be degenerative in nature.

Primary progressive MS (PPMS) appears to proceed to disability faster than other forms, although again there is considerable variation. One large study showed that a quarter of patients with PPMS needed a walking cane by 7.3 years after diagnosis; in contrast, a quarter still didn't need one at 25 years.[144] Other research suggests that this is an overly pessimistic view.[145] In a group of 2837 patients with all forms of MS, only 21 per cent needed a cane fifteen years after disease onset, and by age 50, 28 per cent required a cane. These figures may reflect the effect of MRI in making the diagnosis earlier in people with subtle clinical features, and potentially the effect of disease-modifying drugs now in wide use. People who have CIS with no lesions on brain MRI have a very low rate of progression to definite MS, at least over a five-year period.[146] Having lesions on initial brain MRI at the time of the episode of CIS makes the development of definite MS much more likely.

Other studies have had similar findings. One showed the median time from diagnosis to an EDSS score of 3 was 17 years, and to a score of 6 was 24 years. Twenty years after onset, only 25 per cent of those with relapsing-remitting MS had EDSS scores of 3 or more. The median time from diagnosis to EDSS score of 6 for the secondary progressive groups was ten years and for the primary progressive group was three years. Once an EDSS score of 3 was reached, progression of disability was more likely and more rapid.[147] A larger study of 1844 patients suggested that MS was really one disease with progressive illness, whether primary or secondary, essentially following the same course.[148, 149] It concluded that for most PwMS, disability landmarks were reached at about the same age. For instance, patients required a cane on average at about the age of 63, give or take a couple of years, regardless of the initial course. It also noted, as in previous studies, that women reached these milestones later than men. The authors suggested that age-related degeneration may be an important cause of this progression in PwMS.

Professor George Ebers, winner of the 2013 John Dystel Prize for MS research, has published considerable research in the areas of MS genetics and the course of the illness. Prof Ebers has noted the interaction of environmental and genetic factors in MS, stating that MS can be viewed largely as a preventable disease. Ebers examined the factors leading to development of secondary progressive disease, noting that development of secondary progressive disease is the key determinant of long-term outcome for PwMS. He has been highly critical of the drug industry, which measures relapse rate as the major outcome in its drug trials; very few of the drugs have been shown to have any effect at all on slowing the development of secondary progressive MS (SPMS), which is the major determinant of whether PwMS do well or badly in the long run.[150]

Ebers examined data from 806 people from Canada with relapsing-remitting MS. Over the 28 years of the study, two-thirds of PwMS starting with relapsing-remitting MS had gone into SPMS. By six years from diagnosis, a quarter of PwMS had SPMS; by fifteen years, half the PwMS had SPMS. For each additional year of having the disease, there was a

7 per cent increase in risk of developing SPMS; the risk of developing SPMS doubled after ten years and quadrupled after twenty years. The best predictors of progression to SPMS were an older age at diagnosis (if diagnosed after age 30, one has a 35 per cent greater risk of developing SPMS than someone diagnosed between ages 20 and 30), male sex (men were 41 per cent more likely to develop SPMS during the study than women) and increased frequency of relapses early after diagnosis.

There are many myths about the long-term outlook for PwMS. It used to be said that PwMS did not have a shortened lifespan compared with the general population, and that no one dies of MS. In fact, it is clear that PwMS die considerably earlier than those without the disease—at least if they do nothing about the illness. One Danish study showed that PwMS from 1948 onwards died around ten years earlier than the general population,[151] over half (56 per cent) of them from MS. The excess death rate for those with MS compared with the general population in this study fell by the end of the study to about half the rate it was in the mid-1900s. Again, it is likely that this represented the fact that the diagnosis was being made earlier and in more people by the end of the study, and possibly the effect of the newer disease-modifying drugs. This finding was not supported by a major meta-analysis of all mortality studies in PwMS which showed that the excess death rate for PwMS had not changed at all over the 50 years to 2012.[152] Death due to cardiovascular disease, suicide and infection remained higher for PwMS than those in the general population.

A Welsh study showed that the average age at death for women with MS was 65.3 years, and 65.2 years for men,[153] considerably less than might be expected in the general population. Again cause of death was related to MS in nearly 58 per cent of people. In over a quarter, there was no mention of MS on the death certificate, which may explain why it is so commonly under-estimated as contributing to death.

While these data may be alarming to some PwMS, it is important to know exactly what the natural history of the disease is without any intervention. While we know that drugs make some modest difference to relapse rate, mostly they make little difference to when people develop SPMS. Yet a preventive medicine approach, as recommended by OMS, with attention to lifestyle modification—particularly risk factors around diet, sun exposure, vitamin D supplementation, exercise, stress reduction and so on—is likely to have a significant effect in delaying progression to SPMS, thereby having a major impact on people's lives in the long term.

Prognosis

Despite what many PwMS are told, there is currently no way to predict the course of this disease in individual people. Many PwMS have told me that they were told at diagnosis that they had a very mild form of the illness and shouldn't worry about it. There is actually no basis for making such a statement. Although possibly motivated by a desire not to alarm people about the diagnosis, such an approach is probably unhelpful. At present, we have no way of determining the group into which any particular person with MS falls, from the point of view of prognosis. Although the statistics tell us that people have a worse prognosis if they are older at the onset of the disease, have a progressive disease course, have symptoms at onset that are multiple, motor or balance, and have a short time to their first relapse,[154] these are only generalisations, and don't apply to any individual case.

There is currently no reliable way to predict the course of the illness at the time of diagnosis.

The medical literature makes the observation that the only way to predict how someone will go is to observe the progress of the disease. Those with more severe early attacks with poor recovery are more likely to continue in that pattern.[155] One of the few constant findings in the MS literature is that the 'sooner to cane, sooner to wheelchair'.[144] One group of patients who seem to have quite a benign early course comprises those whose first symptoms are visual—that is, those who get optic neuritis.[156] This group of people seems to develop only mild disability over the ten years after the diagnosis of optic neuritis, but again this applies to a group and can't be used in individual cases for prognosis.

There are several research groups studying novel ways to predict the course of MS. Researchers at Johns Hopkins University in Baltimore have applied a commonly used eye test to PwMS and healthy controls to determine whether the health of the nerve cells at the back of the eye could be used to mirror the health of the brain cells.[157] They studied 164 PwMS and 60 healthy people without MS, using a technique called optical coherence tomography (OCT). This is a relatively simple scan that is radiation free and commonly used to assess the health of the retina (the nerve cell layer at the back of the eye) in people with diabetes. They found a surprisingly strong correlation between the thickness of one of the inner layers of the retina and disease activity in those participants with MS. The thicker the layer at the start of the study, the more likely PwMS were to develop new MRI lesions and relapses during the roughly two years of the study, and the more likely they were to progress in disability.

This is potentially a very important finding for those diagnosed with MS. It implies that the retina can provide a clear picture of the inflammation going on in the brains of PwMS, so that the more inflammation, with associated increased disease activity, the thicker this layer of the retina. Potentially, this means that PwMS could be monitored with this relatively simple eye test to see whether what they are doing about their illness is making a difference. It could ultimately be really useful for people adopting a preventive medicine program to monitor how effectively they are controlling the illness, and whether or not the approach needs to be more rigorous, or whether medication might be necessary. It could also be useful for monitoring the effectiveness of particular medications. Further studies are required before this approach can be confirmed and used more widely, but the results are highly encouraging in terms of monitoring the illness and being able to more accurately predict the disease course.

Pregnancy and breastfeeding

Given that MS is most common in women of childbearing age, it is important to know how pregnancy and MS interact. MS has little or no effect on pregnancy, but pregnancy appears to have a beneficial effect on MS. Women with MS can expect reduced MS activity during their pregnancy, particularly during the last trimester. There is an increased risk for three to four months after childbirth, but the risk of relapse still remains low, and is lowered further with breastfeeding. According to the best available evidence, women with MS can expect normal fertility and normal pregnancy outcomes, although IVF is associated with an increased relapse rate.[158, 159]

Breastfeeding for at least four months after delivery reduces a baby's risk of developing MS by around 50 per cent and also reduces the mother's risk of relapse.[160] The researchers found that virtually all pregnant women without MS breastfed after giving birth, but only around two-thirds of those with MS did. Most of the women with MS (73 per cent) who didn't breastfeed or started early bottle feeding did so in order to start their MS medications again. Women who didn't breastfeed or started bottle feeds within two months of giving birth had a five times higher risk of MS relapse in the year following the birth than those who breastfed. Breastfeeding was even more protective in the sub-group of women with MS who had been on MS medication prior to pregnancy, with those not breastfeeding or starting early bottle feeds having a seventeen times higher risk of relapse than those breastfeeding in this group, in which the women had potentially more serious disease. One study of 201 women in the German MS and Pregnancy Registry showed that exclusive breastfeeding was in effect a modestly effective MS treatment, with nearly double the rate of relapse in the first six months after childbirth for those women who did not exclusively breastfeed.[161] This evidence base seriously calls into question the practice of stopping breastfeeding after childbirth in order to restart disease-modifying therapies.

Breastfeeding for at least four months after childbirth protects the mother against relapses, as well as benefiting the baby.

In keeping with other research showing the benefits of breastfeeding for women with auto-immune disease, one case-control study of 245 women with MS compared with 296 women without MS showed that breastfeeding roughly halved the baby's risk of developing MS in later life.[162] In detailed statistical analysis, the researchers showed that this effect only emerged after four months of breastfeeding. It would seem a sensible recommendation for women with MS to breastfeed for at least this long, given previous research showing a reduction in relapse rates for women with MS while breastfeeding after childbirth.

OVERVIEW

MS is a chronic, progressively disabling disease that is still regarded as incurable. Most of the risk of developing MS is environmental—mostly adverse lifestyle factors—although it only occurs in the small proportion of the population with particular genetic susceptibility. The outlook for people diagnosed with MS today appears better than it has been in previous generations, probably partly because the diagnosis is made earlier and more often than in the past, in people with milder forms of the disease, but possibly also because of new drug therapies. However, it is currently impossible to predict how the disease will progress at the time of diagnosis. It is extremely important for PwMS to tackle this disease early because much of the damage occurs without us being aware of it, and most of the environmental factors responsible for MS progression are lifestyle factors that can be modified.

CHAPTER 2

PREVENTIVE MEDICINE AND CHRONIC WESTERN DISEASE

If the medical profession was as much devoted to the practice of the art of preventing as it is in curing disease, there can be no doubt that many diseases which now decimate communities would disappear altogether . . .

Dr Stephen Smith, President
American Public Health Association 1873

At the heart of preventive medicine is the discipline of epidemiology, a term coined by John R. Paul, of Yale University's School of Medicine, in 1938 to describe the science of exploring the multiple factors contributing to the occurrence of disease in population groups and individuals.[1] Paul's colleague at Yale, Professor C.E.A. Winslow, published a paper in 1942 lamenting the fact that, even at that time, medical practice was dominated by the treatment of disease rather than the promotion of health.[2] These sentiments were echoed by many medical writers through that decade. Today, while population health and epidemiology are robust mainstream specialty areas in medicine, it could be argued that with the dramatic growth of the pharmaceutical industry, there is even more focus on treating disease rather than preventing it through understanding and addressing factors that increase the risk of disease and of its progression.

> *Preventive Medicine is the specialty of medical practice that focuses on the health of individuals, communities, and defined populations. Its goal is to protect, promote, and maintain health and well-being and to prevent disease, disability, and death.*[3]

Preventive medicine is generally divided into primary, secondary and tertiary prevention. Primary prevention is concerned with preventing an individual from ever developing a particular disease—generally through analysis of the factors that increase an individual's risk—and modifying these risk factors. The classic example would be lung cancer. Epidemiological studies going back to the pioneering work of Doll and Hill in the 1950s have documented the strong association between cigarette smoking and the risk of developing lung cancer.[4] Primary prevention of lung cancer involves population-based interventions to convince people who smoke cigarettes to quit, and is highly successful at preventing lung cancer. In most developed countries, lung cancer rates have peaked and are now falling, in parallel with falling rates of cigarette smoking. This has been a major victory for preventive medicine, highlighting the importance of robust epidemiological studies in establishing the association of smoking with lung cancer, followed by public health and health-promotion efforts on a large scale through legislation to prevent cigarette advertising, media quit campaigns and, most recently, plain paper packaging of cigarettes to reduce their appeal.

Secondary and tertiary prevention are aspects of preventive medicine concerned with what an individual can do once diagnosed with an illness to minimise its impact. In the case of secondary prevention, an individual has been diagnosed with the disease but has not yet developed significant symptoms or complications, whereas tertiary prevention refers to the situation where an individual who has the disease, and already has significant symptoms or complications, modifies factors that increase the risk of deterioration to minimise the impact of the disease. Throughout the rest of this book, the term 'secondary prevention' will be used to cover both secondary and tertiary prevention, as the concepts are largely the same for a disease like MS, where many people have persistent symptoms even after the first attack.

Preventive medicine is routinely applied to many chronic Western diseases in most advanced health systems in the world. Examples of primary prevention successes include smoking cessation reducing the incidence of lung cancer, compulsory seatbelt legislation and drink-driving campaigns dramatically reducing the number of deaths from road trauma, and a range of immunisations that have markedly reduced the incidence of particular infectious diseases, or eradicated them altogether as in the case of smallpox. Secondary prevention, where the goal is to halt or slow the progress of disease in its earliest stages, has seen very large reductions in the complications and death rate from heart disease with recommendations of better diet, smoking cessation, exercise, stress reduction and suitable medications, and tertiary prevention is most often seen in the context of stroke rehabilitation programs and patient support groups for a number of conditions.

PREVENTIVE MEDICINE AND MS

In the case of MS, all three avenues of prevention can apply, depending on an individual's circumstances. I will go over this in much more detail in each of the steps of the Recovery Program later, but I want to provide a few examples here. For instance, first-degree relatives of someone with MS—like a son or sister—are at markedly higher risk of developing MS. Studies have now quite clearly shown the link between low vitamin D and an increased risk of developing MS, and research now shows that this risk can be reduced substantially by taking vitamin D supplements. This isn't to say that the risk is abolished altogether; rather, for someone in that position of high risk, the risk can be reduced markedly by taking vitamin D supplements. There will be a fuller discussion of this later.

Epidemiological studies have clearly identified this risk association with low vitamin D, and the reduction of risk with vitamin D supplementation, and this can easily be addressed by taking vitamin D. Another example of primary prevention in MS is smoking cessation. Epidemiological studies have shown the markedly increased risk of developing MS for those who smoke. For someone with a high risk of MS, not starting smoking, or quitting if already smoking, significantly reduces that risk.

This book is focused more on secondary prevention of MS. For those already diagnosed with the illness but not yet experiencing significant symptoms, secondary prevention is a highly effective way of halting or slowing the progress of the disease. Further, for many people, once the disease process has been halted in this way, the body's usual healing mechanisms have an opportunity to heal some of the damage, with associated return of function, just as might occur in heart disease after a secondary preventive approach. For those diagnosed, and already significantly symptomatic or disabled, tertiary prevention applies. By targeting those factors shown to increase the risk of continued deterioration, and using appropriate medications if needed, the disease process can again be halted or slowed, with some return of function—particularly through the medical specialty of rehabilitation medicine.

These preventive medicine approaches are clearly not at all new for many chronic Western diseases. In medicine, we use them all the time for people with cardiovascular disease, stroke, high blood pressure, diabetes, respiratory disease and so on. If a person today was diagnosed with a heart attack in a major hospital in most parts of the world, and was not provided with information about reducing the risk of further heart attacks by reducing saturated fat in the diet, quitting smoking, exercising regularly and looking at a stress-reduction program, the hospital would be seen as simply negligent. What is critically important to the success of such an approach, though, is the painstaking epidemiological study of the particular factors that increase the risk of progression. This is what my research group has been undertaking since 2012 with the Health Outcomes and Lifestyle Interventions in a Sample of people with Multiple Sclerosis (HOLISM) study. Much more on that later.

Sadly, Professor Paul from Yale University was concerned that the very development of preventive medicine as a medical specialty would mean that departments of preventive medicine would be removed from clinical medicine and lead his colleagues to focus overly on medical treatment of disease and forget about prevention.[5] It is pretty clear that this, in conjunction with the commercial interests of industry—particularly in making profits for shareholders of drug companies—has led to repeated failures of modern medicine to utilise important preventive measures in dealing with modern chronic disease. Type 2 diabetes (T2D) is a classic example. There is striking epidemiological evidence that T2D is in most cases caused by lifestyle factors, and its progression is determined largely by risk factors in lifestyle. T2D incidence, for example, exactly parallels the incidence of obesity. There are straight-line relationships with a person's weight and their risk of developing T2D. Yet we now have an industry that has grown around medications for T2D that do little, if anything, about the disease process and simply reduce blood sugar.

MS is a chronic Western disease, with progression influenced mostly by lifestyle; it is particularly suited to treatment with secondary or tertiary prevention.

MS is another example. This book presents the evidence that MS is a chronic Western disease, strongly influenced by lifestyle factors, and that attention to these factors can be a highly effective strategy, both in primary prevention of the disease ever occurring in at-risk individuals— that is, the children and other close relatives of those already diagnosed with MS—and in secondary and tertiary prevention of the disease progressing in those already diagnosed. It is important to note that in MS, just as in heart disease, stroke and kidney disease, this approach is a mainstream medical approach. It has nothing whatsoever to do with complementary and alternative medicine.

While treatment with appropriate medications is part of secondary prevention, managing the illness using medications alone does not utilise all the therapies at our disposal, and is not good medical practice, just as it is not in other chronic Western diseases. Sadly, this drug-only approach has been adopted by many doctors, not only for managing MS, but also for many other chronic Western diseases, despite abundant research showing the great benefits of the broader preventive strategy. As David Suzuki, one of the most important thinkers on our planet, says, 'I was struck by how cardiologists saw her heart in complete isolation from her psychological, physiological, or physical condition. To the heart specialists, the opportunities for treatment consisted of hitting the sick heart with drugs or operating on it. Others things didn't factor into the equation—not the notion that extreme stress . . . not a physiological imbalance from diet, or lack of exercise, not environmental conditions.'[6]

There is a large, congruent literature and evidence base around the particular risk factors that raise a person's chance of being diagnosed with MS, and there is even more evidence about those particular risk factors that increase the rate of progression of the disease. While not widely acknowledged by some doctors treating PwMS, this is well known among researchers and those people actively engaged in their own health after a diagnosis of MS. The European Charcot Foundation Symposium on MS, for example, held in Italy in 2010, focused on a reappraisal of the nutritional and environmental factors responsible for MS development.[7] The keynote address to the symposium outlined the risk factors that can potentially be modified to prevent MS in our children. The role of vitamin D was highlighted, with the experts agreeing that the optimal level to aim for in blood level of vitamin D to prevent MS is at least 100 nmol/L, and that supplementing to this level could dramatically reduce the incidence of the disease. The experts also noted the role of smoking in increasing MS risk, infection with the Epstein-Barr Virus and being overweight. Of course, nothing can be done to reduce one's risk once someone has had glandular fever, but the experts suggested that a vaccine might help in preventing the disease, and hence MS. An obvious omission was any real discussion about diet and saturated fat, and there will be much more about this later.

DEVELOPING THE OMS RECOVERY PROGRAM

For most chronic Western diseases, a preventive approach is more effective than treating complications as they arise. In this context, prevention usually first revolves around identifying risk factors that cause the disease to progress more rapidly, with the development of complications. As we have seen, this is where epidemiology comes in, because it involves studying patterns of disease in populations. Researchers look at data from large populations of people with a particular illness to try to identify factors that increase the risk of progression of the illness. So we compare people whose disease has progressed against those in whom it has not progressed substantially, and see where they are different in terms of their backgrounds or lifestyle to detect risky features in those who have more progressive disease. These risk factors are then targeted in preventive medicine programs.

Let's take heart disease as an example. Heart disease is a good model to use here, particularly with Corthals' theory about MS being a disease of fat dysregulation—much like heart disease.[8] Large studies have now been done over many years, examining the ongoing health of people with heart disease, and correlating whether the disease progresses in line with various risk factors in people's lifestyles. We now know that those who eat a diet containing more animal fats, with a high proportion of calories coming from fats, and who eat more refined foods and fewer fruit and vegetables, have worse outcomes, with higher death rates and more need for treatment with pharmaceutical drugs and medical procedures. People who smoke, exercise less and are overweight also have worse outcomes, as do people in very stressful occupations. The similarities with MS are no coincidence. Having identified these risk factors, public health physicians can use this evidence to build evidence-based guidelines for recommending lifestyle changes to people with, or who are at risk of, heart disease.

Providing advice based on such guidelines has now been considered best practice for many years. People being discharged from hospital now after a heart attack or other cardiac problem without receiving such advice would rightly feel aggrieved. That said, it can still take a long, long time in medicine for such practice to become routine. Recent Australian data showed that fully three-quarters of people discharged from major Australian hospitals after admission for heart disease did not receive such advice.[9]

In MS, there is actually a very large evidence base around the factors associated with developing the disease and its progression. This is to be expected, given the fact that around three-quarters of the risk of developing the illness is environmental, not genetic, and that all of the risk of progression appears to be environmental. As previously noted, a large genome study of PwMS found no genetic markers of disease progression.[10] The evidence base is not nearly as large as that concerning heart disease—and that is perhaps also expected, given how much more common heart disease is. But it probably also reflects the somewhat outdated view of MS as a mystery incurable disease, rather than a typical chronic Western disease like heart disease, type 2 diabetes, high blood pressure and cancer.

Scientists from many countries have studied the risk factors for MS for many, many years. Not least of them was Professor Swank, whose influential paper in the major international journal *The New England Journal of Medicine*,[11] was largely responsible for starting the whole evidence base around the role of food in MS. Another is German epidemiologist Dr Klaus Lauer, who has been researching and publishing in the area for 30 years, with over 40 major international publications on the subject— the most recent summarising knowledge on diet, including protective effects from fish consumption and harms from processed meats, lack of sun exposure, viral infections and cigarette smoking.[12-15] So much is now known about these risk factors, yet most people diagnosed with MS are still not advised about how modification of these risk factors can help reduce the risk of progression of the illness.

It is important to put this in context. We are not talking about a cure for MS here, any more than we are when discussing the lifestyle risk modification approach to treating heart disease. This preventive approach is about modifying risk factors known to accelerate the progression of MS to disability, with the aim of reducing the risk of progression. How complete a lifestyle change is made, and how rigorously one eliminates these risk factors, determines to a large extent how effective the approach is. This seems to be true wherever this approach has been used. For example, in heart disease, Dr Dean Ornish has very elegantly shown, in well-designed studies, that those adhering to an approach almost identical to the OMS Recovery Program—that is, a plant-based wholefood diet plus exercise, smoking cessation and stress reduction—not only halted the progression of their heart disease, but reversed it. His study showed that those adhering most rigorously to the program had the greatest benefit.[16] The blocked coronary arteries of those adhering to the program literally opened up!

In coronary heart disease, because of a primary problem with fat metabolism, fatty deposits accumulate on the lining of arteries throughout the body, but this is particularly important where arteries are small and supply such a vital organ as the heart. So the coronary arteries that bring much-needed oxygen to the heart muscle gradually narrow over time due to the fatty deposits until they are so blocked that not enough oxygen-carrying blood gets through to the heart muscle and people develop chest pain, or angina. If the blockage is complete, they have a heart attack. In Ornish's ground-breaking research, those adhering to these lifestyle changes actually reversed the narrowing,[16-19] so that the vessels gradually opened up over time as the fatty deposits shrank, and blood began to flow normally to the heart muscle, bringing much-needed oxygen and eliminating symptoms. So, while not technically considered a cure, this was prevention at its best, with modification of lifestyle risk factors leading to recovery from the illness. The parallels with MS are striking.

Ornish tried this technique on another common chronic Western disease, prostate cancer, and achieved similarly remarkable results.[20, 21, 22] Men diagnosed with prostate cancer who were assessed as suitable to 'watch and wait' to see whether the disease progressed to a stage requiring treatment were randomly allocated to a standard treatment group or to Ornish's preventive medicine approach. The same lifestyle risk factors were targeted, and again the results demonstrated recovery for the majority of men modifying their lifestyles, with better results for those adhering more strongly to the program. In prostate cancer, it is easier to follow the progression of the illness than in many other common Western diseases, as a simple blood test (prostate-specific antigen, or PSA) reliably correlates with the spread of the disease. So for those adhering rigorously to the lifestyle modification program, PSA levels actually fell somewhat over the course of the study compared with those on standard treatment, the majority of whom ended up needing surgery, radiotherapy or other usual therapies as their PSA levels climbed. Those men adhering rigorously to the diet may not have been able to say they were cured, but they had certainly recovered from the illness, and if they continued adhering to the ultra-healthy lifestyle, they had no further problems with the illness; their PSA results confirmed that the cancer was no longer active.

Interestingly, working with Nobel Prize winner Professor Elizabeth Blackburn, Ornish showed that the lifestyle changes actually made a difference at the level of the participants' DNA! He showed that the expression of genes responsible for cancer is modified by lifestyle factors.[23] Some naysayers who oppose a preventive medicine approach sometimes say that a lifestyle modification program just makes people feel good, and improves quality of life (which is no small benefit in any event), and that there is no underlying physiological reason it should work. This ignores the important work of many scientists over many years, but particularly this recent work showing that lifestyle changes fundamentally alter the expression of a person's genetic structure.

Lifestyle changes make fundamental differences to the way DNA is expressed; preventive medicine is do-it-yourself genetic engineering.

When assessing which particular lifestyle changes need to be addressed for any chronic disease, doctors making the recommendations have to consider the available evidence about risk factors. In medicine, there are relatively standard ways of assessing evidence. The highest level of research is meta-analysis—that is, amalgamation of the results of randomised controlled trials to get an overall idea of the effect of a medical intervention using the largest amount of available data. So testing an intervention—preferably several times—in randomised controlled trials (where one group of people with the disease gets the intervention and the other doesn't, and we assess the difference in outcome between groups) is the most important research, coming after development of a theory and testing an intervention based on the theory in small uncontrolled studies to show that it is safe.

While this book discusses many of the theories about causation of MS, it is important to note that advice to modify certain lifestyle risk factors is backed up with published evidence—that is, it is based on much more than a theory. But, in the case of diet in particular, one important paper noted the strong bias against undertaking dietary research for many chronic conditions including MS because of the difficulties in performing randomised controlled trials on diet.[24] As pointed out in this paper, when we have very strong epidemiological evidence of the benefit of diet (such as the HOLISM study in MS), the purpose of randomised controlled trials is really just to provide some reassurance that the effect is not due to some other confounding factor, but the diet itself.

Angelique Corthals' theory about disordered fat metabolism is one of the more recent and most compelling concepts to emerge, fitting with much more of what we know about MS than other theories. One of the first steps when one comes up with a theory is to check epidemiologically whether it is sound—that is, studies of populations can help us decide whether a theory is worth testing in an intervention study. So with saturated fat being one of the causes and aggravating factors of MS, one can look at population incidence of MS and confirm that the disease is indeed markedly more common where saturated fat consumption is highest, and vice versa. That is what Swank did in his early studies. Following his work in Norway showing that the incidence of MS was six-fold higher in inland parts, where dairy and meat consumption were highest, than in coastal parts where fish consumption was highest, he found that countries where saturated fat consumption was highest had the highest incidence of MS.[25] He then set about testing this with an intervention study. This is the landmark Swank study, where the intervention tested was an ultra-low-saturated fat diet.[26] He studied this meticulously over 34 years, and found that those consuming the lowest amount of saturated fat had by far the best outcomes.

Ideally, we would now have many randomised controlled trials confirming this, but for several reasons we don't. First, by the time this was published in The Lancet in 1990, we had reached the drug therapy era in MS management, and there was strong motivation for investigators to study drugs in MS, as this research was heavily backed by industry, which stood to make billions—and, of course, it has. Second, randomised controlled trials of lifestyle interventions are difficult. The MS research group I head had great trouble studying the effects of live-in educational retreats for people with type 2 diabetes.[27] These are really difficult clinical trials to run.

So there are many theories, and many therapies out there based on the theories. The OMS Recovery Program, however, is the result of an objective weighing up of the evidence for and against all the major theories. The theories often sound very plausible, but if there isn't good evidence from a variety of research methods, the particular intervention generally doesn't make it into the Program. There is the occasional exception to this rule: if a factor has really solid experimental evidence in the laboratory, and sound epidemiological data to back it up—particularly if it is some factor that can be seen as posing a particular risk for PwMS— then the Program will recommend that PwMS avoid it, even if there is no hard clinical trial evidence. This is the case, for example, for smoking and for cow's milk consumption. Some may look at the epidemiological evidence for smoking accelerating the course of MS and ask why health professionals would recommend that PwMS quit smoking and yet, with the same level of evidence for the harm associated with saturated fat consumption, not recommend that PwMS avoid saturated fat. In the case of smoking, in medicine we have always relied on epidemiological evidence to make recommendations about smoking cessation. It is clearly unethical and not reasonable to conduct a study where we randomly allocate some PwMS to a smoking group and others to a non-smoking group. So the recommendations come directly from epidemiological studies showing the strong associations between smoking and worsening disability in MS.

For dietary factors, though, even though the epidemiological evidence is strong, it is feasible to run intervention studies where one group is allocated a particular diet and others are not. It is certainly not easy, but it is feasible. There are many difficulties around people sticking to a particular diet for a study in MS that needs to be of long duration, because it often takes many years to see a difference in disability between people. Thus many would accept that Swank's study, where some people adhered to the diet and others didn't, is strong enough evidence on which to base recommendations. I would agree. This is particularly so when the vast majority of other research on diet supports the same recommendation, including HOLISM study results[28, 29] and research on blood fat profiles funded by MS Research Australia.[30]

In the case of cow's milk, two separate studies from highly ranked international research institutes have shown a specific immune reactivity for PwMS to the protein in cow's milk.[31, 32] Epidemiological studies confirm that in populations where cow's milk consumption is high, the incidence of MS is also high, and vice versa.[33] The world maps of MS incidence and cow's milk consumption are essentially identical. So, for that reason, the Program advocates that PwMS avoid cow's milk products, as the potential risk of ingesting these products outweighs any perceived benefit one might get from eating them, even despite the lack of clinical trial evidence to support the risk. Additionally, it is unlikely that any research funding body will fund large-scale trials of cow's milk versus no cow's milk.

Some may ask why the Program doesn't include the same recommendation for gluten as for cow's milk. While the theories about these possible causes of MS are plausible, at the first pass of checking these theories with the epidemiological data, we find that there is no real population data to support the theories. So for populations eating lots of whole grains, the incidence of MS is no higher than in populations that don't; indeed, the reverse seems to be true. And without any intervention studies to support the theories, it is difficult to recommend that people avoid gluten—especially when avoiding it is an onerous lifestyle change, given how many of our foods we find it in. So while some theories about MS causation and progression will in time be shown to be true and some false, the weight of evidence to date does not support making major lifestyle changes that involve omitting grains, but does support omitting saturated fat as much as possible and not taking the risk of consuming dairy products.

The OMS recommendations are meant to be generic and suitable for most people based on the best available evidence. But for some people there may well be other factors involved, and if the OMS recommendations, rigorously applied, don't seem to be helping, it may be wise to add one of the commonly prescribed disease-modifying drugs (DMDs), or look for other potential triggers. Many people will opt to take one of the DMDs right from the time of diagnosis, without waiting to see whether lifestyle modifications make a difference, and this is a perfectly legitimate choice. While we hope that most PwMS will benefit from the

OMS Program, the journey remains yours, and naturally, after suitable searching and consideration, you may choose to use other modalities to assist in your own recovery. Many of these are mentioned on our website, <www.overcomingms.org>, in the Forum.

> The OMS Recovery Program is based on a rigorous analysis of the best available scientific evidence.

Although the OMS Program is the result of serious consideration of most of the commonly discussed factors involved in MS disease progression, and the recommendations are based on this rigorous analysis, they can change as new evidence becomes available. The first book outlining this general approach, *Taking Control of Multiple Sclerosis*,[34] was published in 2000 and reflected the literature review undertaken in 1999, so is based on the available literature at the time. For instance, in 1999 multivitamin supplementation was recommended, along with supplementation with particular vitamins such as vitamin E. Since the major meta-analyses subsequently showed harm from such supplementation, this position changed—as it often does in science as new evidence becomes available—and in *Overcoming Multiple Sclerosis: An Evidence Based Guide to Recovery*,[35] published in 2010, the recommendation was to avoid these supplements. Similarly, the recommendation in 1999 was for PwMS not to wait for evidence from intervention studies about the potential benefit of sun exposure and vitamin D supplementation, based on compelling laboratory, animal and epidemiological data. It was felt that the risk of waiting was too great, after due consideration of the safety of vitamin D supplementation. Many OMS followers subsequently took vitamin D over many years before the randomised controlled data appeared. While some neurologists still do not advocate the use of vitamin D in MS, most mainstream MS centres now regard it as the standard of care.[36] However, if the data coming in from clinical trials had been neutral or negative, the OMS Program would have moved quickly to change these recommendations.

I don't pretend to have all the answers, as the evidence base in MS, like other diseases, is continually growing, from time to time contradicting previous evidence, necessitating a change in recommendations. This is how science works. The OMS Program recommendations are based on the best available evidence, and may change over time as the evidence grows. So it is possible that some of what is currently recommended may change in the future. For now, the OMS Recovery Program represents a sound plan based on current evidence to enable recovery of good health for PwMS. The OMS website will update with new recommendations where appropriate as new evidence comes in.

VALIDATING THE OMS RECOVERY PROGRAM

Importantly, in this book there is now another very strong level of validation about the OMS Recovery Program. The Program was developed through analysis of the available MS literature in the world's best medical journals—that is, those indexed by MEDLINE, the premier bibliographic database of medical research in the world, housed at the National Library of Medicine in the United States. I used my background in medical science, as a professor in medicine and the editor of a major medical journal, with all the skills and experience that entails, to sort through all the available evidence about what might help a person with MS to stay well—that is, to discover what risk factors could be modified in a secondary or tertiary preventive medicine approach to reducing the risk of progression of the disease.

The literature review required a good deal of detective work; not all the research was published in the neurology journals. The vitamin D and sunlight research, for example, was mostly in epidemiology journals or endocrinology literature; much of the work around the mind–body connection was in the psychology literature, or elsewhere, in what is sometimes termed 'grey' literature. Synthesising the findings into a coherent program of lifestyle risk modification required considerable experience in knowing and understanding the relative strengths of the various research studies.

But now the whole Program has been subjected to its own research evaluation. Both the follow up study of PwMS attending OMS retreats to learn the Program (STudying Outcomes of People attending MS retreats, the STOP-MS study) and the HOLISM study provided a unique opportunity to validate the various parts of the Program and to see how people following it progressed (or otherwise) over time. While the literature review strongly suggested that PwMS attending the retreats would get better, there were really no data to validate this when the retreats started in 2002. Similarly, when the HOLISM study commenced in 2012, there were no studies looking at whether the whole range of risk factors identified in the literature review, when examined in a large international sample of PwMS, would hold up to scientific scrutiny. What my research team at the University of Melbourne undertook was validation of the original tenets of the Program—that is, providing the research evidence to investigate scientifically whether the Program really works. Suffice to say, as we will see, the data are now in, and the Program does work!

This book outlines the Program in seven steps, based first on the evidence supporting each step—that is, the 'Why' behind that step. Then, for each step, it goes into some detail about the 'How'—that is, the provision of detailed suggestions about implementing each step. Feedback from the last edition of *Overcoming Multiple Sclerosis* indicated that there was ample evidence provided to convince PwMS about the various risk factors that needed to be modified to minimise the risk of disease progression, but not nearly enough detail about how to do it. So this book seeks to address that aspect: to not only outline the evidence behind each step, but also be more of a manual on how to implement the Program.

But first it is important to get an understanding of the validation research of the Program that my research team undertook and is continuing with, and how that research has validated the various aspects of the Program. The two main studies comprising the validation research are outlined in detail in the next chapter. Then, under each chapter describing the steps of the Program, the separate parts of the study underpinning that particular step are described. Some parts of the research relate to aspects of health for PwMS that aren't covered by a particular step of the Program, and for those parts—relating to depression, fatigue and engagement—the findings of the research are presented towards the end of the book after discussing the Program in detail.

CHAPTER 3

VALIDATING THE OMS PROGRAM: THE STOP-MS STUDY AND THE HOLISM STUDY

Every great advance in science has issued from a new audacity of the imagination.

John Dewey

INTRODUCTION

In the early 2000s, I was invited to a neurology conference in Sydney, Australia. I received a telephone call from a member of the organising committee who was aware of my personal interest in MS and my first book, *Taking Control of Multiple Sclerosis*. I was invited to talk to a large group of neurologists about the preventive approach I had researched in writing the book and that I had adopted personally since. I accepted the invitation and was asked to send a curriculum vitae (CV) over so that I could be properly introduced. Some weeks later, I received another call, this time from a more senior member of the organising team. He said that he had read my CV and, because I had not actually published (medical research papers) on MS, they had decided to withdraw my invitation.

This was the moment when I realised that I had to do my own research in the field of preventive medical approaches to MS management, or I simply would not be taken seriously. As the years unfolded, and I began to lead live-in retreats for PwMS in the Yarra Valley in Victoria, Australia, and elsewhere, I was acutely aware of the need to study the outcomes of people attending those retreats, and I saw the opportunity to undertake this much-needed research.

 The STOP-MS and HOLISM studies provide strong validation, in a real-world situation, of the benefits of a preventive medicine approach to managing MS.

More recently, as news of the OMS approach spread—particularly with the widespread adoption of social media, and my own forays into that area to try to spread the message—it became clear to me that, while I am not a neurologist, and therefore don't have patients with MS about whom I might have a lot of clinical data like medications and MRI findings, I had to be audacious and employ the services of the very large group of PwMS worldwide with whom I had contact and whose own experiences with the disease I could follow. So I decided to invite them to take part in a unique global study of PwMS, looking for the first time in detail at their lifestyles and how their health was progressing, with the aim of examining whether the various aspects of the OMS Recovery Program—the various lifestyle risk factors that I had identified—were really associated with good or poor health for PwMS in a real-world situation, for thousands of people with the illness internationally.

THE STOP-MS STUDY

From the very first retreat at the Gawler Foundation in April 2002, participants were asked to complete a newly developed but validated questionnaire, the MS Quality of Life-54 (MSQOL-54), built on the SF-36, the Short Form (36) Health Survey that had been widely used since the early 1990s to measure health status in a very large number of research studies. The MSQOL-54 consists of 52 items distributed into twelve scales, and two single items, which give rise to two composite scores: the physical and mental health composites. The tool has been extensively validated and translated in international populations,[1, 2, 3] and in assessing the impact of fatigue,[4] depression[5] and sexual dysfunction,[6] as well as a number of medical therapies.

So the study began collecting ongoing information about the health of PwMS who had attended these retreats over the years. We followed up people attending the retreats who agreed to participate at one year after the retreat, then again at 2.5 years, five years and ten years. Because there were around three retreats a year, continuing until the present day, the numbers of PwMS at each time point gradually grew. We have subsequently published outcomes of the groups as they have reached the one-, 2.5- and five-year time points; these results are outlined in Step 7: Change your life, for life.

Along the way, it became clear that we had to know not only whether people had attended a retreat, but also how closely they adhered to our guidelines. So, like the HOLISM study discussed next, we added a lot of questions about all the various lifestyle factors we had identified as being important. These results are presented later, but in brief they strongly support the OMS Recovery Program and the approach we have taken to disseminating this information via the live-in retreats.

THE HOLISM STUDY

Over the years since my initial realisation that I would have to undertake my own research into these preventive medicine principles, I have gradually developed a suite of resources to accompany the book. A key resource was

the development of the *Taking Control of Multiple Sclerosis* website, named
after the first book, in 2008. In obtaining advice about how to ensure that
the website came to the attention of PwMS, I was advised by a particularly
web-savvy retreat participant that I really needed to use social media such
as Facebook and Twitter to maximise potential traffic to the site. Launched
in 2008, a little after the website, our Facebook page, <www.facebook.com/
MultipleSclerosisManagement>—originally called *Taking Control of Multiple
Sclerosis*—sat fairly quietly for some time. Around 2010, I began posting in
earnest, and in 2013 I changed the name to *Overcoming Multiple Sclerosis*, to
reflect the name of the newer book; in 2015, we passed the 15,000 'likes'
mark. Similarly, I started a Twitter account (@georgejelinek) that passed the
2400-follower mark in 2015. I was posting not only on these sites, but also
on many other websites, blogs and forums, as were many of the PwMS who
had been to our retreats, and others who had read the book and started the
Program without attending a retreat.

So I had a very large group of PwMS worldwide who knew me, and
with whom I regularly communicated about various aspects of the OMS
Program. It became clear to me that this group could form the basis
of another unique study; we had enough PwMS to look very closely
at the factors I had found in researching MS for my first and subsequent books—that is, lifestyle factors like diet, sun exposure, vitamin D,
omega-3 supplementation, exercise, quitting smoking, reducing alcohol
consumption and stress-reduction techniques—and examine their association with the quality of life and health of the people in this group.
Dr Ruth Marrie, Associate Professor in Neurology at the University of
Manitoba, has written that to better understand the roles of various factors
in modifying the course of a disease, careful study will be needed of
'well-characterised populations in which the roles of multiple factors are
considered simultaneously'.[7] This is exactly what we set out to do. Unlike
many other MS studies, I didn't have detailed medical data on file about
these people—like their MRI results or the drugs I was prescribing—as
they were not my patients. Nor could I assess directly how disabled or
not they were, or document whether they were having relapses.

So we had to be a bit more innovative. With the help of Dr Naresh
Pereira, now a doctor at Box Hill Hospital in Melbourne, who first came
to our research unit as a medical student looking to do some voluntary

research work, we trawled through the medical literature trying to find tools that people could use to measure many of these things for themselves, in a way that would translate to similar findings that a treating neurologist could come up with. For instance, Naresh found the Patient Determined Disease Steps scale, where PwMS score their own mobility from 0 (normal) to 8 (bed bound). It is simple and easy to for PwMS to fill in, and is scored consistently by different people. Most important of all, though, it correlates well with the standard measure that neurologists use—the EDSS—and with the widely used multiple sclerosis functional composite; in other words, it has been validated. For our purposes, it was also important that it could be used to assess changes in disability over time,[8] because we planned the HOLISM study to be a snapshot not only of how this large group of PwMS were living at the start of the study, but also at time points over the years after this baseline snapshot. Naresh spent much time finding other tools as well that PwMS could use themselves to score not only their health but also some of the other potential lifestyle risk factors at which we were looking, like diet. Table 1 shows the validated tools that we used in the study.

Table 1: Summary of validated tools used

Outcome variable	Instrument (reference)	Number of items	Authors (reference)
Disability	Patient determined disease steps (PDDS)	1	Hohol et al. 1995[9]
Comorbidities	Self-administered comorbidity questionnaire (SCQ)	13	Sangha et al. 2003[10]
Health-related quality of life	Multiple sclerosis quality of life-54 (MSQOL-54)	54	Vickrey et al. 1995[11]
Dietary habits	Diet habits questionnaire (DHQ), modified	20	McKellar et al. 2008[12]
Physical activity	International physical activity questionnaire (IPAQ)	7	Craig et al. 2003[13]
Social support	Single item measure of social support (SIMSS)	1	Blake and McKay 1986[14]
Fatigue	Fatigue severity scale (FSS)	9	Krupp et al. 1989[15]
Depression	Patient health questionnaire short version (PHQ-2)	2	Kroenke et al. 2003[16]

This was an extremely ambitious study, and completely novel for its time. While I had published my first book back in 2000, no one had since seriously looked at the overall suite of risk factors for worsening disease that I had discovered in my literature search, which I have gone over again in this book. Vast numbers of research studies were being published each year on MS, and large groups of researchers the world over were looking at various aspects of the disease but, amazingly, hardly anyone was looking in any detail at these important risk factors—factors which, if modified, could potentially form the basis of a relatively simple prevention program that could keep PwMS well. And while some groups may have been looking at diet, others at vitamin D and others at exercise, no one was looking at all these factors together, to try to determine which was the most important in modifying disease course.

So I and my research team at the University of Melbourne spent many months painstakingly putting this detailed survey together. We used the common web-based survey tool Survey Monkey, which meant that participants could simply click on the link and then complete the survey online, and the data would instantly be available to us to analyse. Prior to the internet, such studies were orders of magnitude more difficult, and to all intents and purposes were not realistically possible. Senior Australian MS researchers have strongly encouraged the use of such social media resources as novel avenues for better understanding what factors contribute to MS risk and progression.[17]

Having put the survey together, we applied to the relevant Research Ethics Committee for approval of the project. Once it was approved, we tested the survey on seven PwMS who had been to our retreats, to iron out any bugs. We had no idea how many PwMS might want to take part in such a study—after all, the questionnaire was very detailed, taking approximately 45 minutes to complete, and these people all had MS, with many of them quite disabled from the disease, with the usual problems associated with the illness potentially including fatigue, depression and cognitive decline, making a lengthy questionnaire quite an obstacle. Once finalised, my colleague Emily Hadgkiss and I then spent many hours on Facebook, using the networks I had established over the years, and building new ones as we joined new Facebook groups, posting the details of our study and the link to SurveyMonkey to allow participation. Those choosing to participate followed the link and found a detailed participant information sheet, and advice that going on to complete the survey would be taken as consent to the study.

Having posted the explanations and links on the website, Facebook and Twitter, I headed overseas to Laos for a holiday. Internet reception was patchy, but every few days we would find somewhere with wi-fi, and I would check my phone, astounded by the numbers of participants the study was generating. The study was only really possible because of the advantages of the information age. PwMS were sharing the link via their Facebook accounts, tweeting about the study and posting about it on various MS forums. A total of 3053 people consented to participate, seven of whom were pilot study participants, whose data were included in the analysis. Of those who consented, 2519 had been formally diagnosed with MS and therefore met the criteria for study inclusion. All but one of these provided contact details for follow-up (see Figure 1). Of those with confirmed MS, 89 per cent continued to the end of the survey. Of the demographics and clinical characteristics items, there was an average item completion rate of 95 per cent.

We were stunned! The very large number of PwMS in the study made it one of the bigger MS studies in the literature. Importantly, as we began to analyse the data, we noted that the sample of PwMS contained both many people who had been to retreats, read the book or visited the website and were changing their lifestyles, and also a large proportion who had not. In epidemiological terms, this is described as a population with a wide range of exposures. This enabled us to compare health outcomes between those who were using a preventive medicine approach and those who were not. This filled a huge gap in the MS literature; many studies, such as the US Nurses Health Study that examined diet and its effect on MS outcome,[18] really had very few participants who were eating such dramatically improved diets as we saw in our sample, because of the nature of our recruitment techniques. So it was very hard in the Nurses study to compare health outcomes between those eating very healthy diets and those who were not. We realised we had a unique opportunity, and that the data would tell a very important story because of the sample size and make-up in part representing a very major piece of evidence

Figure 1: Breakdown of participants in the HOLISM study

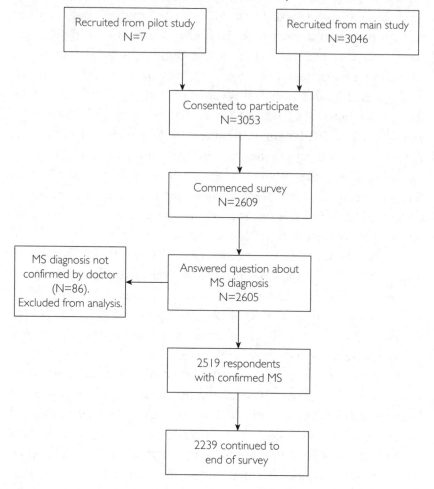

about risk factors for the health of PwMS, in a unique population. What that story was, we had no idea.

The HOLISM study population is unique, comprising a large proportion of people with MS living ultra-healthy lifestyles and a large proportion who were not.

Our first step was to prepare a paper for publication outlining how we conducted this study. In studies of this magnitude, that is critically important. Many journals have word limits for the papers they publish, and they can really limit the amount of information the researchers can provide about the methods they use in the study—in this case, this is particularly important because of the novelty of the study. We prepared our paper and submitted it to the journal *Neurology Research International*, and within a relatively short timeframe, the paper was published.[19]

Our data indicated that we had people from 57 different countries responding, the majority of them (82 per cent) women—a much higher proportion of women than in most MS studies, probably because of our sampling technique, with more women using social media and participating in the forums we sampled. Participants were between eighteen and 87 years of age, with a median age of 46 years. Respondents living in the United States, Australia, the United Kingdom, New Zealand and Canada comprised most (88 per cent) of the study sample. Most (61 per cent) were married, over two-thirds with children. About one-third were in full-time work, with a quarter retired due to medical reasons or disability. The sample was a very well-educated one, with over half having a university bachelor's degree; of these, two-thirds had also completed a postgraduate degree.

Participants had been diagnosed with MS for a median of six years with around half diagnosed within the previous five years. Median age at diagnosis was 37 years. Most (61 per cent) had relapsing-remitting MS. Disability was across the spectrum, but about a third had no symptoms or only mild symptoms that returned to normal after an attack. At the time of the survey, over one-quarter of participants were experiencing symptoms due to a recent relapse. Over the previous year, relapsing-remitting participants reported having an average of 1.09 relapses and over the last five years, an average of 0.97 relapses per year. Nearly one-fifth of the sample screened positive for depression, and two-thirds for clinically significant fatigue.

At the time of the survey, around half of the participants were taking a disease-modifying drug. Very surprisingly, and indicating how many of the PwMS in this study were making significant lifestyle changes, 38 per cent of respondents didn't consume dairy products, 27 per cent didn't consume meat products and 21 per cent consumed neither meat nor dairy. Similarly, only 12 per cent were current smokers, 82 per cent took vitamin D supplements and nearly two-thirds took omega-3 supplements. Meditation practice was undertaken at least once per week by nearly one-third of people in the sample.

There were a number of other findings of interest related to quality of life, disability and depression, but the importance of this paper was that it reported in detail how the study was done prior to a series of studies on the collected data examining the relationship between various lifestyle factors such as diet, omega-3 supplementation, exercise, meditation and smoking, and relapse rate, disease activity and disability. We reported over the next two to three years, in major neurology, psychiatry and general medical journals, the factors associated with disease activity and disability for PwMS in this large sample of people from all over the world. The paper outlining the methods of the study can be found at <www.hindawi.com/journals/nri/2013/580596>. In each of the chapters in Part II outlining the seven steps of the OMS Program, the HOLISM study findings for that risk factor, and how the study validated the original preventive medicine hypothesis, are described.

Of course, our research team plans to follow up this large cohort of PwMS at regular intervals of 2.5 years. We have already collected the data for the first of these time points, and will shortly begin analysing the data at the Neuroepidemiology Unit at the Melbourne School of Population and Global Health, with the help of some of Australia's top epidemiologists and biostatisticians. It will be fascinating to watch the health of these people over time, and to see how it relates to changes in their lifestyles over time.

PART II

THE OMS RECOVERY PROGRAM

STEP 1

EAT WELL

I don't understand why asking people to eat a well-balanced vegetarian diet is considered drastic, while it is medically conservative to cut people open and put them on cholesterol-lowering drugs for the rest of their lives.

Dr Dean Ornish

INTRODUCTION

A very large, congruent evidence base shows that MS is a lifestyle disease, the course of which is largely determined by lifestyle factors, principally diet. The evidence has been assembled painstakingly over nearly a century, with little if any contradictory data. Large-scale epidemiological studies show that the risk of developing MS in a population decreases as the ratio of saturated to unsaturated fat in the diet decreases, as does the rate of progression of the disease. Clinical studies show that PwMS adhering to such diets have far less progression of disability. To better understand why the diet works and is necessary, before proceeding to how to change, some background knowledge is necessary.

WHY

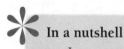

In a nutshell

- Less saturated (animal) fat in the diet has been shown in population and clinical studies to be associated with lower population rates of MS and less progression to disability.
- A poor fat profile in blood, associated with high-saturated fat diets, has been shown to be associated with more rapid progression of MS.
- Many studies suggest a beneficial effect of omega-3 supplementation in reducing relapses.
- Experimental evidence strongly suggests that cow's milk protein harms people with MS.
- The HOLISM study showed that the strongest predictors of good health for people with MS were healthy fat intake, more fruits and vegetables, and more seafood in the diet.
- HOLISM showed no harmful effects of alcohol consumption, except in excess.

Types of fats

Fats and oils are really made of the same thing: fatty acids. The term 'fats' is traditionally reserved for those fatty acids that are solid at room temperature—like fat on a steak—whereas 'oils' is generally used for those fatty acids that are liquid at room temperature—like olive oil—but all fats and oils are made of fatty acids. Saturated fats are those fatty acids found principally in animals, but also in large quantities in coconut and palm oils. The term 'saturated' is a technical one, meaning that all the carbon atoms in the long chains of these fats—often described as the carbon backbone—are connected to each other with single bonds. When the carbon chains of these fats have all the hydrogen atoms they can hold, they are said to be saturated with hydrogen, or simply saturated fats. These fats have high melting points, and so are typically solid or nearly solid at room temperature, except for coconut and palm oils. These latter two oils are not solid because they are a mixture of fatty acids, with much of the mixture being medium-chained saturated fats with lower melting points.

If there is one double bond present between any two carbon atoms, the fatty acid is monounsaturated. The typical example of this sort of fatty acid is oleic acid in olive oil. These fatty acids have lower melting points, and so are liquid at room temperature, but will solidify a little or go cloudy in the fridge. If there is more than one double bond present in the backbone, the fat is polyunsaturated. These fats have the lowest melting points and are liquid at room temperature and in the fridge. Many of these polyunsaturated fatty acids are what we call essential fatty acids. That means they are essential for normal bodily function, but cannot be manufactured in the body; they must be obtained through the diet. They can be thought of in the same way as vitamins.

Polyunsaturated fats are essential to health; they help in MS by making cell membranes more fluid and resistant to degeneration, and omega-3 fatty acids dampen the immune response.

There are two principal types of polyunsaturated fatty acids: those with the first double bond at the third carbon from the omega end of the chain—that is, omega-3 or n-3 fatty acids—and those with the first double bond at the sixth carbon from the omega end—that is, omega-6 or n-6 fatty acids. The omega-3 fatty acids are typified by alpha linolenic acid in flaxseed oil and eicosapentanoic acid (EPA) and docosahexanoic acid (DHA) in fish oil, and the omega-6s by linoleic acid in various cooking oils such as sunflower oil, safflower oil and corn oil. The monounsaturated fats are sometimes called omega 9 fats because their only double bond is at the ninth carbon from the omega end.

Properties and effects of fats

The melting points of these fats determine one of their important properties: their stickiness and flexibility when they are incorporated into the cell membranes of bodily cells. It is important to remember here that body cells are surrounded by an envelope, the cell membrane, that is made up mostly of fats. Our bodily cells are not static objects; they are constantly being remade. Depending on where they are in the body, they may be remade rapidly, like in the gut or the skin, or only very slowly, like in bone and cartilage. But the fats that make up the outer layer or membrane of these cells come from the diet when they are remade.

If the fats in the diet are mainly saturated, cell membranes will be hard and inflexible and tend to stick together. This one fact is really at the heart of the current epidemic in Western countries of diseases due to cells sticking together—diseases due to clots, like heart attacks, strokes and deep venous thrombosis, are all the result of this increased stickiness. And tissues and organs made up of these hard and inflexible cells themselves become hard and inflexible.

So, for instance, in people eating a typical Western diet full of saturated fats, the big blood vessel coming out of the heart, the aorta, usually becomes quite rigid, as do smaller blood vessels in the body, in a process called atherosclerosis, or hardening of the arteries. So when the heart pumps out blood, the pressure rises much higher than if the arteries were soft and flexible. Hence high blood pressure (hypertension) results. If unsaturated fats (monounsaturated or polyunsaturated or both) were the main fats in the diet, the tissues would be soft and pliable instead, and the aorta would be more flexible and pliable, which would mean no high blood pressure. Hard cells are also more prone to degeneration because they are brittle and non-pliable, and break down more easily with normal wear and tear. We know that degeneration is a key part of the development and progression of MS.

In addition to their effects of altering the structure and behaviour of cell membranes, making them more fluid and flexible, and resistant to degeneration, omega-3 and omega-6 fatty acids are converted into immune system messenger chemicals, which act in different, often opposing ways. The immune system produces a range of these chemicals that act as messengers, promoting or suppressing inflammation, or attracting or otherwise affecting other immune cells. Mostly they belong to the classes of cytokines and eicosanoids. Cytokines are soluble proteins produced by cells in response to certain stimuli. They include such chemicals as tumour necrosis factor (TNF), the interleukins (ILs), and the interferons (IFNs). Interferons are now being used in the treatment of MS.

Some of these cytokines promote inflammation—that is, they are part of the Th1 response—and some suppress it (Th2 response). Recent research has shown that PwMS who are challenged with myelin base protein secrete more of the Th1 type cytokines than people without MS.[1] Many of the chemical messengers are made from essential fatty acids. Eicosanoids are a class of unsaturated fatty acids derived from dietary essential fatty acids. They include prostaglandins, leukotrienes and thromboxanes. They are a bit like hormones, but act only in the local area in which they are produced. Again, they can promote or suppress inflammation.

So eating more of one or the other types of polyunsaturated fats can shift the immune response more towards a Th1 or Th2 response.[2, 3, 4] A diet high in monounsaturated fats is essentially neutral for the immune system. One high in omega-6s results in immune chemicals that promote the inflammatory or Th1 response, and one high in omega-3s results in chemicals that suppress the inflammatory response as part of the Th2 response. A review in the British Journal of Nutrition concluded that epidemiological, biochemical, animal model and clinical trial data strongly suggest that polyunsaturated fatty acids have a role in the development and treatment of MS.[5] The authors noted that disturbed essential fatty acid metabolism in MS causes a loss of long chain polyunsaturated fatty acids in cell membranes, causing problems with CNS structure and function. This fits very well with the theory of MS causation of Dr Angelique Corthals.

The pathways in the body for these fatty acids are quite complex. A simple plan of this is presented in Figure 2, showing that the essential fatty acids alpha-linolenic acid (omega-3) and linoleic acid (omega-6) are converted in the body to intermediate fatty acids, which are then converted into a range of eicosanoids. Omega-3 group eicosanoids slow down inflammation and suppress the growth of tumours. The omega-6 group does the opposite.

The typical modern Western diet is heavily over-balanced towards omega-6 fats. By cutting down on omega-6 and increasing omega-3 consumption, shifting the immune balance away from inflammation, not only are auto-immune diseases improved, but many of the typical Western diseases in which inflammation plays such an important role are improved as well. These include diseases such as coronary heart disease,

Figure 2: Pathways in the body for omega-3 and omega-6 fatty acids

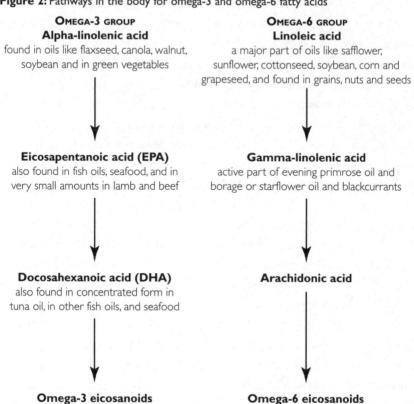

OMEGA-3 GROUP	OMEGA-6 GROUP
Alpha-linolenic acid	**Linoleic acid**
found in oils like flaxseed, canola, walnut, soybean and in green vegetables	a major part of oils like safflower, sunflower, cottonseed, soybean, corn and grapeseed, and found in grains, nuts and seeds
Eicosapentanoic acid (EPA)	**Gamma-linolenic acid**
also found in fish oils, seafood, and in very small amounts in lamb and beef	active part of evening primrose oil and borage or starflower oil and blackcurrants
Docosahexanoic acid (DHA)	**Arachidonic acid**
also found in concentrated form in tuna oil, in other fish oils, and seafood	
Omega-3 eicosanoids	**Omega-6 eicosanoids**

asthma and cancer. These are the unexpected beneficial side-effects we can get from cutting saturated fats out of our diet and supplementing with flaxseed oil. Not only are we likely to live longer and not be so disabled from MS, but it is also a comfort to know that we are less likely to get the other common diseases associated with ageing in our society. This is particularly important as we know that PwMS have more heart and blood vessel disease than those without MS.

The effect of essential fatty acid intake on these eicosanoids has been studied in great detail in PwMS. Gallai and colleagues showed that there was a marked decrease in the chemicals that promote inflammation after only four weeks' supplementation with fish oils. IL–1beta, IL–2, IFN-gamma and TNF-alpha were all significantly decreased.[6] The decreases were even more pronounced after three and then six months. The pro-inflammatory eicosanoids PGE2 and LTB4 were also decreased. This is important because these chemicals have been shown to be involved in causing relapses in MS patients.[7, 8] The patients in this study were taking quite large doses, of the order of 5 g per day, of EPA plus DHA. In most fish oil capsules, only 30 per cent of the oil is EPA and DHA, so about sixteen or seventeen of the 1000mg capsules a day is the equivalent of the dose used in the study.

The authors noted that to get a similar level of suppression of the immune system to that achieved with fish oil, it would be necessary to use a standard chemotherapy agent, such as steroids and cyclosporine A. These powerful drugs have many toxic effects, particularly with long-term use. Omega-3s in the diet are clearly a preferable way of achieving such beneficial immune system changes.

Researchers have examined the effects of differing amounts of omega-3 and omega-6 in diets of children over a year old who were at increased risk of developing type 1 diabetes.[9] This type of diabetes is the auto-immune type, and is very similar to MS as a disease except that the target of auto-immunity is the insulin-secreting cells of the pancreas rather than the myelin sheaths of nerve cells in the brain. In this study, they showed clearly that infants with higher amounts of omega-3 fatty acids in their diets were 55 per cent less likely to develop auto-immunity to their pancreatic cells, as evidenced by development of one of the three measured auto-antibodies to pancreatic cells; for children with at least two of these three measured antibodies—that is, those at highest risk of developing diabetes—the risk was reduced by 77 per cent for those consuming larger amounts of omega-3s. This association was confirmed by showing that, in a sub-set of this group of children who had the fatty acid composition of their red blood cells measured, those with higher amounts of omega-3s in their membranes had a lower risk of developing auto-immunity to pancreatic cells.

Changing the balance of fats in the diet to that in the OMS diet works in two main ways. First, it changes the membranes of our bodily cells, reducing saturated fats and increasing the polyunsaturated essential fatty acid content of those membranes. The fats get taken up into the cell membranes of nerve cells in the nervous system, making nerves more pliable and more resistant to immune attack and degeneration. They also get taken up into the immune cells themselves, and every other cell of the body, improving their function, reducing degeneration and decreasing cancerous change. Second, the production of pro-inflammatory omega-6 eicosanoids is reduced, thus diminishing inflammatory attacks. So, while there is probably little difference between omega-3 and omega-6 fatty acids in terms of membrane pliability and function, the suppression of immune system activation achieved by omega-3 fatty acids makes them the supplements on which to concentrate for replacing saturated fats.

Research has suggested a number of theories about why vegan diets plus fish oil and vitamin D may be of wide-ranging benefit to people's health, largely through their effects on the immune system,[10, 11] and UK scientists have added new experimental evidence for the benefits of fish oil in regulating inflammation.[12] There has also been extensive evidence about the anti-inflammatory effects of fish-based Mediterranean type diets.[13, 14, 15] Fish oils are the omega-3 fatty acids most people know about. However, there are plant-based omega-3s as well. Alpha-linolenic acid is the plant form, and this is found in abundance in linseeds (otherwise known as flaxseed) and their oil extracts, but also in canola or rapeseed oil and some nuts, mainly walnuts and pecans, and their extracted oils. As can be seen from Figure 2 above, the plant omega-3s are converted in the body to the fish form (EPA and DHA). Many authorities say that this is not always an efficient mechanism, and is blocked by saturated fats and the absence of certain vitamins and minerals. Possibly less than 10 per cent of alpha-linolenic acid gets into the EPA and DHA forms. For this reason, many people prefer to get these substances directly from fish oil and bypass the conversion in the body. It is likely, however, that the plant form—typically taken as flaxseed oil—is just as good as fish oil in its immune effects. More on that later.

Studies of fats in cells and blood

Several studies have examined the fatty acid composition of the membranes of cells in PwMS. Comparing fourteen PwMS and 100 people without MS, scientists found that the cells of PwMS contained significantly less polyunsaturated fatty acids, which had been replaced in the cells by saturated fatty acids.[16] Two other studies showed deficiencies in omega-3 fatty acids in cell membranes of PwMS.[17, 18] Importantly, further research has now shown that the higher the cell membrane concentration of saturated fats becomes, the worse the outcome.[19] In a separate paper, the same authors showed that the membranes of cells in PwMS were less fluid, and that this correlated with increased saturated fatty acid composition of the membranes.[20]

Researchers at Buffalo University have noted a connection between high cholesterol and disability in PwMS.[21] Further, they studied a group of people with their first demyelinating event who were part of one of the drug trials, looking at their fat profile in blood and brain lesion development on MRI scanning.[22] Their study found that worse fat profiles, with high cholesterol levels typically associated with a high-saturated fat diet, were associated with worse MRI measures of lesion activity—that is, more brain lesions. They noted that early intervention with dietary, exercise and lifestyle modifications shown to reduce cholesterol might be useful for managing MS progression. Typically, these modifications are exactly those recommended in the OMS Recovery Program.

A bad fat profile in blood and cell membranes, reflecting a high saturated fat diet, is associated with more rapid progression to disability in MS.

High-quality Australian research following a group of PwMS in southern Tasmania has also found significantly less disability over time for people with better fat profiles in their blood.[23] People with a bad fat profile—generally associated with high animal fat consumption—had considerably more disease progression over the 2.5 years than those with a healthier lipid profile—usually associated with consumption of more unsaturated fat–containing foods. Lead investigator Dr Ingrid van der Mei said at <www.msra.org.au/bad-fats-major-culprit-ms-progression>, 'Our new findings confirm that dietary measures to control fats in the blood is also another important measure Australians living with MS should act upon.' A diet low in saturated fat and high in unsaturated fat is optimal for improving blood fat profiles. For instance, even just increasing almond intake has been shown to progressively improve the profile of fats in the blood of volunteers[24] and people with high blood cholesterol,[25] with quite marked falls in levels of cholesterol and bad fats.

Evidence about dietary fats from population studies

Much of our current knowledge of the benefit of a change in dietary fats for PwMS began with the lifelong work of Professor Roy Swank, a North American neurologist. Swank was a highly respected, leading academic neurologist. He was born in 1909 in Washington state, received a Bachelor of Surgery at the University of Washington in 1930 and an MD and PhD in 1935 from Northwestern University in Chicago. He founded the Swank MS Clinic in Oregon, taught at Harvard from 1945 to 1948 and the famous McGill University from 1948 to 1954, and was Professor and Head of the Neurology Division at the University of Oregon Medical School from 1954 to 1976. Swank was clearly no lightweight! He published six books and 170 articles in his field and received numerous honours. He died in 2008 at the age of 99, just a few months short of his 100th birthday. He was one of the world's leading academic neurologists. Swank initially proposed his theory about saturated fats causing and worsening MS in 1950. Initially, he showed that MS was less common in coastal Norway, where fish consumption was high, than in inland areas of Norway where people ate a lot of beef and dairy products.[26]

Later, bigger international studies have strongly supported these findings.[27] Analysing mortality data from twenty countries, Knox suggested a causal relationship between total fat intake and MS. Studies of people of similar Danish genetic backgrounds living in the Faroe and Shetland Islands had similar findings.[28] Those on the Faroe Islands maintained a fishing lifestyle with high fish consumption—that is, a diet high in omega-3 fatty acids—and had a low incidence of MS. Those on the Shetland Islands adopted the agricultural diet of their English counterparts, and had a high incidence of MS.

Professor Swank noticed a higher incidence of MS where saturated fat consumption was high; later research has confirmed this.

The most important population study examined fat consumption in 36 countries, assessing the impact of diets with differing amounts of animal, fish and unsaturated fats on rates of death due to MS.[29] Higher saturated fat consumption correlated strongly with higher MS mortality. Table 2 is a modified list of countries in descending order according to death rate (among women). Populations with high fish oil consumption had lower MS mortality, unless it was overbalanced by very large animal fat consumption, such as in Denmark. These findings were highly significant. The higher the ratio of polyunsaturated to saturated fats, the lower the mortality, and similarly with the unsaturated to saturated fat ratio (not shown). This evidence, from very large populations in a large number of countries, is very strong.

More recent research has shown that PwMS consuming fish and alcohol regularly reduced progression to disability by about 40 per cent (in smokers, progression accelerated by about 35 per cent).[30] One of the few studies in the area not to find evidence for a dietary influence in MS was the US Nurses Health Study.[31] However, saturated fat consumption is extremely high and going up in the United States, and there was probably not enough of a difference in saturated fat consumption between the highest and lowest intakes to detect a difference in MS progression.

Another notable physician who has dedicated his career to discovering the factors behind the increasing incidence of MS is neuro-epidemiologist Dr Klaus Lauer. Lauer has published a large suite of epidemiological studies in MS, particularly concentrating on dietary factors. He has particularly identified the likely role of processed meats—especially hot dogs and sausages—in the development of MS.[32] Lauer cites the nearly nine-fold increase in prevalence of MS in Kuwait over 30 years from 1980, and attributes this to the large increase in hot dog consumption in that country, as in most of the Arab world. He has recommended a diet based on reduced consumption of red meat, and increased seafood, fruit and vegetables, and believes studies published to date support such a recommendation for prevention and treatment of MS.[33]

Evidence from case-control studies

Case-control studies involve researchers recruiting people with a certain disease—in this case, MS—and randomly choosing a similar number of people without that disease carefully matched to be very close to the disease group in terms of sex, age and so on. Both groups are then care-

Table 2: Fat consumption 1979–81 by country, in order of highest to lowest MS mortality

Country	SFA (%E)	PUFA (%E)	P/S	AF–FO (%E)
Denmark	16.6	5.9	0.36	33.4
United Kingdom	14.7	6.5	0.44	27.2
Switzerland	16.7	6.9	0.41	29.1
Poland	12.8	4.2	0.33	23.6
Czechoslovakia	13.2	4.5	0.34	24.5
Norway	15.1	6.9	0.46	24.6
Netherlands	17.3	6.9	0.40	31.8
West Germany	14.1	6.6	0.47	26.0
Sweden	16.5	6.1	0.37	29.9
Belgium	16.0	7.0	0.44	30.1
New Zealand	17.8	4.3	0.24	32.7
Austria	14.1	7.4	0.52	25.5
Canada	14.5	6.8	0.47	27.8
United States	13.9	8.6	0.62	25.0
France	14.6	7.0	0.49	27.8
Finland	16.9	4.6	0.27	30.3
Yugoslavia	8.6	6.3	0.73	16.6
Australia	12.1	4.7	0.38	25.0
Italy	9.9	6.3	0.64	17.4
Greece	9.4	5.1	0.54	14.4
Argentina	10.4	7.4	0.71	20.9
Portugal	7.7	7.6	0.99	13.1
Spain	9.5	7.6	0.80	16.7
Israel	9.2	9.0	0.98	12.9
Japan	6.5	7.1	1.09	9.5
South Korea	3.4	3.1	0.91	5.2

Abbreviations

%E = per cent of total energy including alcohol

SFA = saturated fatty acids

PUFA = polyunsaturated fatty acids

P/S ratio of PUFA to SFA

AF – FO = animal fat minus fish oil

(Modified from Esparza et al)[29]

fully questioned about various lifestyle factors of interest. For instance, if the theory is that sunlight prevents MS, the researchers may take 100 PwMS (cases) and 100 people without MS (controls) and compare the estimated amount of time spent in the sun during their lives prior to developing MS. They might break the amount of sun exposure down into four groups, ranging from say an average of 30 minutes a day in the sun to an average of two hours in the sun for the highest sun exposure. Looking at how many people in the 30 minutes a day exposure group had MS or didn't have MS, they might find that 50 per cent of those people with lowest exposure had MS; looking at the two hours per day group, they might find that 10 per cent of those people had MS. So less sun exposure would seem to increase the risk of developing MS. Researchers express this as an odds ratio (OR); in this case, the odds of developing MS comparing the lowest to highest sun exposure is 5:1, that is an OR of 5.0, or five times the risk.

This is one way that scientists discover possible risk factors for particular diseases. For instance, comparing people who smoke cigarettes with a group of those who don't, and finding that in the smokers 20 per cent got lung cancer and in those who don't smoke only 1 per cent got lung cancer would produce an odds ratio of 20:1 for smoking causing lung cancer. In the case of smoking and lung cancer, we would accept that result as constituting proof, because it is clearly unethical to conduct a randomised controlled trial, randomly allocating people to smoking and not smoking, and see who develops lung cancer! The parallels with dietary studies are pretty clear. Trying to allocate people to a smoking group would be very hard, as would trying to allocate people to a particular diet. Generally, people make those lifestyle choices for themselves.

Even if one allocated some people to the better dietary group, the chances are that they would fall back into old habits during the study, and be no different to the usual diet comparison group. Similarly, many people entering the study allocated to the usual diet group might read the study information, notice that the researchers were hypothesising that the better diet would result in better health, and take up the diet during the study. In effect, this would ruin the group comparison. One might end up in the same position, as we will soon see that Professor

Swank did, and simply compare those who stuck to the diet to those who didn't, even though it was a randomised controlled trial. This is one of the reasons we should carefully consider the results of epidemiological and case-control studies when looking at the role of diet in MS, because that might be the best level of evidence we can actually obtain.

Many case-control studies have been performed in MS. One showed higher risk of MS for increased animal fat intake, with roughly a doubling of risk for every extra 33 g of animal fat intake.[34] Nutrients shown to be protective included vegetable protein and fibre. Another showed that higher meat and dairy consumption, and low fish consumption, increased the risk of MS.[35] Another showed that people consuming more full-fat milk were over twenty times more likely to have MS than those who did not, with similar results for lard and meat. Another found that the most significant risk factor for MS was a predominant meat-based versus vegetable-based diet.[36]

Clinical trials

Population and case-control studies provide good evidence of an effect of dietary fat intake on MS development and progression that builds on our basic science knowledge of the effects of fats on the immune system and degeneration. Stronger evidence to enable a dietary recommendation in MS is what happens when such a dietary change is adopted by PwMS. So clinical studies are needed in which we actually test the effect of the dietary intervention in real life.

Professor Swank's low-saturated fat study

Beginning in 1949, Professor Swank enrolled 150 PwMS in a long-term study of the effects of a very low-saturated fat diet.[37, 38] He followed them with meticulous examination and recording of dietary fat consumption for 34 years. Many of the patients were unable to stick to the diet, allowing comparison between those who did and those who did not. The study was supported by independent grants from the MS Society of Canada, the Montreal Neurological Institute, the Department of Health and Welfare of Canada, the MS Society of Portland and other grants. The resulting paper in *The Lancet* reported results for the 144 patients who completed the 34 years of the study. A drop-out rate of only six patients (4%) is remarkably low for medical research studies of such duration. Of the 144 patients, 72 stuck to the diet (good dieters), consuming less than 20 g/day of saturated fat. The other 72 consumed more saturated fat. The patients' neurological disability was graded using a neurological disability scale devised by Swank, from 0 (essentially unimpaired) to 6 (deceased). Point 4 on the scale represents wheelchair needed, and point 5 represents confined to bed and chair. Swank's scale essentially used two points on Kurtzke's EDSS scale to every one point on his.

Swank's 34-year study of a low-saturated fat diet in treating MS reported dramatically better health outcomes for those sticking to the diet.

Regardless of level of disability at entry to the trial, good dieters deteriorated a little but not very significantly. Good dieters at level 1 on entry had an average final grade of 1.9 when examined 34 years later. Good dieters starting the study at level 2 had a final level of 3.6, and those at level 3 or worse a final level of 4. The results were best for those who started with minimum disability, with 95 per cent surviving and still physically active 34 years later, excluding those who had died from non-MS diseases. The benefits occurred in all three groups; even people with significant disability markedly slowed the progression of the disease if they stuck to the diet.

Poor dieters had terrible results. Poor dieters with minimum disability at entry ended with an average grade of 5.3—that is, wheelchair and bed bound. This outcome was in line with the outcomes of most PwMS at the time. Those with moderate disability also ended up at 5.3, and those with severe disability had a grade of 5.6. Only 7 per cent of patients who did not stick to the diet remained active. The death rate among the poor dieters was extremely high: 58 of the 72 (81 per cent) were dead by 34 years, 45 from MS-related causes (see Table 3). The statistics were very strong. The main features of these results are reproduced below. Swank differentiated between 'fats' and 'oils', with 'fats' representing hard saturated fatty acids and 'oils' representing liquid unsaturated fatty acids.

Table 3: Results for participants in Swank's saturated fat study

	Good dieters		Poor dieters	
Minimum disability (grade 1)				
Number	23		6	
Mean duration of MS (years)	31		25.9	
Before trial	2.4		3.5	
Average final neurological grade (change)	1.9	(0.9)	5.3	(4.3)
Deaths: all other causes	5	(21%)	5	(83%)
Deaths: MS only	1	(5%)	4	(80%)
Mean fat intake	17.1		35.7	
Mean oil intake	16.3		11.0	
Moderate disability (grade 2)				
Number	25		33	
Mean duration of MS (years)	32.0		28.0	
Before trial	4.9		5.3	
Average final neurological grade (change)	3.6	(1.6)	5.3	(3.4)
Deaths: all other causes	10	(40%)	25	(76%)
Deaths: MS only	8	(34%)	16	(66%)
Mean fat intake	15.4		46.1	
Mean oil intake	18.2		10.2	
Severe disability (grades 3–5, average 3.2)				
Number	24		33	
Mean duration of MS (years)	33.8		29.9	
Before trial	6.2		10.4	
Average final neurological grade (change)	4.0	(0.8)	5.6	(2.4)
Deaths: all other causes	8	(33%)	28	(84%)
Deaths: MS only	5	(21%)	25	(75%)
Mean fat intake	15.8		36.5	
Mean oil intake	18.1		10.5	

(Modified from Swank and Dugan[38].)

Figure 3 shows the dramatic fall in relapse rate after commencement of the diet, from around one relapse per year pre-diet to about 0.05 per year once stable on the diet. Although the fall in relapse rate occurred quite quickly, down to 0.3 relapses per year within a year, patients did

Figure 3: Relapse rate (number per year) before and after going on a low-fat diet

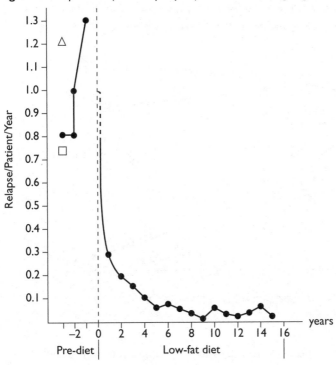

Source: Reprinted with permission from Elsevier Science, from Swank 1991.[39]

not achieve complete stability for around three to five years. This is an important point for those tempted to 'try the diet' and give up because nothing seems to be happening.

Figure 4 shows that, regardless of the level of disability on commencement of the diet, for those who adhered to the diet there was some deterioration but it was relatively minor over the course of the study. For those who did not adhere to the diet, disability was severe by the end of the study and the death rate was extremely high (78–91 per cent depending on initial level of disability). Patients who adhered to the diet actually consumed 16 g of saturated fat per day on average, whereas those who did not adhere to the diet consumed 38 g/day. Even for the 'poor dieters', this was a marked reduction from the probable 80 g/day or so that they were consuming prior to the study. But this was not enough to stop deterioration. Close enough was not good enough. An important

Figure 4: The effects of fat consumption on early, mildly disabled (0, 1, 2; solid line), and late seriously disabled (3, 4, 5; broken line) patients in the Swank study

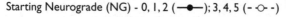

Starting Neurograde (NG) - 0, 1, 2 (—●—); 3, 4, 5 (- ○ -)

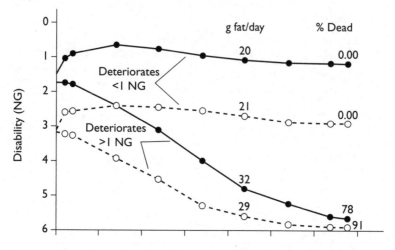

Source: Reprinted with permission from Elsevier Science, from Swank 1991.[39]

observation by Swank was that people who defaulted on the diet—even many years after beginning it—soon relapsed, and if they stayed off the diet, deteriorated to disability.

At 50 years after the commencement of the study, Swank attempted to follow up the 63 patients surviving at the end of the 34-year study.[40] Not surprisingly, the great majority of the surviving 63 patients (47) had adhered to the diet; only sixteen survivors had not adhered to the diet. Fifteen patients were contacted, and personally interviewed and evaluated. All fifteen had remained on the low-saturated fat diet for 50 years. The ages ranged from 72 to 84. Of these fifteen, thirteen were physically normal and walked without difficulty. The other two required assistance with walking. Swank concluded that if PwMS can rigorously follow the diet, with no more than 10–15 g of saturated fat per day, they can expect to 'survive and be ambulant and otherwise normal to an advanced age'.

An editorial on this follow-up study by Swank in the same journal attempted to provide a biochemical explanation of why the diet should work in MS.[41] It concluded with the intriguing question, 'The big question is: If their results are so stunningly impressive, why haven't other physicians, neurologists, or centers adopted this method of treat-ment?' It is an important question, and one that has never been answered satisfactorily. Swank had his theories on why the diet wasn't widely taken up by the profession, which can be read at <www.drmcdougall.com/res_swank.html> in an interview with his colleague Dr McDougall.

Swank's intervention study represents important confirmation of the basic science and population study evidence about the potential benefit of a change in fat consumption. Many researchers would consider such significant findings sufficient to make broad-based recommendations about diet for PwMS. Yet this did not occur following publication of the findings. One must wonder why.

There has only been one major criticism of Swank's work pub-lished.[42] The authors argued that the neurological assessments of the patients—that is, determining how they progressed—were not blinded. This means that the investigators knew which patients were sticking to the diet when they tested them to see how the disease had progressed. While this may have introduced some bias into the assessment, it is very hard to argue that there is bias in assessing whether someone is bed bound, confined to a wheelchair, or dead, as most of the poor dieters were. Another criticism was that the good dieters had more cases of short duration and very mild disability than the other group. Despite the criticisms, the authors argued in favour of further study of the dietary fat hypothesis. Given the very poor outcomes of this disease documented in countless natural history studies, it is difficult to understand why diet was not recommended as part of secondary preventive medicine advice after publication of the paper.

Sadly, Swank's paper was accompanied in *The Lancet* by an anony-mous editorial that cast doubt on the validity of the findings. Most journals have a policy of publishing commentary on important papers in the same issue.[43] The unnamed author criticised the paper for not being randomised—that is, the patients were not randomly allocated to low and usual fat groups in the study. Rightly, the editorial author suggested that those patients who relapsed would be more likely not to follow the diet. However, in summing up, this unnamed author wrote that 'the role of lipids in MS must remain not proven'. Carrying with it the impres-sive and prestigious stamp of *The Lancet*, this was a powerful message.

A casual read of the editorial and paper may have led many clinicians to discount the highly significant findings in Swank's study.

> The duration of Swank's study of 34 years was ironically its weakness; standards of proof in medicine had changed by the time of publication, and there was little interest in his extraordinary findings.

It is ironic to note that the great strength of Swank's study—its duration of 34 years—was also its great weakness. It is rare to find any clinical trials in the medical literature of such duration. When Swank started his study in 1949, the standard of proof in medicine was to test a new therapy out on patients and assess whether they got better or not. Because of the duration of Swank's study, by the time it was published in 1990, the standard of proof in medicine had changed dramatically. Randomised controlled trials had become the accepted level of evidence. Another reason for the lack of adoption of his findings into practice was that by the time of publication of the results, pharmaceutical agents for the treatment of MS were just being brought to the market by drug companies. Ironically, this major piece of research potentially could have won Swank a Nobel Prize had it been published at the time he started it; by the time it was finished, it was consigned to the 'unproven' basket despite its great strengths and remarkable findings. This is despite the fact that the disease was considered incurable, at the time had no other therapies that were effective, and the only side-effects of treatment with Swank's diet were positive.

The size of the benefit found in Swank's study for those consuming a low-saturated fat diet was stunning, and compares more than favourably with any therapies currently available. The diet was clearly associated with dramatically slower progression of disability, something for which medicine has been searching with modern pharmaceutical agents, but that it has still not found after decades of research.

Other clinical trials on low-saturated fat diets

Other studies of low-saturated fat diets support the work of Swank. One small randomised controlled trial on dietary fat in MS, of one year's limited duration, compared people with relapsing-remitting MS assigned to a low-fat diet (15 per cent of calories) supplemented with fish oil to similar PwMS allocated to the standard American Heart Association heart diet, in which fat makes up 30 per cent of calories, supplemented with olive oil.[44] Only around two-thirds of the participants were able to stick to their diets. Relapse rates fell significantly from pre-trial rates, more so for the fish oil group. In fact, the fish oil group had a mean relapse rate of 1.14 relapses per year in the year prior to the trial, and dropped by 0.79—a reduction of 69 per cent. The olive oil group had a pre-trial rate of 1.17, which dropped by 0.69—a 59 per cent reduction (personal communication, Bianca Weinstock-Guttman, 2008). These findings were statistically significant despite the small numbers of participants. The drop of 69 per cent for the low-fat plus fish oil group is very similar to the relapse rate reduction in the first year of Swank's study (see Figure 3 above).

The authors concluded that, despite the study limitations, a low-fat diet supplemented with omega-3 fatty acids may complement the beneficial effects of concurrent disease-modifying therapies, because virtually all PwMS in this study were on disease-modifying drugs. Dr John McDougall, trained by Professor Swank, recently published the results of a very small randomised controlled trial examining a plant-based wholefood diet for PwMS.[45] The aims were simply to determine whether PwMS could stick to such a diet and whether it was safe. The study was under-powered to find any differences in relapse rates or MRI lesion numbers. (Under-powering means that there were too few subjects in the study to find a significant difference in these outcomes.) With the numbers of PwMS in this study, 22 complying with diet and 27 not on the diet, the difference between the two groups in terms of number of MRI lesions and relapses would have to be very large to be significant. They found that those on the diet had a drop in low-density lipoprotein of 12.4mg/dL and in cholesterol of 16.2, compared with those not on the diet of 5.6 and 4.7 respectively, and that those complying with diet lost 16.3 lbs (7.4 kg), whereas those not on the diet gained 1.6 lbs (0.7 kg). As we have previously seen, these better fat profiles in blood and more normal body weight have been associated with better health outcomes for PwMS in previous research.

The authors concluded that the safety of the diet had been demonstrated—although one wonders who might question this—and that compliance with the diet was achievable. They noted that they really couldn't find a difference in outcome with a short, small study like this, in which some subjects were also on disease-modifying therapies. So the study achieved its aims, but one could argue quite reasonably that there was no need for it; the diet is safe and people adhere to it without much difficulty once they understand the potential benefits. So the researchers could and should have gone straight to a large study with many hundreds of PwMS that could have answered the much more telling question of whether the diet actually works in terms of reducing relapses and preventing disease progression.

Essential fatty acid supplements

Clinical trials have shown that by simply adding polyunsaturated fats to the diet, there is a tendency towards slower progression of MS. This might well be expected, given that the addition of unsaturated fats to the diet improves blood fat profile, and fat profiles have been shown to affect rate of progression of MS. Three randomised controlled trials from the 1970s examined this in detail, but all were relatively poor quality studies.[46, 47, 48] None reduced saturated fat intake, and it is known that saturated fat competes with unsaturated fats for uptake into cell membranes and in biological pathways. Optimal improvements in blood fat profile come from a combination of reducing saturated fat intake and increasing unsaturated fat intake.

The control groups also did not really take an inactive substance. They were given oleic acid, or olive oil, which has been shown to reduce the severity of the animal model of MS, experimental auto-immune encephalomyelitis.[49] Countries like Italy and Greece, where the olive oil intake is high, have a low incidence of MS. Oleic acid gets taken up into cell membranes like the polyunsaturated fatty acids, and is flexible and pliable, unlike saturated fatty acids. Finally, the numbers were too small in each individual study to get a statistically significant effect. However, meta-analysis of the studies (pooling the results) revealed a significant decrease in rate of deterioration with essential fatty acid supplementation for those with minimal or no disability at entry to the study.[50]

Another trial in the 1980s looked at the effects of nutritional counsel-ling on outcome.[51] These investigators were working on behalf of a group called Action for Research into Multiple Sclerosis (ARMS). The group was formed by a number of PwMS distressed about the lack of available therapies offered to them after diagnosis. Judy Graham, who wrote the excellent book *Multiple Sclerosis: A Self-help Guide to Its Management*,[52] was one of them. Two hundred PwMS entered the study. There was a high drop-out rate, as the diet, testing and analyses were quite rigorous. Eighty-three remained in the study for 34 months. They were coun-selled to decrease saturated fat intake and increase polyunsaturated fats, as well as increasing antioxidants. This is where the fat part of the diet differed from Swank's. Unlike Swank, patients were able to eat saturated fats, but had to ensure that the ratio of polyunsaturated to saturated fats remained high. For those who complied with the recommendations, as judged by rigorous dietary analysis, there was no significant deterioration in disability; for the poor dieters, the disability worsened significantly. The investigators showed that the good dieters did modify their diet by monitoring levels of the fats in the blood.

A more recent blinded randomised controlled trial of fish oil supple-mentation in Norway did not find any benefit from supplementing with omega-3s on disease activity in MS.[53] The study enrolled 92 PwMS from several centres in Norway randomised to two groups. PwMS in the active treatment group received 7 g of fish oil daily and people in the other group a placebo capsule containing corn oil, which contains a large pro-portion of linoleic acid, previously shown to reduce the progression of disability when used at a higher dose of around 17–23 g/day in the studies discussed above from the 1970s. Both groups also used interferon-beta therapy, and were followed up for two years. No difference between the groups was found in appearance of new lesions on MRI, disability, disease progression, fatigue or quality of life scales.

This study was not very helpful in that previous studies in a variety of diseases have emphasised the need to reduce saturated fat intake in addition to omega-3 supplementation for optimal benefit; the dose of omega-3 supplementation was around two-thirds lower than that used by Gallai and colleagues, who demonstrated dramatic anti-inflammatory effects of high dose fish oil in PwMS; and the control group was taking a placebo previously shown to reduce disease progression. So the only real conclusion of the study is that, at low doses, omega-3s appear to have no additional benefit over the known beneficial effects of omega-6 supplementation in MS.

Another small study compared omega-3 supplements with omega-6 in PwMS.[54] Again, there was no avoidance of saturated fats; rather, the patients were 'given dietary advice to encourage a low intake of animal fat and a plentiful intake of omega-6 fatty acids'. The omega-3 group did substantially better, although the results were not quite statistically significant.

One review concluded that fish oil may be beneficial in MS, both through its immune mechanism of action and through structural effects within the nervous system.[55] The UK National Health Service National Institute for Health and Care Excellence (NICE), which produces guidelines for doctors managing PwMS, recommended for many years that 'PwMS should be advised that linoleic acid 17–23 g/day may reduce progression of disability',[56] although this recommendation was removed in the 2014 revision.[57] Evidence is starting to emerge that polyunsaturated fatty acids play an important protective role in the CNS,[58, 59] and some researchers in the field are starting to call for a reappraisal of the role of fats in the development of MS.[60]

 Despite relatively scant research in the area, supplementation with omega-3 polyunsaturated fatty acids may be helpful for people with MS.

The findings of these studies on essential fatty acid supplementation, although relatively poorly designed, with small numbers and poor choice of placebos, support the population-based evidence presented earlier. The OMS recommendation is for PwMS to supplement with omega-3 fatty acids. Whether to use plant-based or marine-based omega-3s is a question that has not really been studied in the previous literature, although the HOLISM study undertaken by our OMS research group has looked at that and the other dietary factors important to PwMS in detail.

HOLISM study findings on diet

The HOLISM study enabled a detailed exploration of whether or not some of the lifestyle habits related to diet and omega-3 supplements predicted the health of the roughly 2500 PwMS in the study. We knew that this study would help determine and potentially validate whether such elements of lifestyle could be considered risk factors for relapses, the progression of the disease and other factors like fatigue and depression. No other study in the MS literature had ever been able to answer these questions so thoroughly and with such robustness. We started our study with great excitement in 2012; little did we know how dramatic the findings would be, and how much the findings would validate the work of Swank and others on healthy fat intake for PwMS.

To study diet in detail, we needed a validated tool that had previously been used to examine dietary habits. This is a difficult area of research; numerous tools have been developed—many of them exceedingly complex—including daily food diaries. For our study, we were asking questions about so many different lifestyle habits and behaviours that we needed a tool that was relatively simple and quick to complete, but reproducible and valid, and that relied only on the participant completing it. We ultimately chose the Diet Habits Questionnaire (DHQ), a 24-item instrument used to assess the dietary habits of an Australian cardiac population.[61] This tool and its scoring system were originally developed according to the National Heart Foundation of Australia's Nutrition Recommendations and the National Health and Medical Research Council (NHMRC) and Commonwealth Department of Health and Ageing's Dietary Guidelines for Australian Adults, and take into account the type and quality of fat consumed. This was an important consideration for us, in order to be in a position to evaluate Swank's key research.

For example, in the DHQ, healthy fruit and vegetable intake would be considered to be at least five vegetable and two fruit servings per day, and regular consumption of legumes and raw nuts or seeds. Healthy fat intake would include fish consumption, the selection of avocado and mono/polyunsaturated oils for salads and spreads, minimal use of oil in cooking and infrequent consumption of processed or fatty meats, full-fat milk, cakes, biscuits and takeaway foods, among other items.

The questionnaire considers both the type of food and the method of its preparation. Each item scores between 1 and 5, with a score of 1 indicating very poor dietary behaviour and a score of 5 indicating healthy dietary behaviour. These items produce ten dietary sub-scores: cereals, fruit and vegetables, omega-3 fatty acids, food choices, food preparation, takeaways and snacks, fat, fibre, sodium and alcohol. We excluded four items from the survey—three regarding salt intake and one on alcohol—as we were assessing that much more rigorously with a dedicated alcohol assessment measure. The removal of these items did not affect the calculation of the remaining eight dietary sub-scores, but was convenient because it led to a total score out of 100.

Of the roughly 2500 PwMS in the study, we were amazed to find that 38 per cent didn't eat dairy products and 27 per cent didn't eat meat.[62] This made our sample of PwMS unique in the medical literature. No other study has ever reported such a high proportion of people not eating meat or dairy, and for many previous studies, this has limited their ability to detect any differences between the health of those eating and not eating meat or dairy, as the numbers in these groups were too small for any meaningful comparison. In contrast, we had very sizeable numbers of PwMS in these groups, and very sizeable numbers overall with very healthy dietary habits, reflecting the educated, engaged group of PwMS who responded to our survey. For the first time in medical research history, this enabled us to really make meaningful comparisons between ultra-healthy and unhealthy dietary lifestyles and their effects on the health of PwMS. This was confirmed in initial analysis, where we showed that those with a higher level of education were markedly more likely to report healthy dietary habits, while those who were overweight or obese reported much lower DHQ total scores.

The very healthy dietary habits of many people with MS in the HOLISM study did not appear to make them miserable, as is common perception, but rather were associated with a markedly better quality of life.

We started by examining quality of life. People who are unwilling to change poor dietary habits often ask how they can give up their 'pleasures', as it will only make their lives miserable. We found exactly the opposite. Those PwMS in our study reporting healthier habits in relation to fruit and vegetables and fat were significantly more likely to have a better quality of life. Those who didn't eat meat and those who didn't eat dairy had significantly better physical and mental health quality of life than meat and dairy consumers. When we did sophisticated regression analysis of our data, we found that for every one-point increase on the 100-point diet scale towards a healthier diet, physical and mental health quality of life went up by around half a point on that 100–point scale. Better diet meant a better life! The most important dietary predictors of better physical and mental health were healthy fruit and vegetable intake, and healthy fat intake (see Figures 5 and 6).

Figure 5: Physical health quality of life by dietary factors

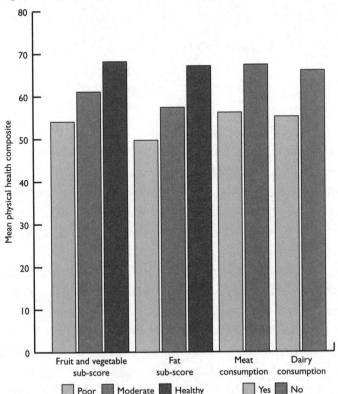

Figure 6: Mental health quality of life by dietary factors

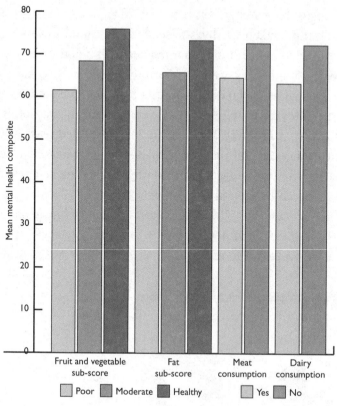

There were similar findings for disability, with better diet associated with lower levels of disability, and to a lesser extent for relapse rate. For every one-point increase towards a better diet on the 100-point DHQ scale, there was a 1.2 per cent drop in relapse rate over the previous twelve months, although this finding was not significant on the more sophisticated regression analysis.

So, overall, every ten-point increase on the DHQ total score towards a healthier diet predicted nearly a six-point increase in physical and a five-point increase in mental health quality of life, and 30 per cent less likelihood of being more disabled. While fruit and vegetable intake was an important factor in both quality of life and disability, the biggest differences were for those PwMS in the healthy fat group. Those in the healthy fat group had nearly a twelve-point increase in physical health and over an eight-point increase in mental health, and 42 per cent less likelihood of being more disabled. But having a fat intake that was moderately healthy wasn't associated at all with disability. This really suggested to us that a more rigorous approach to dietary fat was required, which strongly supported the work of Swank, which showed that saturated fat had to be reduced to an absolute minimum for the greatest health gains.

Separately, we studied the association of fish consumption and omega-3 supplementation.[63] We took the data on fish consumption from the DHQ, categorising frequency of consumption as less than once weekly, one to two days weekly, and three or more days weekly. For omega-3 intake, we looked at whether participants took fish oil, flaxseed oil or both, and how much they took.

Again, our results reflected the exceptionally healthy and educated group of PwMS who volunteered for the study, with approximately 30 per cent consuming fish three or more times weekly. Once again, those with the healthiest lifestyle behaviours—in other words, consuming fish three or more times a week—had a dramatically reduced risk (nearly 70 per cent) of being disabled. Those taking flaxseed oil had a 42 per cent lower risk of being disabled, and those taking fish oil had a 29 per cent lower risk. Quality of life across the board was similarly better for those consuming fish more frequently (see Figure 7) and taking omega-3s, with flaxseed oil superior once again. But it was in relapse rate that flaxseed oil had the strongest associations in sophisticated regression analysis. Here, those PwMS taking flaxseed oil regularly had over 60 per cent fewer relapses than those not taking it (regardless of how frequently they were eating fish), and those eating fish three or more times a week had over 50 per cent fewer relapses than those eating fish less frequently. Interestingly, fish oil had no significant association with relapse rate. This may reflect the results of clinical trials of fish oil in MS, where there have been somewhat divergent results.

People with MS in the HOLISM study consuming a diet like the OMS Recovery Program diet had dramatically better health across the board compared with those eating poor diets.

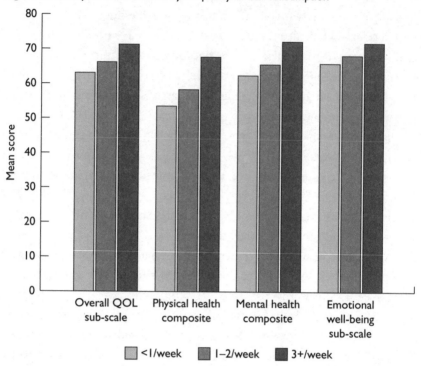

Figure 7: Quality of life outcomes by frequency of fish consumption

We concluded that there is a strong and significant association between better dietary habits and MS health outcomes, in particular quality of life and level of disability—particularly related to healthy fat intake, and a higher intake of fruit, vegetables and fish. This, of course, is the basis of the OMS Recovery Program diet. We also noted the great differences between flaxseed and fish oil; these findings strongly suggest that flaxseed oil should be used as the preferred omega-3 supplement. Really, such strong validation of the findings of Swank, which came from a study using a totally different methodology, should convince many who still doubt the benefits of diet in MS. In epidemiology, we call this consistency, and it is one of the hallmarks of a causative effect. So we recommended that clinicians consider providing advice to PwMS around the potential importance of a healthy diet, given the observations from this study and others, and the clear general beneficial effects on health. It is hard to imagine what downside there is to such an approach—particularly as it has significant benefits for quality of life as well.

Other dietary factors

Altered fats

At the time Swank began his interest in dietary fats in MS development and progression, in the mid-twentieth century, the food industry had not yet begun manipulating fats to any great extent. Scientists at Procter and Gamble in the United States were the first to chemically alter vegetable oils to change their physical properties, such as melting point. They began by tampering with cottonseed oil so that it could be stored as a solid substance rather than a liquid, producing the first Crisco oil (crystallised cottonseed oil). Over the course of the twentieth century, there was an explosion of altered fats with modified physical and chemical properties; Simopoulos credits the explosion of chronic disease in Western countries over that period to many of these changes.[64] To put it simply, many of these human-modified fats did not exist in nature prior to our tampering with them, and once absorbed into the body and into cell membranes and biological pathways, they can have entirely unpredictable effects, although we can surmise that these effects are largely harmful. Evidence from basic science strongly suggests that it is important to avoid human-refined and human-made fats.

Oils can be altered in many ways. The least-dramatic alteration—although it is still worrisome—is the process of producing refined oils. Many are unaware of how oils are modified in this refining process. 'Refining' oils basically converts fragrant nut or seed oil extracts into colourless, tasteless, odourless oils that don't resemble the original food. This begins with mechanical pressing, involving cooking the nuts or seeds for around two hours at temperatures up to 95°C, and then mashing and filtering the oil, which is sold as natural, unrefined oil. Mostly, though, the oils are subjected to solvent extraction, in which the oil is treated with powerful acids and alkalis, deodorised and bleached and sold as pure refined vegetable oil. By now it is full of trans-fatty acids, cyclic compounds, dimers and polymers that are not found in nature.

More drastic changes are now commonly made to oils to alter their structure and properties. In manufacturing new altered fats, liquid oils are converted to semi-solid fats in order to prolong their shelf life and allow them to be used in products like biscuits and shortening. These fats are known as hydrogenated fats and trans-fatty acids. These fats are the result of major food processing practices that have really transformed our diets. In hydrogenation and trans-fatty acid production, commercial processes heat unsaturated fats to high temperatures in the presence of certain metallic catalysts, and cause chemical changes in the fats to prolong their shelf life or alter their spreadability.

Trans-fatty acids are created by heating the original oils with certain catalysts, to create mirror images of the original fat; unlike the original, they are hard, have higher melting points and stick together. As little as 5 g a day of trans-fatty acids increases the risk of heart disease by 25 per cent.[65] There are likely to be similar effects on other degenerative diseases. The Australian Consumers Association has tested a variety of popular fast foods. They found that trans-fats make up from 0.8 to 22.5 per cent of total dietary fats, yet no laws require labelling of the trans-fat content of Australian foods.[65] The Food and Drug Administration in the United States has stated that there is no safe level of trans-fats, and is trying to phase them out of the American diet. These altered fats have extremely harmful effects in the body.

Altered fats have unpredictable and dangerous effects when eaten.

Trans-fats have been implicated in a wide range of Western diseases such as cancer, heart disease and immune dysfunction. They make cell membranes more rigid and dysfunctional than saturated fats, and should be avoided completely. Swank didn't know much about these altered fats, but trans-fats and hydrogenated vegetable oils are worse than saturated fats. They worsen the fat profile in blood, raise cholesterol and compete with essential fatty acids for inclusion in cell membranes, and in making the eicosanoid chemical messengers. Membranes containing trans-fatty acids are like those made of saturated fats, but even more rigid and less pliable. Yet a leading nutritionist estimates that Americans are now consuming 5–10 per cent of all their calories as trans-fatty acids. Expert reviews have suggested eliminating hydrogenated oils and trans-fats from the diet to protect against heart disease—a disease with similar risk factors to MS.[66]

Cow's milk

There is a strong correlation between cow's milk consumption and MS all around the world.[67, 68] This has been known for many years. Countries where cow's milk consumption is high have high rates of MS; within countries, regions where cow's milk is consumed in large amounts have higher rates of MS. More recent laboratory work from Germany and Canada provides a possible explanation.[69, 70] A number of cow's milk proteins have now been shown to be targeted by the immune cells of PwMS. Injecting them into experimental animals has caused lesions to appear in the CNS of the animals. Other researchers have demonstrated how certain proteins in cow's milk mimic part of myelin oligodendrocyte glycoprotein, the part of myelin thought to initiate the auto-immune reaction in MS.[71]

 Consuming cow's milk products is best avoided for people with MS.

There is likely a similar causative role for cow's milk in type 1 diabetes, also an auto-immune disease. Indeed, medical researchers are now so concerned about this that a worldwide study has begun in which children are being kept off cow's milk to see whether diabetes can be prevented.[72] This involves a major collaborative international study group of 78 clinical centres in fifteen countries, with the aim of recruiting 2032 children into the study. Enrolment for this study concluded in 2006, and there will now be a waiting period until sufficient time has passed to see what rates of diabetes are found in the groups.

A number of papers have reported interesting results from the study. One looked at 230 infants at high risk of developing diabetes detected by their immune system markers of risk and at least one family member with diabetes.[73] They randomly allocated them to receive cow's milk or a substitute formula whenever breast milk was unavailable, and observed the children up to ten years of age. They then looked at whether they developed auto-antibodies indicative of developing type 1 diabetes. Almost twice as many of the group receiving cow's milk developed these antibodies as those receiving the formula, suggesting an important role for cow's milk in triggering diabetes.

The Trial to Reduce IDDM in the Genetically at Risk [TRIGR] study was in part triggered by a randomised controlled trial from the University of Helsinki that studied 242 newborn infants who had a first-degree relative with type 1 diabetes and a genetic predisposition to diabetes.[74] They found that avoiding cow's milk formula provided significant protection from developing the auto-immunity associated with diabetes compared with the infants who did get cow's milk.

Another study into the degenerative neurological disorder Parkinson's disease found that people who consumed more dairy products had two to three times the risk of getting the disease.[75] This study involved over 135,000 men and women in the United States, and used stringent methods for collecting data on food consumption. The researchers speculated that dairy products may have a generally toxic effect on nervous tissue.

Cow's milk is not a very healthy food, and one wonders why it is consumed so widely in Western communities. After all, cow's milk is the breastmilk of another animal; while suitable for calves until they are weaned from the breast, it is hard to understand why it would be considered suitable for adults of another species. After all, one in five Australian adults of British descent, two in five of Mediterranean descent and four in five of Aboriginal or Asian descent have lactose intolerance, and can become quite ill from ingesting milk products. This can be in the form of mild or more severe bloating, flatulence, stomach cramps and diarrhoea. There are many good reasons not to drink cow's milk, particularly for PwMS.

Researchers have analysed the long-running Nurses Health Study, looking for the effect of vitamin D intake during adolescence on the incidence of MS. As cow's milk is fortified with vitamin D in the United States, possible beneficial effects of adolescent vitamin D intake through dairy products might be counteracted by harmful effects of milk on MS development. So the authors looked at milk consumption as well as vitamin D intake. Nurses who consumed three or more servings of whole milk a day in adolescence were 47 per cent more likely to develop MS in later life than those who did not.[76]

Salt

There is evidence to support a high-salt diet being harmful for PwMS. American researchers followed 70 PwMS for two years, looking at the amount of sodium they were excreting—a marker of their salt consumption.[77] They found a positive correlation between relapse rates and salt intake in quite sophisticated statistical modelling. The relapse rate was nearly three times higher in people with medium salt intake, and four times higher in people with high salt intake compared with the low-intake group. Those with high salt intake had a 3.4 times higher chance of developing a new lesion on MRI and about eight more lesions on MRI. They confirmed this relationship in an independent sample of 52 PwMS.

This confirms earlier basic science research showing that high sodium (salt) concentrations markedly boost the activity of particular T cells involved in the immune response, effectively promoting the Th1 response and increasing inflammation.[78] Other research in the animal model of MS showed that higher salt intake affected the integrity of the blood–brain barrier and, in animals with certain genetic backgrounds, worsened the MS-like disease in females.[79] Despite the limited research, there seem to be good reasons for PwMS to reduce their salt intake, and a number of authorities are already recommending this for PwMS, despite the paucity of research to date.

Alcohol

One of the most common questions asked at the OMS retreats is whether alcohol is harmful for PwMS. For many years, there was very little literature on which to base any recommendation about this. In the past, the best advice in the absence of anything specific to MS was to refer PwMS to the NHMRC guidelines for alcohol consumption and general health. These essentially were giving the message that low to moderate alcohol consumption with alcohol-free days was the safest option to minimise alcohol-related harm.

There have been mixed findings about drinking habits of PwMS and the development of MS.[34, 80, 81] One survey has shown a clear association between alcohol use and lower disability scores in people with relapsing-remitting MS and progressive MS.[82] A recent study again showed that greater alcohol consumption was associated with less disease progression among those with relapsing-onset MS.[30] However, drinking alcohol moderately for longer has been linked to more disability and MRI changes, with reduced disability among those consuming alcohol for fifteen years or less but greater disability among non-drinkers or longer-term drinkers.[83]

HOLISM study findings on alcohol

The HOLISM study provided the opportunity to formulate evidence-based guidelines for PwMS related to alcohol consumption. Given the mixed previous research, it has been tricky framing any recommendations for PwMS who want to aim for optimal health. Interestingly, we have solid data for another auto-immune disease, rheumatoid arthritis, about the protective effects of moderate alcohol consumption.[84] And there have simply been no data available to date about whether quality of life is positively or negatively affected by alcohol consumption, although many of us have suspected a beneficial effect.

HOLISM changed all that. Of nearly 2500 PwMS worldwide, most of those who drank alcohol reported consuming alcohol less than once a week, and most were categorised as having low consumption, which in our study was a very low amount—less than 15 g of alcohol per week.[85] This is only one and a half standard drinks a week, which is one and a half small bottles of beer, or one and a half 100 ml glasses of wine. Fewer than 1 per cent engaged in binge drinking, and fewer than 1 per cent consumed high levels of alcohol. Low alcohol use was more common in those from Canada and the United States, and less common in those from New Zealand or the United Kingdom. Moderate alcohol use was defined as up to 30 g of alcohol a day for women—that is, three standard drinks a day—and for men up to 45 g/day, which is 4.5 standard drinks. This is a higher level than many places regard as moderate, but definitions vary so much from country to country that we had to choose a level that would cover most countries. Moderate drinking was higher for those in New Zealand or the United Kingdom, and lower in those from the United States.

Our findings about the relationship between alcohol consumption and disease outcomes such as disability, relapse rate and quality of life are important, as it is possible to base recommendations on them. Most doctors would accept that this is probably the highest level of evidence that we can obtain about alcohol consumption and health for PwMS, as it is highly unlikely that it will ever be possible to randomly allocate people to groups with differing alcohol intakes and expect them to adhere to this research plan.

In our study of the real-life situations of all these PwMS from all over the world, those with moderate alcohol use were more likely to have normal physical ability or some disability, and those with a low alcohol use were more likely to require major mobility support. Similarly, quality of life was significantly better across the major areas surveyed for those who consumed moderate levels of alcohol compared to those with low consumption (see Figure 8). Although their numbers were small, PwMS who engaged in binge drinking had significantly lower levels of mental health-related quality of life than all others. There was no relationship between amount of alcohol consumed and relapse rate for those with relapsing-remitting MS.

Moderate alcohol intake by people with MS is associated with better quality of life than low or high intake.

Figure 8: Quality of life outcomes by level of alcohol use

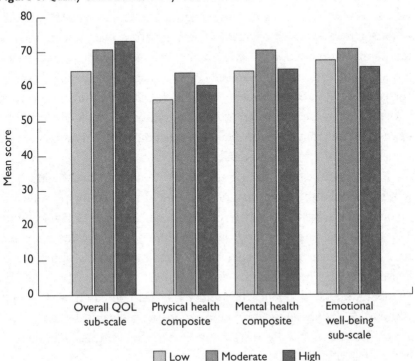

Overall, we showed that PwMS with moderate alcohol consumption had better health in terms of a lower level of disability and better quality of life compared with those with low alcohol intake. This fits well with what we know from previous research about the potential benefits of moderate alcohol use by people with other chronic diseases.

Gluten

Some researchers contend that, in an evolutionary sense, legumes and gluten in cereals are relatively recent additions to the human diet, and may be implicated in auto-immune diseases, including MS. The most severe form of gluten intolerance is coeliac disease. Here, people develop serious digestive system disorders due to an immune response to the gluten in wheat. One might expect, if gluten was a key ingredient in the diet to be avoid by those with MS, that PwMS might have a higher than usual incidence of coeliac disease or, vice versa, that people with coeliac disease might have a higher than expected incidence of MS. A large population study examined 14,000 people in Sweden with coeliac disease and compared them with 70,000 other people without the disease, acting as controls.[86] One would have expected a higher rate of MS (or other CNS degenerative disease) in those people with coeliac disease than in the controls if gluten was involved in causing these diseases. In fact, the researchers found no statistically significant association between coeliac disease and subsequent multiple sclerosis, Parkinson's disease, Alzheimer's disease, hereditary ataxia, the symptom ataxia, Huntington's disease, myasthenia gravis or spinal muscular atrophy. This is very strong evidence that there is no link with gluten.

If there was a link, one should at least expect to find PwMS have more antibodies to gluten than other people. In one study of 95 PwMS, no one had elevated antibody levels.[87] Another study of 49 PwMS found 12 per cent had raised antibody levels to gluten; however, this compared with 13 per cent of unselected blood donors, so it was unlikely that PwMS had any special sensitivity to gluten.[88] Another study of 166 PwMS found no difference in antibody levels compared with people without MS.[89] Other research found no one with coeliac disease-related antibodies among 217 PwMS, but one case in the controls.[90] This person had coeliac disease.

Only one study I have been able to find, of 72 PwMS and their first degree relatives compared with 123 people without MS, found a suggestive difference.[91] In this study, seven of the PwMS had antibodies suggestive of coeliac disease, versus three of the healthy controls. These antibodies to gluten were more common in the first-degree relatives of PwMS, with 23 of 126 relatives being positive. The authors then did gut biopsies—a more definitive test of coeliac disease—and found that eight of the PwMS had biopsies suggestive of coeliac disease. The authors recommended increased efforts at detecting coeliac disease in PwMS and, for anyone found to have coeliac disease, a gluten-free diet, as one would expect. The numbers in this study were small and, while the prevalence of coeliac disease was several times higher in PwMS than those without, because of the small numbers it is hard to give much weight to the findings, particularly as they contradict the remainder of the research findings to date.

There is insufficient evidence to recommend excluding gluten from the diets of most people with MS.

Using an alternative approach to investigating this problem, researchers fed a gluten-free diet to animals with the experimental form of MS, EAE. The animals did not improve, and initially had a more severe disease course.[92] While they later seemed to have less disability than the other animals, their initial deterioration makes it difficult to be definite about any effect either way.

In all, these papers do not provide clear evidence of a link between gluten intolerance and MS, but for some people it may be an issue, and a trial of a gluten-free diet may be warranted. Alternatively, testing for antibodies to gluten might be sensible for those who are concerned.

Supplements
Vitamins
In addition to diet, Swank placed all of the patients in his studies on a multivitamin tablet each day. But is there evidence to support the use of

vitamin supplements? While we have known for centuries that a diet rich in micronutrients—specifically vitamins, minerals and antioxidants, like the OMS diet—is helpful for preventing a range of diseases and slowing down the ageing process, it has not been clear whether extracting those nutrients, concentrating them and taking them in supplement form has any benefits. Like essential fatty acids, many of these compounds cannot be made in the body and must be ingested in the diet. A diet rich in fruit and vegetables is likely to have its great health-giving benefits because of the combination of all the nutrients in the whole package. It is hard to imagine that eating badly and then supplementing with one, two or more of the individual nutrients can replicate the value of the original food.

Until recently, there has been little evidence—despite much interest and research in the area—that multivitamins make any difference at all to health. It was assumed that, even if they had no benefit, at least they were doing no harm, and so could be taken almost as a form of insurance against an unhealthy lifestyle. Several major studies published in the early 2000s have now cast serious doubt on this assumption, raising the likelihood that taking antioxidant and vitamin supplements probably does real harm.[93–99] These studies were well-conducted systematic reviews or meta-analyses of all the published randomised controlled trials on multivitamins and antioxidant supplements in various diseases, and their effect on overall mortality.

High-quality evidence shows that taking multivitamin supplements causes real harm.

One meta-analysis of seven randomised controlled trials of vitamin E and eight of beta-carotene supplementation versus placebo or no intervention in heart disease[99] involving around 220,000 patients showed no effect from vitamin E supplementation, but beta-carotene supplementation resulted in a 7 per cent increase in deaths overall, and a 10 per cent increase in deaths from heart disease. Another looked at various supplements in the prevention of cancers of the digestive system.[94, 95] The researchers examined trials involving over 170,000 people, and found no benefit of beta-carotene, vitamin A or vitamin E in reducing the incidence of these cancers. Again, however, they found an increase in the overall death rate of the people who took these supplements versus those taking placebo. For beta-carotene and vitamin A combination supplements, there was a 29 per cent increase in mortality, and for beta-carotene together with vitamin E, there was a 10 per cent increase.

Another meta-analysis examined nearly 136,000 people in nineteen clinical trials, taking either vitamin E alone or in combination with other supplements.[98] They found an increase in the overall death rate of those taking high-dose vitamin E (400 IU or more per day), with a clear dose–response relationship—that is, the higher the dose the more likely it was that death was the outcome. The size of the increase in risk was alarming, with an extra 39 deaths per 10,000 people taking the high-dose supplements compared with those not taking vitamin E.

One large study looked at the relationship between multivitamin use and the five-year risk of prostate cancer in over 295,000 men in the National Institutes of Health Diet and Health Study who were cancer free at enrolment in 1995 and 1996.[97] They found a 32 per cent increased risk of advanced prostate cancer and a 98 per cent increased risk of death in those men taking multivitamin supplements more than seven times a week. Another meta-analysis examined the risk of taking antioxidant vitamin supplements in 68 trials with nearly a quarter of a million participants, looking at the death rate from all causes for people taking supplements versus no treatment.[93] They separated the trials into those of high and low quality. The high-quality trials showed an increase in risk for those taking the supplements, with a 4 per cent increase in death rates for those taking vitamin E alone, 7 per cent increase for those taking beta-carotene and 16 per cent increase for those taking vitamin A.

These results are of great concern, particularly as it has been shown by the 1987, 1992 and 2000 National Health Interview Surveys in the United States that vitamin and mineral supplement use increased from just under a quarter of all adults in 1987 to over one-third in 2000.[100] This is probably similar in most developed countries.

One accompanying editorial summed up the situation by asking, 'Why is it not possible to take a vitamin pill to obtain the same effect as a balanced diet?'[101] The author stated that, 'Antioxidant supplements in pills are synthetic, factory processed, and may not be safe compared with their naturally occurring counterparts.' In effect, antioxidant and vitamin supplements are the ultimate in processed food, in that we refine the food down to its tiniest active component and eat that, while throwing the rest of the food away.

A recent review examining the evidence around dietary supplements only found evidence for a benefit from vitamin D and omega-3 supplementation—exactly the two recommended supplements on the OMS Recovery Program.[102] It reinforced the potentially harmful effect of taking beta-carotene, vitamin A or vitamin E supplements. The very influential Nurses Health Study in the United States, looking at the development of MS in over 176,000 US nurses, found no association between the intake of the antioxidant vitamins C or E, or dietary carotenoids (such as beta-carotene) and the development of MS, either taken as vitamin supplements or calculated from the foods participants ate.[103]

Overall, the data indicating the harms from multivitamin use in massive studies are compelling, providing a high level of proof. This is one of the most studied areas in medicine, and the results are uniform and very disturbing. It is simply too dangerous to take these vitamins.

Calcium

Some authorities seem to suggest the calcium supplements are useful for PwMS. A number of well-designed trials and meta-analyses have, however, raised serious doubts about the safety of calcium supplementation. A major randomised controlled trial examined 1471 post-menopausal women, 732 randomised to calcium supplementation and 739 to placebo.[104] Heart attacks were over twice as common in the calcium group than in the placebo group. The investigators also looked at the combined end point of heart attack, stroke or sudden death, and found that this was also nearly twice as common in the calcium group.

Some might consider this increased risk acceptable if the benefits of calcium supplementation were very marked. But recent work has raised doubts about whether there is really any benefit in terms of bone health from supplementing with calcium. Researchers have shown that calcium supplementation increased hip fracture risk by 50 per cent.[105] A meta-analysis reported that randomised controlled trials showed no reduction in hip fracture risk with calcium supplementation, and that an increased risk was possible.[106] For other fractures, there was a neutral effect. In another meta-analysis of randomised controlled trials, researchers found that for every two fractures we prevent by giving calcium supplements to prevent osteoporosis, one person taking the supplements has a heart attack.[107] This is clearly an unacceptably high figure, and reinforces the message that it is sun exposure and vitamin D supplementation that are safe and useful for fracture prevention, rather than calcium supplementation. The calcium supplementation industry in Western countries is a product of our avoidance of adequate sunlight.

It really is time for a reappraisal of the whole calcium–vitamin D issue in health. This is covered in much more detail in Step 2 but, briefly, vitamin D is very important for a variety of reasons, not least its helpful effects on mood, muscle strength, cancer, vascular and auto-immune disease.[108] The doses used in supplementation are, however, generally too low. The blood level needs to be at least 75 nmol/L for any benefit to bone health,[109] and probably twice that to really get the full health benefits for other conditions. For example, a level of 100 nmol/L or so is the threshold level above which there is a great protective effect against developing MS.[110]

For calcium, like many other heavily marketed supplements, the evidence suggests that it pays to be very selective about what supplements to take. Supplements need to be taken for a good reason, with a therapeutic aim in mind, and utilising the best available evidence to support their use. For people with adequate vitamin D levels (and for people in most geographic regions, this means supplementation with relatively large doses of vitamin D in winter), calcium supplementation is unnecessary. For those who avoid the sun or cannot get much sun in winter, and those with osteoporosis, supplementation with around 5000 IU of vitamin D daily, rather than with calcium, is recommended. On the basis of current evidence, calcium supplementation poses too great a risk to human health, and is not recommended.

Potentially helpful supplements
Apart from vitamin D and omega-3 fatty acids, which are discussed in separate sections, a number of individual supplemental vitamins may

be of value in MS, according to the available evidence. This, however, generally only applies to situations where blood levels of that particular nutrient are found to be low.

Vitamin B12

Vitamin B12 is an important nutrient. It is a B group vitamin found primarily in meat—especially liver, eggs and dairy products—but also in large quantities in seafood of various types, particularly sardines. No plant foods can be relied on as a definite source of vitamin B12. It is necessary for the maintenance of a healthy nervous system and plays a key role in the metabolism of fatty acids essential for the maintenance of myelin. Prolonged B12 deficiency can lead to nerve degeneration and irreversible neurological damage. But deficiency is more commonly caused by failure to absorb B12 from the intestine rather than a dietary deficiency.

MS and vitamin B12 deficiency are similar diseases in terms of their inflammatory and neurodegenerative processes. Decreased levels of vitamin B12 are also fairly common in PwMS. In addition to its role in myelin formation, B12 has important immunomodulatory effects and stimulates nerve growth—a bit like vitamin D. Researchers have raised the possibility of B12 causing MS, and suggested close monitoring of vitamin B12 levels in PwMS, as well as B12 supplementation.[111]

People with low levels of acid in the stomach are susceptible to deficiency. Deficiency is also well known to occur in vegans. As many people are taking drugs that lower stomach acid levels, like ranitidine or omeprazole, if they are also on a vegan diet, there is a real risk of B12 deficiency. It can take many years for deficiency disease to develop after changing to diets low in B12. Vitamin B12 deficiency is surprisingly common, even in people who are not on vegan diets or have low acid levels in their stomachs. One study showed that about 23 per cent of people aged over 50 had low vitamin B12 levels.[112]

Fortunately, vitamin B12 is essentially non-toxic, so it is unlikely that one can do any harm by taking supplements. PwMS on vegan diets (without seafood) may consider taking regular vitamin B12 tablets, of the order of 250 to 1000 µg per week, although this should be guided by occasional blood testing to see whether it is necessary. B12 is effective when taken by mouth and does not require injection,[113–15] contrary to popular belief; it is also quite cheap.

> If people with MS wish to take a supplement, the B group vitamins are recommended.

The B group vitamins are extremely important, particularly to normal brain function. They are involved in a multitude of chemical reactions within the body, including the metabolism of fats. They are quite cheap and readily absorbed. People who drink alcohol regularly need a good intake of B group vitamins. The B group also includes folate. Folate deficiency has been shown to be involved in causing Alzheimer's disease. Folate is intimately related to normal nerve cell development, as shown by the reduced incidence of spina bifida in babies born to mothers taking folate supplements.[116] It also reduces homocysteine levels, which are associated with degenerative disease. More recently, it has been shown to reduce the incidence of stroke.[117, 118]

Vitamin B3 (nicotinamide) has been shown in the animal model of MS to prevent degeneration of axons, and thereby to protect the animals against the usual progression of the disease if given before the disease is induced, and to improve the disease once present.[119] There is potential here for treatment of MS, but research is still required in humans to support these findings. These data support the view that if any vitamin supplements are likely to be helpful in MS, they are the B group vitamins.

Flavonoids

The best-known source of flavonoids is grapes, hence the well-documented health benefits of low to moderate consumption of red wine. Ordinary tea also contains chemicals called polyphenols that are powerful antioxidants. Asian green tea has higher concentrations again. Studies of people drinking only two or more cups of tea a day have shown major reductions in heart disease, stroke and other degenerative diseases.[120] Drinking too much, though, can cause problems because of the caffeine intake. But taking flavonoids as supplements rather than in food, like vitamins, is not recommended.

Iron

Many PwMS are concerned that they will become iron deficient on a vegan-plus-seafood diet. This is a theoretical risk, as a good vegan diet has a reasonable amount of iron in it. It can be an issue for women, particularly those who have heavy periods. If this applies, it is possible to get iron levels checked periodically, or to take a small supplement. Excess iron is quite toxic, and it is certainly better to be getting a small amount rather than a lot. Researchers have noted that abnormal iron accumulation is common in a variety of neurodegenerative diseases, including MS, and there is evidence that iron plays a role in promoting inflammation.[121] They have shown that the common Th1 pro-inflammatory cytokines were more toxic to nerve cells if they had high levels of iron. Another study examining iron metabolism in 20 PwMS compared with ten healthy controls concluded that iron overload may play a part in the development and progression of MS.[122] Concerns about iron deficiency for people on a vegan-plus-seafood diet are probably unwarranted. Certainly there is no case for taking a regular iron supplement without first checking iron status.

Glucosamine

Glucosamine is an extract from the shells of shellfish that has been shown to be helpful in arthritis. In experimental animals, it produces a shift in the balance of the Th1/Th2 immune response towards a suppressive Th2 response, and to significantly suppressing the animal form of MS, EAE, in the laboratory.[123] The authors of this study suggested a potential use for glucosamine, either alone or in combination with disease-modifying drugs to enhance their benefit and reduce their doses in MS and possibly other auto-immune disorders. Other research suggests that the N-acetyl form of glucosamine is likely to be more effective in MS.[124]

Coenzyme Q10

Coenzyme Q10 (CoQ10), also known as ubiquinone, is a vitamin-like substance found in high concentrations in the mitochondria, small energy-producing parts of each bodily cell. CoQ10 is essential for this production of energy in the body to occur. Small trials have suggested it reduces oxidative stress in PwMS;[125] oxidative stress is known to be associated with relapses. In a double-blind placebo controlled trial of CoQ10 for twelve weeks in PwMS, fatigue and depression were improved in those taking the CoQ10.[126] More recently, scientists in New Zealand have synthesised a form of this substance that concentrates particularly in mitochondria when taken by mouth. Mitoquinone, or MitoQ, is available commercially and may have advantages over CoQ10.[127] This supplement appears to have beneficial neuroprotective effects in a model of Parkinson's disease.[128] It has not yet been studied in MS, and it is quite expensive.

HOW

Introduction

So how does one put all this evidence together to come up with a recommended nutritional program that can help PwMS recover? Many PwMS are confused by the number of diets they see for MS when browsing the internet, so how do we know that the nutritional approach recommended on the OMS Recovery Program is the preferred one? And how do we go about implementing it in real life?

In a nutshell
- Eat plant-based wholefoods plus seafood, the optimal nutrition to prevent MS progression.
- Embrace this as a permanent life change rather than a diet, which implies it is temporary.
- Empty out the pantry of all the old foods and start with a clean slate.
- Substitute healthy foods for the unhealthy ones that contain dairy products and saturated fats.
- Regularly add cold-pressed extra virgin flaxseed oil to food after cooking and before eating.
- Do not count grams of saturated fat in foods.
- Avoid frying with oil; instead, dry fry, stir fry with water or steam.

Considering the evidence

The combined weight of evidence, drawn from a variety of studies across the medical literature, with varying methodologies from basic science through population studies to clinical trials, clearly and strongly shows that saturated fat consumption, and hence fat concentrations in cells and blood fat profiles, is a key determinant of the rate of developing disability for PwMS. The evidence is clear, congruent, consistent and of good quality. As a result, it forms the basis of the OMS Recovery Program. The evidence accumulated from countless research articles and summarised in this book has now been validated by the HOLISM study, which provides strong confirmatory evidence of these benefits.

The evidence shows that saturated fat consumption needs to be minimised to prevent disability in MS. Yet it appears that it is not enough to modify one's diet so that the amount of saturated fat is reduced somewhat. From the available evidence, that may only slow the disease a little or not at all. Swank's work shows that the 'bad dieters' reduced their saturated fat intake markedly, yet this was not enough to alter the disease course. The HOLISM study showed strong associations of good health for PwMS with a very healthy fat intake, but not a moderately healthy fat intake. Hence the OMS diet uses an all or nothing approach—that is, saturated fat is eliminated from the diet as much as is possible, not just cut down. Not eating meat at all is important for this reason, as meat is the major source of saturated fat in most people's diets.

The evidence also shows that achieving a good fat profile in blood is important for the same reason. Sound population studies, including the HOLISM study, show that fish consumption is associated with better outcomes for PwMS, both in disability and quality of life. Regular omega-3 fatty acid consumption is also likely to prevent progression to disability, particularly if saturated fat consumption is minimal. Other evidence, not specific to MS, shows that altered fats, including trans- and partially and fully hydrogenated oils, should be avoided—especially frying breakdown products. Similarly, fruit and vegetable consumption needs to be increased for most people, and does appear to be associated with better outcomes for PwMS. Cow's milk should be avoided by PwMS as it appears just too risky to consume dairy products based on the available evidence. Evidence about general health benefits of diet suggests strongly that more fibre is helpful, and processed food is harmful to health. Excess salt should probably also be avoided.

Developing an ideal diet for PwMS

So what is the best way to go about achieving all of these aims? Rather than simply adhering to an existing diet, like the Swank diet or the Paleo diet, or some other diet that targets one or more aspects of these requirements, I used the best available evidence to develop an OMS nutritional approach that targeted all these aspects: a program to provide the best possible chance of minimising risk of progression of MS and potentially allow recovery. The Swank diet, for example, suggests that low-fat dairy products are fine, along with deep-fried fish and other foods that do not satisfy all the requirements outlined above. While the Swank diet produced dramatic results in slowing the rate of deterioration of PwMS in that study, on average people in each group of disability still deteriorated—albeit much more slowly than those who ate more saturated fat.

The Paleo diet has not been specifically studied in PwMS; indeed, there are very few papers in the medical literature about the Paleo diet as treatment for any condition. Its recommendations for liberal use of coconut products is at odds with the work of Swank and others, as these products contain the highest known dietary concentration of saturated fats. It also recommends eating meat, including grass-fed organ meat, but also bacon. Bacon is particularly high in saturated fat and is definitely not on the menu for those hoping to recover from MS. The Mediterranean diet has been widely studied, and is perhaps the most intensively researched and proven diet in the medical literature. It has great benefits for a variety of common Western diseases and for brain function.[129-135] But it does not satisfy most of the objectives outlined above that come from a thorough review of the optimal dietary strategies for PwMS.

The OMS diet is based on rigorous analysis of the best available evidence.

The OMS nutritional approach, on the other hand, is designed to incorporate all the best medical evidence about diet from all possible sources. Analysing the medical literature on diet, one is struck by the better health outcomes achieved by people following plant-based diets. Similarly, there is ample evidence that processed foods are unhealthy, and that they contribute to chronic disease. Reading widely around this subject, one encounters the work of expert nutritionists and physicians who have dedicated their careers to illuminating the evidence about healthy nutrition. Drs T. Colin Campbell, Caldwell Esselstyn, Dean Ornish and Artemis Simopoulos, among others, are remarkably congruent in their research findings and recommendations about what constitutes the optimally healthy diet.

Dr T. Colin Campbell is a nutritional biochemist who grew up on a dairy farm and was an avowed carnivore until conducting his now well-known China Study (the book of this name[136] makes very interesting reading). Essentially, he demonstrated, in elegant population studies of rural Chinese villages, that a plant-based wholefood diet is associated with very low rates of the common degenerative Western diseases like heart disease and common cancers. He has authored over 300 research papers on the subject, was involved in the hit documentary *Forks Over Knives*, and has sat on several US National Academy of Sciences expert panels on food. Like Swank, he is no lightweight. Over 80 years old himself, he has eaten a plant-based wholefood diet since undertaking the China Study.

Dr Caldwell Esselstyn is a surgeon who is also widely known for his role in *Forks Over Knives*. His book *Prevent and Reverse Heart Disease*[137] influenced a very ill former US President, Bill Clinton, to take up a plant-based wholefood diet and reverse his own heart disease. Esselstyn has long argued the benefits of a plant-based wholefood diet, arguing that heart disease does not need to exist, because it is a food-borne disease.

Dr Dean Ornish is a physician who has revolutionised the treatment of heart disease in the United States following a series of influential studies showing that narrowing of the coronary arteries to the heart could be reversed with a plant-based wholefood diet.[138-141] He also showed that prostate cancer could be controlled with the same diet.[142, 143, 144] His heart program has been rolled out through US hospitals and is Medicare funded.[145] He took these findings further, publishing with Australian Nobel Prize winner Professor Elizabeth Blackburn, showing that dietary and lifestyle changes actually changed the expression of a person's DNA: that someone isn't actually stuck with their genetic make-up for life, but can change it.[146] This was ground-breaking research.

Dr Artemis Simopoulos, who initially trained in paediatrics, proceeded to work with the National Institutes of Health in the United States, ultimately advising the US President on nutritional matters. She has published over 300 research papers, mostly on nutrition, and her book *The Omega Plan*, advocating healthy fat consumption—particularly increasing the intake of omega-3 fatty acids—was a worldwide best-seller.[64]

A plant-based wholefood diet

The clear message from an analysis of the outputs of such luminaries in the field of nutrition and diet is the congruence and consistency of their findings that the optimal diet for human health is a plant-based wholefood diet, with a concentration on healthy fat consumption—particularly omega-3s. That means, where possible, eating food that is whole rather than processed or refined. There is now a very powerful food-processing industry that produces substances (I hesitate to call them foods) that are becoming increasingly removed from their actual food sources. Reading the labels of some packaged food in supermarkets, one has to wonder whether they are actually food or a chemistry experiment with us as the guinea pigs. The basis for any nutritional approach to overcome most chronic conditions needs to be a plant-based wholefood diet. This sits well with Swank's work, in that a plant-based wholefood diet is very low in saturated fat.

 A plant-based wholefood diet is the optimal diet for human health.

A series of articles in 2012 in the *Medical Journal of Australia*, Australia's premier medical journal, outlined the strong case for a plant-based diet to improve the health of the community as well as the planet. The series tackled and dispelled common myths about vegan and vegetarian diets:

that one cannot get enough iron or zinc on these diets; that there is not enough protein; that supplements are needed; and so on. It additionally provided evidence that such diets are likely to significantly improve health. The series should reassure those PwMS considering these dietary recommendations that such a diet is mainstream and that they will not be taking any risks with their health—indeed, quite the reverse is true. The authors also provided some practical tips for preparing such meals.[147] The series is open access, so is freely available for download. It can be viewed at <www.mja.com.au/open/2012/1/2/plant-based-diet-good-us-and-planet>.

Interestingly, using Swank's method of counting saturated fat, where he didn't include the fat in vegetables, nuts or grains, a plant-based diet really produces a minimal number of grams of saturated fat per day. So eating a plant-based wholefood diet also obviates the need for counting grams of saturated fat. An important factor in devising the optimal nutritional program for PwMS is not only making sure it accords with the best available evidence of what works in improving MS, but also ensuring that the approach is sustainable. So it needs to be health-giving, but also tasty, varied and able to be sustained in the long term. Counting grams of fat is not really a sustainable way of eating; a plant-based wholefood diet eliminates the need for that counting.

Including seafood

There is ample evidence—not just from Swank's work, where fish and other seafood were recommended instead of meat, but also from many population and case-control studies—that increased consumption of fish and other seafood is associated with better outcomes for PwMS. That is probably at least in part due to the omega-3 fatty acids contained in seafood, but the findings of the HOLISM study strongly suggest that seafood and omega-3s each have helpful effects for PwMS in their own right.[63] Certainly omega-3 supplementation is helpful, judging from the best available evidence. So a plant-based wholefood diet plus seafood and omega-3s ticks all the boxes. That diet forms the basis of the OMS Recovery Program. Once people engage with such a dietary change, they love it! There is no end to the list of delicious, colourful and, most importantly, healthy recipes based on a plant-based wholefood diet plus seafood and omega-3s. In the information age, if one is ever stuck for something to prepare, a casual Google search will usually find a tasty recipe. Try typing in 'vegan chocolate mousse' or 'vegan chocolate cake', for example, and prepare to be delighted with the outcome.

So a plant-based wholefood diet plus seafood and omega-3s is optimal for PwMS, avoiding refined products as much as possible. A plant-based wholefood diet plus seafood and omega-3s, avoiding meat and dairy, is very low in saturated fat and has an abundance of healthy omega-3 oils. But, as we have seen, that is not the whole story. Additionally, it is important to avoid altered fats, and not to fry food. People following such a nutritional approach will have very healthy fat profiles in blood with low cholesterol levels, mostly without needing to take medication to achieve that—unlike a sizeable proportion of the rest of the population. And they will be very unlikely to develop any of the common, serious chronic conditions that beset Western countries in epidemic proportions in the twenty-first century, largely due to modern food industry practices.

 Adding seafood to a plant-based wholefood diet adds additional benefit for people with MS.

While most of the evidence in the context of MS is about frequency of fish consumption as opposed to other seafood, all seafood is a good source of protein, making up for omitting meat as well as having similar oil in it. The actual amount of fish oil in seafood varies markedly, though, from high concentrations in oily fish like mackerel (around 14 per cent per cent), sardines (11 per cent), herring (9 per cent), salmon (6 per cent) and anchovies (5 per cent) to very little (less than 1 per cent) in white fish and much seafood, like lobster and prawns. As a result, evidence from studies showing that increased frequency of fish consumption is beneficial for PwMS is extrapolated to all seafood in the OMS diet. Because the actual fish oil in seafood is around 30 per cent saturated fat, those oilier fish with higher concentrations of fish oil are best eaten in moderation, whereas most other seafood—particularly white fish, crayfish, squid and prawns—can be eaten whenever desired. It is also important to eat low on the food chain, which means the smaller fish and seafood, as pollutants like mercury are concentrated in the bigger fish at the top of the food chain.

Implementing the diet

So the first step in the OMS Recovery Program is to adopt a plant-based wholefood diet plus seafood and omega-3s. Given early evidence of the potentially harmful effects of excess salt consumption, one should also be careful to minimise salt intake, and early evidence of the harmful effects of being overweight suggests that maintaining a normal body weight is also important. In any case, eating in this way tends to lead to weight loss for most people, because most of the empty calories that we commonly eat are no longer in the diet; it is common for PwMS on the OMS diet to get in touch via the website and ask what strategies they can use to put on weight! There are many, many people who would dream of having that kind of problem.

So how does one go about implementing this nutritional program? Many people find just working out what is involved with such a dietary change very daunting. And it is not just a diet, which implies a temporary change; this is a permanently different way of living—a change for life. Importantly, it is much easier to stick with this approach if one makes a decision to really embrace this lifestyle change, rather than feeling it is being imposed from outside. But many people say they don't like particular foods, or just can't give up meat, or cheese, or chocolate. It can help to think first about why we eat.

There are many reasons we eat what we do. Sometimes it is from hunger—although uncommonly in developed countries. It can be because of our culture of origin: people growing up in Greek families, for instance, often eat very differently from those growing up in Vietnamese families. It can be social: we take what we are offered at an afternoon tea. It can be for the taste. Or for health. If we sit and analyse why we eat, we can come up with a very long list of reasons. One that always comes up is habit. For many of us, we have just settled into a comfortable habit of eating certain foods—a bit like where we sit at the dinner table. We say we like certain foods because we are used to eating them. Changing those habits, while daunting for many people, is actually very simple. Like the Nike advertisement says, the best way is to 'Just Do It'. It is remarkable how one can respond negatively to eating something new, but after eating it a few times, one gets a taste for it. I recall visiting some Asian countries as a young man and finding the food daunting. Asian food is now one of my favourite cuisines.

Changing dietary habits

Dietary habits are interesting. We cling to our old eating habits, but once we decide to change them, and they become a new habit, we cling just as hard to the new habit! For those who used to have sugar in their coffee or tea, remember how awful a cup of coffee or tea tasted without it; many of us have given that up for health reasons, and now couldn't possibly drink a cup of coffee or tea with sugar! It is a diametrically opposite taste, yet the new habit is just as hard to break as the old one. This is actually exactly the same situation as reducing salt intake: once one no longer adds salt at the table, the food actually starts to taste better. Adding salt is also just a habit.

So finding the motivation to change the habit becomes the key ingredient, because once changed, the new habit sticks. While fear of becoming disabled is a pretty powerful motivator, it is interesting that the longer PwMS spend on the OMS diet, the more this motivation changes from fear of what will happen if MS progresses to the joy of living well and of enjoying really good, healthy food. Moving health higher up the rankings in terms of motivation is also useful. My experience of many men on our OMS retreats is that when first confronted by a green juice, they screw their faces up, start to gag when they drink it and generally resist ingesting it in any way possible. Once one focuses on the goodness in the juice—the incredible array of vitamins and antioxidants—and imagines what a change they will make to cells in the body that are not functioning well, the whole experience of drinking it can change.

An interesting facet of changing our diet is the attitude we take into such a change, and the language we use to describe what we are doing—both to other people and, more importantly, to ourselves. An attitude of

embracing the change wholeheartedly helps, in contrast to an attitude
of restriction or of only being 'allowed' certain foods. Saying 'I can eat'
or 'I can't eat' certain foods implies some external authority telling one
what to do and setting limits. Most of us find it hard to be constantly
told what to do. To use language that simply states 'I eat' or 'I don't eat'
implies that it is your own choice to eat or not eat certain foods—which,
of course, it is. Many people who choose to embrace the OMS nutritional
approach develop a passion for food and for cooking that they never
knew they had. Finding exciting new recipes, discovering new flavours
and making the most healthy creations are actually great fun when you
become passionate about food.

Making a start

A good way to go about the change is to devote some time at the beginning of the diet to becoming really knowledgeable about what is really
in various foods and getting to know in detail the fat composition
of common foods. Many people choose to clean out their cupboards of
all the old food and start afresh, going down to the supermarket and
spending half a day just browsing the aisles, reading the ingredients on
tins and packets of foods they commonly ate, getting to know exactly
what they are putting in their mouths. You will soon be exposed to a
range of terms that are unfamiliar—things like xanthan gum, casein,
whey, emulsifier and soy lecithin. It can be useful to have an electronic
tablet or smartphone handy to check what these things are. Xanthan gum,
for example, is a product of bacterial fermentation of various sugars, and
is used to thicken foods—commonly ice cream.

But it is important to discover these things for oneself, deciding what
one is going to choose to eat and what one is not. It is interesting to
find out how many names there are for milk protein, for example—and,
as noted earlier, milk protein is to be avoided by PwMS. Noticing how
many of the foods we used to eat are really just a concoction of various
chemicals can be a powerful stimulus to giving them up and moving to a
wholefood diet. Most packaged foods in supermarkets now have a nutrition facts box on them. I go into this in detail later, but usually there is a
sub-heading under the fats for saturated fat content. This is a useful way
of checking the amount of saturated fat in the food.

Becoming an expert on what is actually in your food can have great health benefits.

An important point to remember is that all oils contain some saturated fat, monounsaturated fat, and polyunsaturated omega-3 and omega-6 oils. It is just that the relative concentrations vary from food to food. So red meat does contain omega-3, omega-6 and monounsaturated fats, but it predominantly contains saturated fat, and for that reason should not be eaten. The oil in fish, on the other hand, while containing all of those types of fats, has mainly omega-3, omega-6 and monounsaturated fat; despite the 30 per cent or so of saturated fat in fish oil, it can be eaten— and should be—to get the health benefits of the omega-3 fatty acids it contains. So all oil in food contains all the types of fats; PwMS need to concentrate on those with more in the unsaturated part of the spectrum, and avoid those principally containing saturated fat, like meat, cheese and coconut products.

What to eat and what not to eat
Up to this point, a lot of the discussion has been somewhat theoretical. But what foods are actually best not eaten? What should PwMS eat? The following list might help to begin deciding which foods are actually harmful for PwMS.

Foods that should not be eaten
The following foods are not to be eaten:
- meat, including processed meat
- eggs (except for egg whites)
- dairy products, including low-fat dairy
- biscuits, pastries, cakes, unless fat-free
- commercial baked goods unless the ingredients are in line with the diet
- prepared mixes (cake mix, pancake mix and so on)
- snacks like chips, corn chips, party foods
- margarine, shortening, chocolate, coconut and palm oil
- fried and deep-fried foods, except those fried without oil

- most fast foods
- altered fats and oils.

This list concentrates on the foods that must be omitted, but doesn't indicate that the foods that are left are very healthy and enjoyable. Omitting these foods means that remaining foods consist of all vegetables, fruits, nuts, seeds and grains, seafood, egg whites and so on, where possible in a wholefood form, and from these ingredients one can make an enormous variety of tasty, satisfying and above all healthy meals. Table 4 summarises the foods that PwMS should eat as often as they like, in moderation because they are oily and part of that oil is saturated fat, and never because they contain harmful substances.

There is some debate about chocolate's role in good health, as cocoa (from which it is made) is full of good antioxidants; however, most chocolate is also loaded with saturated and altered fat, so it should be avoided. In most countries, the cocoa butter used to make chocolate can contain up to 15 per cent altered fat, making chocolate a relatively concentrated source of altered fats. Cocoa, however, is a natural vegetable product (a legume) with only a little saturated fat, and can be used liberally in baking and desserts. Cocoa is a very healthy vegetable product

Table 4: Foods to eat and foods to avoid

As often as desired	In moderation	Never
Vegetables	Avocado	Dairy products
Fruit	Olives	Meat
Grains (wheat, rye, barley, oats, quinoa, etc.)	Nuts, seeds	Egg yolks
Legumes (beans, lentils, cocoa, etc.)	Oily fish	Commercial cakes
Soy products	Alcohol (two standard drinks a day, at least two alcohol-free days a week)	Most fast food
White fish and most seafood		Margarine
		Foods fried in oil
		Palm oil, 'vegetable oil', coconut products

turned into junk food when used to make chocolate. Chocolate is to be completely avoided by PwMS; however, making foods containing cocoa provides the same flavour in a healthy way.

Substituting

When adopting the OMS diet and making changes, many PwMS find that they quickly become experts at which healthy foods can be substituted for the old unhealthy ones. There is a very large range of plant-based 'milks' that substitute well for cow's milk, all with different properties and therefore different potential uses in cooking. Soy, oat, rice, almond and other grain and nut milks are perfect for recipes where one might previously have used cow's milk. Soy and almond milks have more protein, and so are better suited to baking, where one is aiming to have some 'setting' of the finished product. Rice milk is much lighter, with little protein, and many people find it suits cereals very well. Oat milk is somewhere in between. It may take some experimenting to find the most suitable option for individual tastes. I used rice milk for years on my muesli, but now prefer a mixture of rice and oat milk. It is a very individual thing. But it is interesting how, once that habit has changed, most people find it impossible to go back to cow's milk. Mostly they find the taste and consistency disgusting!

Recipes that call for eggs can easily be modified so that two egg whites are used in place of one whole egg. Egg whites are where the protein is concentrated, and all the fat is in the yolk. So the whites are excellent for binding foods, and can be used in cakes, or in dry-fried fish patties to hold them together. Egg frittata with egg whites and various vegetables under the grill is delicious—and, of course, very healthy.

 There are many healthy foods that can be substituted for unhealthy ones.

Table 5 shows which foods can be substituted for the unhealthy foods to keep within the nutritional guidelines advocated here. For recipes using these guidelines, go to our website at <www.overcomingms.org>. You may also want to sign up to the Members' Forum, where people

Table 5: Healthy substitutes for unhealthy foods

Food	Substitute food
Cow's milk:	
drinking, over cereal	Rice, oat, almond, soy milk
baking, cooking	Soy or almond milk
Dairy yoghurt	Soy yoghurt
Butter:	
on toast	Flaxseed oil
baking, cooking	Extra virgin olive oil
Vegetable oils	Extra virgin olive oil
Meat	Tofu, tempeh, fish
Eggs	Egg whites
Refined sugar	Honey or no sweetener
White bread	Wholemeal bread
Commercial biscuits	Fat-free biscuits
Refined cereals	Homemade muesli
Salt	Herbs
Chocolate (in desserts, drinks)	Cocoa
Sweets, lollies	Dried fruit
Potato chips	Nuts
Snacks	Vegetable sticks, dried fruit, nuts
Soft drink	Water, vegetable or fruit juice
Fast food (burgers, etc.)	Sushi, salad wraps (falafel, if desired)
Ice cream	Sorbet

following this lifestyle exchange recipes. Alternatively, the *Overcoming Multiple Sclerosis Cookbook*, published by Allen & Unwin, with crowd-sourced recipes collated by Ingrid Adelsberger from New York, who came to our first British OMS retreat in 2013, is a wonderful source of recipes tried and tested by PwMS.

These guidelines mean that foods like margarine are out, and so are pies, biscuits and particularly fast foods like chips. It is important to look carefully at labels. If the words 'hydrogenated vegetable oil' or 'partially hydrogenated vegetable oil' appear, leave the product on the shelf. Indeed, 'vegetable oils' should be avoided, as they are likely to contain the cheaper saturated vegetable oils like coconut and palm oils. The only freely available oil that is not subjected to the above refining processes, and can be used as a general, all-purpose oil, is extra virgin olive oil. It is called extra virgin because it is made from the first cold pressing of the olives. Virgin olive oil is made from later pressings and olive oil is refined oil.

Oil supplements

In place of saturated fats in the diet, we need to substitute essential fatty acids, with the balance tipped heavily in favour of the omega-3s over the omega-6 fatty acids. While the dietary change to a plant-based wholefood diet plus seafood will result in a major increase in the quantity of essential fatty acids ingested with food, most of them will be omega-6 fatty acids, unless one concentrates the diet heavily on oily seafood. Swank recommended between 20 g and 50 g a day of these unsaturated oils, mostly ingested with food. He unfortunately didn't differentiate much between omega-3s and omega-6s, and at that time there were far fewer omega-6 fats in supermarkets. Swank noted that if people did not take in enough unsaturated fats to replace the saturated fat they were omitting from their diets, they often became very tired and listless. Although it is important to reduce the amount of fat that is saturated, it is still crucial to get enough of the essential fatty acids for incorporation into bodily cells and manufacture of chemical messengers. So this nutritional approach is not no fat—there is quite a bit of fat, but it is good fat.

Plant versus fish omega-3s

Omega-3 fats can be plant-based or fish-based. The best plant source is flaxseed oil, otherwise known as linseed oil. Because it is relatively unstable and prone to oxidation, flaxseed oil needs to be cold pressed and packed in the absence of oxygen and light. Several brands satisfying these conditions are on the market, and most health food stores carry a range in the refrigerator section. Interestingly, many pharmacists also stock flaxseed oil in their refrigerated section, recognising that it is not only a food but also a medicinal product. Flaxseed oil needs to be used within about six weeks of being bought, and it should be stored in the fridge. It is time to use it on wooden furniture rather than eat it when it starts to develop a slight but characteristic bitter taste. My own flaxseed oil never lasts long enough to develop that rancid taste.

The flavour is very pleasant, and many PwMS find it very tasty on salads or pasta, but added only after the meal is cooked and ready to serve. Others may prefer to mix it with orange juice or spoon it over cereal. It is also very tasty on toast before putting on the jam or, in Australia, Vegemite. It is also relatively inexpensive. If bought in advance, it can be frozen without affecting its chemical structure or effectiveness and allowed to thaw out in the fridge when needed. It is interesting to note that Swank recommended 'raw linseed oil' (which is, in fact, flaxseed oil) for people who couldn't tolerate cod liver oil in his study. One wonders how he stumbled upon this, given how little was known then about omega-3 fatty acids.

In contrast, fish oil capsules are available in all health food shops, but are expensive, and our HOLISM data suggest fish oil is not as effective as flaxseed oil. Indeed, we could find no significant benefit for fish oil supplementation at all. Cod liver oil is less concentrated in the amount of fish oils it contains; the proportion of omega-3 oils in cod liver oil is around two-thirds lower than in fish oil and the proportion of saturated fat higher, so it is not really a substitute for fish oil. It contains vitamin D, around 400 IU per 5 ml dose, but also around 3000 units of vitamin A. In high doses, vitamin A is very toxic, with skin changes and mental deterioration the commonest effects. Quite a large dose is needed to get these effects—perhaps of the order of over 50,000–500,000 units a day. We now know that taking vitamin A as a supplement, even in low doses, is associated with an increased risk of death. So cod liver oil should not be taken as a supplement instead of fish or flaxseed oil.

It is quite inexpensive to get fish oil in a tin of sardines. John West sardines in spring water, for example, contain 110 g of sardines with 16.7 per cent fat, or fish oil. So this is 18.4 g of fish oil, or roughly eighteen and a half capsules. It is best to get seafood-based omega-3s through food if possible. There is currently great concern about whether fish oil capsules actually have as much omega-3 in them as they claim, and about pollutants in the oil.[148] They are also often oxidised—that is, the fish oil in them is going rancid. This may explain why there are such variable results in clinical trials of fish oil, as some trials probably use capsules sourced from reputable manufacturers, and others not.

 Flaxseed oil is preferred to fish oil for omega-3 supplementation, right from the beginning of the diet.

Flaxseed oil would appear to be superior to fish oil when choosing an omega-3 supplement. Given that our oceans are gradually becoming more polluted, particularly with heavy metals like mercury, and that heavy metals are known to cause neurological problems, and with the problems with fish oil capsules alluded to above, it is good that a plant-based oil like flaxseed oil can provide all our omega-3 needs. Some raise the issue that the fatty acid in flaxseed oil, alpha-linolenic acid (ALA), needs to be converted in the body to the fish oil fatty acids, eicosapenanoic acid (EPA) and then docosahexanoic acid (DHA). Various figures are put on this conversion—mostly up to 10 per cent is converted, dependent on general health, saturated fat consumption, alcohol consumption and a number of other variables.

However, in his excellent book *Fats that Heal, Fats that Kill*,[149] Udo Erasmus disputes this. While Erasmus quotes only a figure of 2.7 per cent per day of the ALA being converted to EPA, and says that this figure is likely to be higher for people getting all their essential nutrients from diet and supplements, he notes that once the ALA is stored, much more is available for conversion to EPA and DHA than is ingested. Most people's fat deposits contain about 2 per cent ALA, but this figure is quite a bit higher for those following the OMS Program. This is about 200 g of ALA, which could make about 5400 mg of EPA (equivalent to about 30 1000 mg capsules of fish oil). If there is no ALA in one's fat deposits at all (taking no omega-3s in the diet whatsoever), then just taking two tablespoons of flaxseed oil would supply enough ALA to make only about 378 mg of EPA, equivalent to two 1000 mg fish oil capsules.

So most people have enough stored if they are supplementing with ALA every day to make quite adequate amounts of EPA and DHA. Apart from the likelihood that flaxseed oil works better, the advantage of doing it this way rather than taking it as fish oil is not only related to chemical toxins like mercury in fish oil and to questions about the sustainability of our fish stocks, but also to the fact that the EPA made this way is fresher, produced in the body every day.

At least two dessert spoons of flaxseed oil should be eaten each day (20 ml), and up to four dessert spoons. One feature of flaxseed oil is that it also contains 17 per cent linoleic acid, so there are omega-6 essential fatty acids as well. The HOLISM study data suggests that it is fine to start the OMS diet with flaxseed oil, with no need to take fish oil at any stage, as it appears less effective than flaxseed oil. The HOLISM study also shows that there is no need to omit flaxseed oil on days when one is eating seafood. Both the oil and seafood have beneficial effects in their own right.

Oily fish can be eaten fresh or tinned. Many PwMS have a can of sardines or mackerel or similar for lunch, either in a sandwich or salad or on their own. For most common good brands of canned fish, this will supply close to the required 20 g of fish oil. It is interesting to note that the cheaper the tin of sardines, the lower the fish oil content, probably because they are processed and the fish oil is extracted to be sold separately.

Most people get a good balance of unsaturated oils in their diet in this way, with omega-6s mainly from food, and omega-9s from the small amount of olive oil in cooking and over salads or for dipping bread. Most of the unsaturated oil in the OMS diet comes from nuts and grains. Nuts are very high in monounsaturated oil (oleic acid, the same as in olive oil), and to a lesser extent so are grains like oats. Raw rather than cooked nuts are preferred because heating oils damages them. Of the nuts available, raw almonds have the lowest saturated fat content.

Calculating fat consumption

For those keen to count grams of saturated fat in their diet, this can be very confusing. Swank's estimation of saturated fat was actually quite inaccurate. He didn't account for the fact that all oils are a mixture of unsaturated and saturated fats, including all the good oils like flaxseed and olive oil. It can be quite confusing to read on the label of an olive oil bottle that it contains 12 per cent saturated fat, and many people wonder whether they should count that in their daily quota of saturated fat. Any oil bottle label will show that it contains a proportion of saturated fat. Swank did not include these low levels of saturated fat in his calculations of daily intake. He also encouraged eating fruits, vegetables and grains, but didn't count the saturated fat found in all of these products that contain any oil. So avocadoes, for example, contain around 15 per cent fat, some of it saturated (as all oils are). Saturated fat makes up around 2.1 per cent of an avocado. So eating a 200 g avocado adds 4.2 g of saturated fat to the daily intake of saturated fat.

But Swank didn't count this, so he said that someone eating the minimal amount of saturated fat per day—say, 5 g—could eat an avocado and still count the total saturated fat for the day as 5 g. They might, for example, additionally have a bowl of porridge for breakfast. Oats contain around 7 per cent fat, with 1.1 per cent saturated fat. So if they had 100 g of oats in soy milk, they would get another 1.1 g of saturated fat from the oats and 0.5 g of saturated fat from a 250 mL cup of standard soy milk. So their total would already be 6.6 g of saturated fat from very healthy, OMS-friendly plant-based products. Had Swank counted these, his recommendation to stay below 20 g of saturated fat per day would have been more like ingesting 30 g per day.

Likewise, Swank recommended that his patients consume as much bread as they liked. Most bread has around 2.9–3.4 per cent fat in it, and the ingredients often list 'vegetable oil' rather than one of the recognised oils, meaning this is probably palm oil—that is, saturated fat. Had Swank counted these fats, his figure for daily saturated fat consumption would have been even higher.

 There is no need to count grams of saturated fat on the OMS diet.

While some saturated fat is worse for us than others—for instance, long-chain saturated fats are worse than medium-chain saturated fats—it simply gets too confusing to try to analyse not only how much saturated fat is in everything we eat, but also what length carbon chains make up those saturated fats. So counting saturated fat has to go. That is one of the many reasons we recommend a plant-based wholefood diet plus seafood. As previously discussed, there is ample evidence that this is the healthiest diet available for general health. It is also the lowest saturated fat diet around.

One could, of course, argue that ultra-lean meat such as kangaroo or turkey actually has less saturated fat than, for example, an avocado. While that is true, and some people following the OMS Recovery Program do choose to eat these meats, it is a much more sustainable proposition to simply no longer eat meat. Human nature being what it is, having some meat that is 'allowed' and other meat that is 'not allowed' eventually leads to slippage on the diet, and incorporation of other meats into the diet. Effectively, it puts meat on a pedestal, as if it is some kind of special food. Additionally, there may well be issues with meat protein that are harmful to health in general and also in MS. German epidemiologist Klaus Lauer's lifelong work on environmental risk factors in MS has shown key risks for such foods as hot dogs, pork and smoked meats for PwMS.[150] Unlike these meats, the MS literature consistently shows a health benefit for PwMS with increased fish consumption. A plant-based wholefood diet plus seafood is thus ideal, and completely removes the need for counting saturated fat.

That said, it remains sensible to know exactly what we are eating and be aware of those foods that fit the OMS Program but are relatively high in saturated fat, like avocadoes and oily fish, and limit their consumption, as shown in Table 4 under foods to consume in moderation. Someone following the OMS Program will be well within Swank's 20 g daily limit of saturated fat if they follow these guidelines. So it seems sensible to do as Swank suggests, and eat bread as and when desired. However, I try to minimise the saturated fat consumption by buying bread either without oil in the ingredients, such as some of the pita breads and sour-dough loaves, or bread made with a named oil such as olive oil. Most supermarket-brand breads, for example, are made with canola oil rather than unnamed vegetable (palm) oil. While canola oil is a refined oil and so has been altered, and is originally low erucic acid rapeseed oil (in fact, modified rapeseed oil) and so is not ideal, it is better for our health than palm oil. Italian ciabatta loaves use olive oil.

The crux of the eating change is to cut out animal fat, dairy products and 'hidden' saturated fats in apparently vegetarian products like cakes, pastries and potato chips. This is where the bulk of the saturated fats in the Western diet now reside. If in doubt when buying something, it is important to study the label carefully. Usually the label will show the saturated fat content.

Cooking and oils

It is important to change habits around cooking as well as eating. Frying with oil results in the formation of highly toxic frying breakdown products. These chemicals are even more harmful than saturated fats. So alternative methods of cooking need to be explored. It is sensible to understand the science behind this when looking at these cooking methods. Steaming, of course, uses steam that is at a constant temperature of 100°C. This temperature, for the time it takes to steam most foods, will not result in denaturing of the oils the food contains. So steaming can be done in the old-fashioned way of having one pot of water with a pot over it with holes in the bottom and a lid on top. There are plenty of these steamers on the market. But some more fancy steamers that are like small ovens actually have the capacity to steam at lower temperatures.

Some foods are better cooked at lower temperatures, so if you are planning to go down this route, it would pay to invest in a good book about steaming. Steamed vegetables are great, and can be finished off with some flaxseed oil drizzled over the top before serving. Fish and seafood are also wonderful steamed. Some varieties of fish work better than others, but fish only takes six to eight minutes in a steamer to be cooked, and remains very juicy and tender. Before serving, various flavours can be added with soy sauce, sesame oil or other exotic flavours. Or the seafood can be marinated for some time before steaming to give it more flavour. Boiling is also an option, and one can be sure that the temperature of boiling water never goes above 100°C. However, many nutrients from the food leach out into the water when boiling, so steaming is the preferred option.

Next up from steaming is baking. Most baking of vegetables or seafood is at around 180°C, and at that temperature, for the time it takes to bake vegetables and seafood, the oils will not be significantly denatured. Some people like to brush on some extra virgin olive oil before baking vegetables. This makes the vegetables crisper and browner. Others prefer to simply bake without oil and then add flaxseed oil before serving, just to be absolutely sure they are getting the oils in perfect condition. Similarly, cakes that have oil as an ingredient can be baked in the oven at these temperatures without worrying about the oil denaturing. It is preferable to use extra virgin olive oil if one is adding oil, although other unrefined extra virgin oils would also be suitable.

Frying with oil should be avoided; dry frying with a non-stick pan is an alternative.

Frying with oil is to be avoided. The temperature at the interface between the food and the pan, where the oil sits, can get very high—certainly high enough to cause significant breakdown of the oil, forming toxic products. Many people get confused by the subject of the smoke point of oils. In general, that is not an issue for those following the OMS Program, as oils shouldn't be used in frying. Dry frying is perfectly acceptable, however. So, for example, fish that is coated with some flour can be fried on a good quality non-stick fry-pan, or on baking paper on the pan. While the food doesn't brown up in quite the same way as if it was fried with oil, with practice it is easy to make very tasty and appealing fried fish in this way. Teflon-coated pans are not recommended. Teflon is a polymer that coats many non-stick fry-pans, but unfortunately it can be scratched off and get into food during cooking, with unpredictable but likely harmful results. It also isn't completely stable, and breaks down at around 200°C, giving off poisonous fluorocarbon gases. Another problem is that the bonding agent that binds the Teflon to the pan can also break down at high temperatures and end up in the food, again with harmful results.

Similarly, oil should not be used for stir-frying. Stir-fries can be made quite easily just using water, or soy or oyster sauce—perhaps with some sweet chilli sauce. For people who find they just have to have some oil when frying, it is best to use the smallest amount possible, and to add a little water while frying. This keeps the temperature of the oil down to acceptable levels and avoids so many frying breakdown products forming. Ideally, though, it is best to learn to do without the oil altogether.

It is important to remember that the highly unsaturated omega-3 and omega-6 oils are too unstable to cook with—particularly flaxseed oil. Heating them rapidly causes oxidation, and conversion to fat breakdown products that are harmful for health. While the supermarkets are full of these oils and promote them as suitable for frying, they are not. It is best, in fact, to avoid the commercial so-called cooking oils altogether. These products are now so refined, bleached, deodorised, heated and tampered with that they bear little resemblance to the foods from which they originally came.

Extra virgin olive oil, on the other hand, is relatively stable. Generation upon generation of Mediterranean people have used olive oil for cooking with remarkably low rates of the common degenerative Western diseases, including MS. But trying to avoid cooking with it altogether is so much better, as all oil degenerates to some extent with heat. Olive oil can be used in many other ways. Rather than using margarine, a small dipping bowl of olive oil with balsamic vinegar has been served to accompany bread for centuries. The oil sits on top and the black vinegar on the bottom. Or extra virgin olive oil can be used alone. Lots of people already love the taste of extra virgin olive oil, but there is a range of flavours from robust to mild for those not so in love with the flavour. Many others now are using extra virgin cold pressed flaxseed oil as their dipping oil for bread. While it may take a little while to get used to, it is absolutely delicious, although it is important to find a good brand. In Australia, there is none better than Stoney Creek oil, which has a deep golden colour and a wonderful nutty flavour. The general all-purpose oil around the kitchen should be extra virgin olive oil. It is one of the few unrefined vegetable oils that is available commercially. Ordinary olive oil is treated in much the same way as the other refined vegetable oils, and is probably best avoided.

By substituting olive oil for most of the fats in recipes, such as butter and margarine, and by using only the whites of eggs (roughly two whites for one egg) and substituting soy milk for cow's milk, it is possible to make a range of cakes and desserts that contain very little saturated fat but taste wonderful. It is sensible to use as little as possible: moistness in cakes can often be achieved by substituting fruit juice for the suggested oil if preferred. Just because saturated fat is out, food doesn't stop being tasty—quite the reverse. It is possible to make a wonderful passionfruit soufflé with egg whites only and olive oil, and a range of cakes like banana cake and chocolate zucchini cake (using cocoa, sugar and a small amount of olive oil instead of chocolate).

Other oils can be used as well. Sesame oil, for instance, is wonderfully fragrant and can give an Asian dish a superb aroma and taste, but can simply be added over the dish at the end of cooking prior to serving, rather than being used in the cooking process. Most people prefer to take their flaxseed oil supplements in this way as well. There are extra virgin oils made of many seeds and nuts, and all can be quite tasty—although they should not be heated if possible. The oils should preferably be stored in the fridge, where they will last longer. As all contain some saturated fat, it is best not to use too much of them.

An upper limit of unsaturated oils

Swank's advice was to only sparingly eat foods very rich in unsaturated fats, so as not to go over 50 g per day. He didn't specify why, but it is likely that he was concerned that all oils contain saturated fat, and this recommendation minimises the overall load of saturated fat, which could become a problem if the intake of unsaturated oils like fish oil was not restricted. Typically, oily fish have the highest unsaturated fat content. A can of sardines containing 110 g of fish has around 18 g of fish oil, of which about 4 g is actual omega-3 fatty acids. The can of sardines also contains 5–6 g of saturated fat, and this is the reason to limit their intake. Canned sardines with fresh tomato on bread is certainly an inexpensive and tasty way to get essential fatty acids. The fish with the highest omega-3 content are fresh and canned salmon, sardines, canned mackerel, fresh tuna, anchovies and canned herring. Australian salmon has a much lower omega-3 content than Atlantic salmon.

Restaurants and eating out

Many people are concerned that all of this can make going out to friends' places or restaurants a little difficult. Some people at our retreats have even said they eat the meat dishes their friends serve them so as not to make a fuss. Given how critical the right food is to the health of a person with MS, this is not a sustainable or acceptable solution. There is nothing wrong with being very up-front with friends about one's eating habits. At the retreats, we sometimes recommend that when people get home, they consider telling all their friends about the changes they are making to their habits and their lives. While some PwMS feel that this is imposing on their friends, it is often seen by true friends in a different way. Once good friends find out that you are being proactive about MS and changing your diet, it is more common for them to want to help, to prepare and serve food in ways that will assist you in getting better. Some of these friends, once the whole situation is explained to them, will choose to change their own diets, both for their own better health and as a show of solidarity with you.

 It pays to phone ahead and let restaurants know of your eating choices.

Some of our friends use the term 'inclusive eating' to describe what happens when they cater for a group that includes people overcoming MS. Inclusive eating means that if, say, eight people come over for dinner, and two are overcoming MS, all the dishes they serve will be able to be eaten by everyone there. In other words, they will all be OMS-friendly. After all, how hard is it for the average person to have spaghetti marinara, rather than spaghetti bolognese, for example, or a chilli prawn stir-fry rather than a chicken stir-fry? A vegan chocolate mousse for dessert or a vegan chocolate cake will be as delicious as one cooked with animal products, and everyone will be able to eat it.

Similarly, when going out for a meal, there is a lot to be gained from giving the restaurant a heads-up about one's eating preferences when making the booking. How one phrases this is a personal choice, but sometimes it is simplest to say something like 'I am vegan but I do eat seafood', and ask whether they will be able to cater for that. Of course, this doesn't stop them suggesting a green prawn curry full of coconut milk, so one may wish to be a bit more specific. These days, most restaurants are eager to know about dietary preferences or allergies, and most will cater for them without question. One of our retreat participants coined the term 'vegaquarian' for seafood-eating vegans. Some people find it easier to say they are allergic to animal products. Everyone seems to understand what an allergy is. If a difficult waiter says a meal wouldn't be the same without the cheese, it may be helpful to ask whether anyone on the kitchen staff knows CPR!

I am also very up-front with my work colleagues about my dietary choices, as I have been about the MS diagnosis. My colleagues tend to put

'George-friendly' food at my end of the table at functions. It is surprising how many people tend to come down to my end to eat.

Travelling overseas can be seen by many as a bit of a problem because of these dietary choices. I have never found this to be so. Interestingly, from a dietary point of view, travelling is almost always easier in developing rather than developed countries. This is because the food in developing countries is always less refined and more plant-based. In parts of South-East Asia like Cambodia and Laos, where my wife and I love to travel, it is really easy to find simple plant-based dishes, often with rice, and seafood is plentiful both along the coast and inland because of the many rivers that cut through these countries. While language barriers can make things difficult at times, there are usually ways around that. Probably the only real issues in these places are the use of coconut products and palm oil. Hence ordering soups, salads, and steamed or grilled dishes is usually best. Contrast that with, say, Paris and other places in central Europe where dairy is very pervasive; restaurants can have trouble understanding the concept of certain meals being served without cream or cheese! Further south, around the Mediterranean, it is much easier, due to the liberal use of olive oil instead of butter and frequent grilling of food.

Most restaurants everywhere have a range of meals that contain no or very little saturated fat. Italian restaurants are usually easy, as are Japanese, with their focus on raw fish and other seafood. Once you are used to pizzas without cheese, you will end up wondering how you ever ate them with cheese.

Eating in

It is easy to create tasty, nutritious meals based around a no-saturated fat diet. With Google these days, it is easy to find recipes. Our website, <www.overcomingms.org>, and our *Overcoming Multiple Sclerosis Cookbook* feature a large number of recipes that I have assembled over many years; just sign up and you will get access. The recipes are broken down into the meals of the day, salads, soups, sides and so on. It is really easy, for example, to make one's own muesli. Rolled oats, other grains such as barley or rye, sultanas, diced dried fruit and linseeds or other seeds like pumpkin or sunflower are mixed together. The fats in this are mostly unsaturated but, as always, there is some saturated fat from plant sources, so Swank would not have counted it.

It is easy to make really good vegetable soups using vegetable juices as a stock, or a commercial vegetable stock—although checking ingredients is important here, as partially or fully hydrogenated vegetable oils are added to some stocks. Pumpkin, sweet potato, potato and leeks are all great. More simple snacks or light meals are easy too. A lunch consisting of a bowl of sultanas covered in soy yoghurt, with linseeds sprinkled over the top and passion-fruit pulp or mixed berries on top is absolutely delicious. There are now lots of recipes available using this approach. They include vegetable curries, vegetable stir-fries with or without tofu or prawns, using oyster sauce, soy sauce, blackbean sauce or sweet chilli sauce, depending on the desired flavour, and simple pastas with an extra virgin olive oil base.

Making one's own soy yoghurt is simple. Most supermarkets these days seem to stock yoghurt makers. There is nothing special about these; they are just insulated containers that have a heater built in so that they can keep the yeast culture warm overnight, as the yeast doesn't grow well in the cold. It is best to use really high-quality soy milk, like Bonsoy, as it makes the thickest and tastiest yoghurt. It is also best to make it plain, without flavourings, as it can then be used on savoury dishes like Indian curries, or combined with berries or fruit later to make it sweet. Incidentally, the issues with high iodine content in Bonsoy have now been sorted out, with the removal of the seaweed additive that was present in earlier years.

Finding foods that don't contain saturated fats is actually really easy. Foods on the shelf in the supermarket are now labelled with every ingredient, in many cases down to the types of fats contained. It really is straightforward to find non-fat foods. The added bonus of giving up these saturated fats and substituting omega-3 fatty acids is, of course, a longer, healthier life, with less chance of cancer, heart disease and most modern Western-style diseases.

Reading labels

Today, in most countries, it is a requirement that packaged food is labelled with nutritional information. It is helpful to get some expertise in reading these labels. Typically they are headed 'Nutritional Informa-tion', and contain the number of servings per package and the size of each serving—usually in grams. Below is a typical one for a packet of Japanese miso soup with spinach and mushroom. Somewhere around the box with the detailed information, either just under or just above, one typically finds the list of ingredients. In this case it says:

Ingredients: soya bean paste (soya bean, rice, salt) 60%, spinach 10%, shitake mushroom 1%, salt, sugar, bonito.

Nutritional information

Servings per package   1

Serving size   12g

	Quantity per serving	% Daily intake* (per serving)	Quantity per 100g
Energy	142kJ 34 Cal	2%	1183kJ 283Cal
Protein	2.7g	5%	22.5g
Fat Total	Less than 1g	<1%	4.8g
Saturated	Less than 1g	<1%	Less than 1g
Monounsaturated	Less than 1g		1.0g
Polyunsaturated	Less than 1g		2.9g
Trans	Less than 0.01g		0.03g
Carbohydrate Total	4.4g	1%	
Sugar	2.1g	2%	
Sodium	946mg 41.1mmol	41%	7882mg 342.7mmol

*Percentage daily intake based on an average adult diet of 8700kJ. Your daily intakes may be higher or lower depending on your energy needs.

So this information is what one sees on a typical nutrition information panel. It is based on the daily energy intake for an average adult male diet of 8700 kJ, or a little over 2000 calories. A person's individual dietary requirements may be higher or lower than this, depending on several factors including gender, body-mass index (BMI), age and amount of physical activity.

It helps to become an expert at reading food labels.

The column labelled percentage daily intake shows the daily levels of consumption of each of the listed nutrients that meet the nutritional needs of most healthy people. Values are dependent on age and gender. It is important to check the recommended serving size. If the product is listed as being for eight serves, but you divide it up into four, you end up with twice the amount listed per serve. So when one reads this nutrition information, it is important to check the number of serves claimed, as this may be quite unrealistic. It is worth looking at the per 100 g column, as this standardises the amount and can be used to compare energy, fat or carbohydrate content between different foods.

The recommended energy intake for a person varies considerably based on age, BMI, gender and amount of physical activity undertaken. Older women, for instance, need to reduce their energy intake by about 500 kJ per day, and older men by considerably more, about 1300 kJ, but by less than this for those who are very physically active. People who undertake moderate physical activity regularly can take in about 30 per cent more energy.

There is considerable debate in the literature about how much protein is recommended. While men need more than women, and many authorities put this figure at about 60 g/day, Colin Campbell in the China Study recommends considerably less. Certainly, for most of us in developed countries, there is no problem with adequate protein intake. A vegan diet actually provides adequate protein, particularly if it is rich in legumes and grains, but for those on the OMS Recovery Program, who also eat seafood regularly, the possibility of inadequate protein intake is essentially non-existent.

It is interesting that most health authorities are now suggesting that fat should make up a maximum of 30 per cent of total energy intake, or about 70 g/day, but that saturated fat should represent less than 10 per cent of the total energy intake, or less than 24 g/day. This is not much above Swank's recommendations for stabilising MS; it really reinforces how mainstream Swank's guidelines were.

In the case of the miso soup, reading the label carefully reveals that while the amount of fat in one serve is less than 1 g, in 100 g there is 4.8 g of fat. However, the proportion of this that is saturated fat is less than 1 g per 100g. The fat is predominantly unsaturated, being 1 g of mono- and

2.9 g of polyunsaturated fat per 100 g; looking at the ingredients, we can see that there is no added fat, so this fat is the fat in the soya beans, a very healthy fat for PwMS, and a tiny amount from the bonito, again a healthy fish oil. This sort of detailed reading and interpretation of food labels is really useful, particularly early on in the Recovery Program, until one is familiar with the composition of all the various foods one usually buys and whether or not they fit with the principles of the Program.

Salt

As we have seen, basic science research, confirmed by a small study in PwMS, strongly suggests that high salt intake is a particular problem for PwMS and that salt should be avoided. Authorities generally say an adequate sodium intake is around 460–920 mg/day, but with a suggested upper limit of 1600 mg. This latter target is about half of what the average Australian currently consumes, so most of us need to markedly reduce our intake. In general, intake above 2300 mg/day is considered likely to cause harm, but levels much lower than this may cause harm in MS. In the example above, of a single sachet of miso soup, the salt intake is 946 mg. Miso and other soy products like soy sauce can be very high in sodium, and this is one of the many reasons it is important to look carefully at labels. That said, not adding salt to meals at the table is the preferred way of avoiding high salt intake, as well as choosing lower sodium foods.

 High salt intake is best avoided for people with MS.

Alcohol

Our HOLISM data, on top of the small amount already known about alcohol consumption by PwMS, indicates that not only is moderate alcohol consumption not harmful for PwMS, but also health outcomes are probably better for those who consume alcohol in such moderate amounts compared with those who have only a small amount of alcohol, or those who drink a lot.[85] So what constitutes moderate alcohol consumption? In our study, up to 30 g/day for women and 45 g/day was considered moderate, in line with international literature and guidelines. Remember that this is an average, so with more alcohol on some days and less on some days, one reaches this average, always remembering that the literature strongly suggests at least two alcohol-free days per week. In Australia and many other parts of the world, a standard drink is said to be 10 g of alcohol; this equates to a 330 ml can of beer (4 per cent alcohol) or a 100 ml glass of white wine. On any given day, though, it is wise not to drink heavily, even if the average over a week is still within these guidelines.

OVERVIEW

While eating a plant-based wholefood diet plus seafood can seem daunting, many PwMS find it not only gets easier with time, but also becomes an end in itself. Creating wonderful food, eating for health, inspiring our family and friends to become healthier by example—it is no wonder that eating the OMS way is so strongly associated with better quality of life in our studies, not to mention its clear benefit for good long-term health. Eating this way is not hard; changing old unhealthy eating habits to new healthy ones is easy once you make a start. Embrace the change: your body will thank you for it over the many long healthy years of your life.

STEP 2

GET ENOUGH SUN AND VITAMIN D

Sensible sun exposure, in moderation, is very important for good health. We should appreciate the sun for its benefits, and not abuse it.

Professor Michael Holick

INTRODUCTION

Adequate sun exposure and vitamin D are important in both the primary prevention of MS—that is, stopping people from developing the illness in the first place—and in the secondary and tertiary prevention of MS— that is, stopping the illness from progressing, or progressing so rapidly. But some people may see encouraging people to get more sun as controversial. After all, haven't we been told to stay out of the sun because it causes skin cancer?

Since excessive ultraviolet light exposure was first shown to cause malignant melanoma in the 1970s, public health authorities have conducted campaigns designed to reduce people's risk of this deadly skin cancer by encouraging them to avoid sunlight. Now accumulating research clearly shows that regular sun exposure is actually essential for optimal health. Much of this research started with its benefits in MS. There is now no doubt that inadequate exposure to sunlight—particularly in winter—increases the chances of susceptible people developing MS, as well as other diseases. Additionally, taking vitamin D—the hormone produced in the body by exposure to sunlight—has clearly been shown to reduce the risk. Similarly, data are accumulating that disease progression is slowed by higher vitamin D levels in blood and vitamin D supplementation; vitamin D has a clear secondary preventive role.

WHY

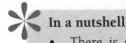

In a nutshell
- There is substantial consistent evidence that adequate sun exposure and vitamin D intake prevent MS.
- Lack of sun in childhood and adolescence—especially in winter—increases the risk of developing MS.
- There is growing evidence that vitamin D supplementation has beneficial effects for the health of people with MS.
- Low vitamin D levels are consistently associated with more relapses in a range of studies.
- The HOLISM study showed better quality of life for people with MS supplementing with vitamin D, with a graded response to increasing doses.

Sun exposure and vitamin D

Sunlight is made up of electromagnetic radiation of different wavelengths. We know that visible light actually comprises a range of wavelengths representing the visible colours of the rainbow, through red, orange, yellow, green, blue, indigo and violet. There are many wavelengths of electromagnetic radiation longer than the red spectrum; next longest is infrared radiation, with which many of us are familiar as the light that is used in many remote-control devices and similar gadgets. At the other end of the spectrum, with shorter wavelengths than violet, is ultraviolet (UV) light. The wavelength of UV is about 400 nm down to about 10 nm. Under some conditions, UV light can actually be seen by humans.

UV light comprises three bands, UVA (400–315 nm), UVB (315–280 nm) and UVC (280–100 nm). Most UV light from the sun—around 95 per cent or more—is UVA. About 5 per cent is UVB, as most UVB is absorbed by the ozone layer, and all UVC is filtered out by the ozone layer before it hits the Earth. A number of different chemicals absorb UV light; some of these are put into sunscreen for just that reason. Ordinary glass also blocks out most UVB light, although UVB can get through water.

When UVB hits the skin, it starts a chemical reaction, resulting in the formation of vitamin D in the body (Figure 9). Vitamin D is the hormone responsible for absorbing calcium from our food. Skin colour plays an important role in this; people with darker skin need more UVB exposure than fair-skinned people to make the same amount of vitamin D. In fact, there are many papers showing that humans originated with darker skin closer to the equator, and the development of fair paler skin was an

Figure 9: UVB from the sun acting on skin to make vitamin D

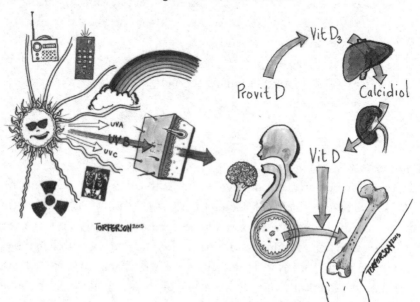

adaptation to moving to colder climates further from the equator, where there was markedly less UV exposure. Those humans who had fairer skin had a better chance of survival as they produced more vitamin D, and vitamin D is essential for human health. Lack of vitamin D causes rickets (soft bones), as well as loss of muscle strength and poor balance. We used to see these diseases commonly in coal miners who were rarely exposed to sunlight, but today we are seeing more and more osteoporosis and even rickets due to people being overly zealous about public health warnings to avoid sun exposure.

Vitamin D is made in the body from the action of UVB light on exposed skin.

Excessive UV exposure can certainly be harmful to health. The skin and the eyes are very sensitive to UV exposure in the lower part of the UVB spectrum. Exposure to UVB in this spectrum causes sunburn and skin cancer, the latter probably by direct damage to our DNA, and can cause cataracts in the eyes.

When UVB light hits the skin, it converts a chemical in the skin, 7-dehydrocholesterol, to cholecalciferol, or vitamin D3. Cholecalciferol is in turn acted on by the liver to form 25-hydroxycholecalciferol, or calcidiol. This in turn is activated by the kidney to form 1,25-dihydroxy-cholecalciferol, or calcitriol, the most active form of vitamin D responsible for calcium metabolism.

How much vitamin D is made from sun exposure?

The amount of vitamin D that is made from the action of UVB light on the skin depends first on the amount of UVB. The UV Index is the internationally accepted standard for the amount of UV radiation that exists on a particular day and time in a particular place. The UV Index is a linear scale—that is, it increases in exact proportion to the amount of UV radiation. Each point on the scale represents 25 milliwatts of power per square metre of skin. So a UV Index reading of 14 means that there is twice the UVB about as with a UV Index of 7. The UV Index varies depending on season, time of day and amount of cloud cover. So in Melbourne in winter, the UV Index dips down to a reading of just 1, or even less on a cloudy day, but in summer can be as high as 12. This is higher than it once was because of depletion of the ozone layer in that part of the world. If there is a lot of cloud cover, a UV Index of, say, 12 could be reduced to 6 or 7. And the time of day is very important. These UV Index figures are quoted for approximately midday when the sun is at its highest. At 10.00 am or 2.00 pm, the figure is about two-thirds of that, around 8 for a UV Index 12 day. At 8.00 am or 4.00 pm, the level would be much lower, around 3–4.

When sunlight of a UV Index of 7 acts on a person with completely exposed skin—that is, they are nude—then around 1000 IU of vitamin D is produced for every minute spent in the sun. But that stops after about fifteen minutes when, in simple terms, all the 7-dehydrocholesterol available for conversion to vitamin D has been used up. So the maximum amount of vitamin D one can get in a single exposure, regardless of how long is spent in the sun, with the body completely uncovered, is 15,000 IU. If, say, half the body is covered up with shorts and a singlet, only 7500 IU is made. If only face and hands are exposed for that length of time—about 5 per cent of the body surface area—then only 750 IU is made, no matter how long one stays out in the sun. If it is a UV Index of 7 day, and one has on shorts and singlet (50 per cent less skin exposure), and it is cloudy (50 per cent less UV), and one stays out for 15 minutes at 10.00 am (around a third less UV), then about 2,500 IU of vitamin D3 is made. It is a common misconception that exposing a smaller amount of skin—say, face and hands—can be compensated for by staying out for longer, but that is not true. After 15 minutes, no more vitamin D is made from that area of exposed skin. If one takes off more clothes, then more vitamin D will be made.

Because vitamin D is made in the body from the action of sunlight, it should not really be considered a vitamin, but a hormone. While we can't live without vitamin D, vitamins usually have to be ingested in the diet. Vitamin D was first called a vitamin because we noticed that if children with rickets (caused by not getting adequate sun exposure) were given cod liver oil, they got better, and it was thought there must be a vitamin in such oil that was essential for health. We do, in fact, get some of our vitamin D through our diet—mostly from oily fish. This is one of the explanations for Japanese people having low rates of MS; they should have a high incidence because Japan is a long way from the equator and doesn't get much sun, but their fish consumption is extremely high, and they therefore get considerable amounts of vitamin D in their diet. But we all get the great majority of our vitamin D from the sun.

Sunlight is by far the most efficient way of getting vitamin D. Professor Colleen Hayes, from the Department of Biochemistry, University of Wisconsin, Madison, says:

> Contrary to popular belief, you cannot get enough vitamin D to meet your biological needs by ingesting fortified foods. Urged by the fear of skin cancer, individuals are avoiding sun exposure and using sunscreens. Somewhere, there is a balance between too much sun and melanoma risk or too little sun and auto-immune disease.[1]

An interesting point to make here is that it has long been known that regular, moderate sun exposure, as opposed to getting sunburnt periodically, may actually protect against melanoma.[2] The fear of skin cancer with small, regular amounts of sunlight exposure may, in fact, be quite irrational.

Blood levels of vitamin D

Blood levels of vitamin D are measured in nanomoles per litre (nmol/L) in Australia, New Zealand and the United Kingdom, but in nanograms per millilitre (ng/mL) in the United States. The conversion factor is 2.5, so a level of 150 nmol/L in Australia equates to a level of 60 ng/mL in the United States. The generally accepted normal levels in blood are 75–250 nmol/L, but many, many people in our societies are vitamin D deficient because they avoid the sun in an attempt to prevent skin cancer. If one's level is low, it takes months before the level stabilises at a higher point through ingesting a regular daily supplement. Vitamin D is a fat-soluble hormone, which means that once it is formed or taken as a supplement, it is rapidly stored in fat tissue in the body. Because of this storage, it takes quite a while for vitamin D levels measured in the blood to come up after regular sun exposure, or after taking an oral dose of vitamin D. So, for a person without MS, if the level is low some doctors would simply start a supplement, and the blood level would eventually come up to normal over a period of months. For PwMS, however—particularly those just diagnosed or having a relapse—it is critical to get the blood level up quickly if it is low, as a persistently low level increases the likelihood of the disease being more active.

Raising the blood level of vitamin D quickly is quite easy, and can be achieved by taking what is called a megadose of vitamin D. Now many people get concerned with this concept of taking a very large dose of anything. However, a megadose of vitamin D for people with low vitamin D levels has been shown to be perfectly safe. For people with initial levels indicating severe deficiency (less than 12.5 nmol/L), a one-off megadose of 600,000 IU in one study raised levels to an average of only 73 nmol/L.[3] This is still probably half the minimum level to aim for in MS, but it can be seen that even large doses of this vitamin are quite safe. After the megadose, it is important to keep getting regular sun exposure or to take regular supplements, or both, as over weeks to months, the levels fall away again quite slowly.

 A one-off megadose of vitamin D is a perfectly safe way to raise low blood levels of vitamin D quickly.

The action of vitamin D being formed from skin exposure to UVB is important because it is now known that vitamin D plays a key role in the development and progression of MS. For many years, vitamin D was thought to be responsible only for regulation of calcium levels in the body; however, some decades ago, scientists discovered vitamin D receptors on immune cells, and realised that vitamin D plays a key role in modulating the immune system. While intimately involved in immune system function, vitamin D also directly affects brain function.[4] Vitamin D has protective effects and immunomodulatory effects (the ability to affect or change immune system function, in this case towards a Th2 response) in the brain, and is useful in neurodegenerative and neuroimmune diseases, typified by MS. Researchers have concluded that its immunomodulatory potency is equivalent to other currently used immunosuppressant medications, without their typical and sometimes severe side-effects.[5] Recent work has shown that high-dose vitamin D promotes an anti-inflammatory state in PwMS.[6]

Other immune system effects of sun exposure

There is now a very comprehensive literature relating lack of sun exposure to the risk of developing MS, and a growing evidence base behind the potential for vitamin D supplementation to both prevent MS and reduce the relapse rate in people diagnosed with MS. But does the sun work in other ways than just through raising vitamin D levels and possibly having an effect on melatonin levels? Researchers from Professor Fiona Stanley's Institute for Child Health Research in Western Australia have now summarised the literature showing that sun exposure has profound effects on modulating the immune response independent of vitamin D.[7] We know that vitamin D is a marker of how much sun exposure one has, and so it has been tempting to think that just correcting that low level through supplementation will correct the immune problems caused by lack of sun exposure. However, while it does appear that vitamin D supplementation is helpful for PwMS, it seems likely that sun exposure is required as well for the optimal immune benefit.

There are a number of possible ways in which sunlight might improve MS. Professor Michel Dumas, of the Institut d'Epidémiologie et de Neurologie Tropicale in Limoges, France, feels that there may be five factors involved, acting through modulation of the immune system by the ultraviolet light in sunlight.[8] These are decreased production of certain cells in the skin involved in the immune response; reduction in certain proteins on the cells necessary for activating immune cells; increased production of interleukin-10, an anti-inflammatory cytokine; reduction of interleukin-12, a cytokine responsible for immune cell activation; and vitamin D3 production interfering with the function of certain immune cells in the skin.

 Sun exposure is helpful for people with MS in other ways than just through production of vitamin D.

Researchers at the Karolinska Institute, in a large case-control study of over 1000 PwMS, examined the risk of developing MS in relation to sun exposure habits and vitamin D levels.[9] Confirming the huge literature that now exists on the increased risk of MS with low levels of exposure to sunlight, they showed roughly a doubling of the risk (2.2 times) for those with the lowest levels of reported sun exposure compared with those with the most sun exposure. Interestingly, they also looked at the relationship with vitamin D levels, and while they found an increased risk of MS with lower D levels, the effect was not as strong (1.4 times) as the effect for sunlight. This implies that there are other protective factors derived from sun exposure than just vitamin D.

The changing paradigm about sunlight and health

Medical journals are now full of scientific papers suggesting that we have overdone sun avoidance in Western society, and that sun avoidance may be more harmful than over-exposure.[10] A number of authorities are now pointing out that, due to sun avoidance, Americans are in the middle of an epidemic of vitamin D deficiency[11, 12] and that, paradoxically, vitamin D deficiency is emerging as a major public health issue even in sunny countries like Australia.[13] The problem is so great that it has been described as a pandemic.[14] It has been estimated that in 2004 sun avoidance cost the United States US$40–56 billion in terms of the cost of its health consequences.[15]

It would appear from the available evidence that the risks of sun avoidance greatly outweigh the risks associated with sun exposure.[16] Sun avoidance increases the risk of a range of diseases. The evidence is clear about vitamin D deficiency causing bone problems like osteoporosis and fractures, now in almost epidemic proportions in Western societies, but it also increases the risk of falling in the first place.[17] This is particularly true in winter when vitamin D levels are lower because of a lack of sun exposure. In Geelong in south-eastern Australia, it has been shown that falls and fractures are more likely in winter when vitamin D levels are at their lowest.[18] One large study showed that supplementing people with vitamin D reduced the incidence of falls by around 50 per cent.[19]

But there is a much wider problem with sun avoidance and vitamin D deficiency. Muscle weakness, depression, high blood pressure,[20] cardiovascular disease[21] and auto-immune diseases like rheumatoid arthritis and diabetes[22, 23, 24] are also linked to low vitamin D levels. High-quality epidemiological data and meta-analyses have shown that type 1 diabetes, an auto-immune disease similar to MS but attacking the pancreas, becomes considerably more common as ultraviolet light exposure from sunlight falls,[25] and can be reduced in incidence by about 30 per cent with vitamin D supplementation.[26]

> We have overdone public health messages about avoiding the sun; regular low-dose sun exposure is essential for good health.

Additionally, certain cancers—particularly cancers of the breast and ovary—seem to be associated with sun avoidance.[27] This effect appears to far outweigh the known effect of too much sun causing skin cancer. Dr William Grant has concluded that for every melanoma prevented by public health messages about sun avoidance, the population incurs six to seven internal cancers. Overall, one meta-analysis of all the studies on vitamin D supplementation showed that people supplementing with even small doses of vitamin D had on average a 7 per cent reduction in death rates from all causes during the studies.[28]

One study examining vitamin D levels in over 13,000 American adults found that people in the lowest quartile of vitamin D levels (under 44 nmol/L in their study) had a 26 per cent higher death rate from all causes than those with the highest quartile of vitamin D levels, independent of other factors.[29] The long-running Harvard University cohort studies, the US Nurses Health Study, Health Professionals Study and Physician Health study have examined in great detail the health outcomes of these professional groups related to various risk factors. In relation to vitamin D supplementation or maintenance of adequate vitamin D levels, these studies have shown that the risk of various cancers was reduced for pancreatic cancer by 41 per cent, breast cancer by 28 per cent and bowel cancer by 33 per cent.[30] For MS, there was a 65 per cent reduction in risk, for hip fractures a 37 per cent reduction, and for heart attacks a 2.1 per cent reduction in risk for every 2.5 nmol/L increase in vitamin D level in the blood. The authors concluded that, based on the findings from the Harvard cohorts as well as many other studies, the risk of various chronic disease end-points is minimised at a circulating vitamin D level of at least 30 ng/mL (75 nmol/L). I recommend that people who actually have one of these diseases should maintain the level at 150 nmol/L or higher to provide the best chance of a good outcome.

Vitamin D also stimulates production of small molecules in immune cells that kill bacteria and viruses; influenza and the common cold are more common in winter when vitamin D levels are lower, and high levels have a protective effect against these common infections.[31] One study looking at common viral illnesses suggested that maintaining a blood level of vitamin D of 95 nmol/L or more could prevent around half of the viral infections—such as colds and flu—that we regularly see in winter and autumn.[32] This is particularly important for PwMS, where there is good evidence that viral infections can trigger relapses. So vitamin D may well have both direct and indirect protective effects in MS. Many PwMS notice that once they get their vitamin D levels up, they stop getting colds and flu.

An epidemiological study of cancer rates in Europe showed that lack of adequate exposure to sunlight was likely to result in a large increase in the rates of cancers other than skin cancer. Indeed, the suggestion was that around 25 per cent of breast cancers are due to lack of sun exposure. The *Medical Journal of Australia* reported that sun avoidance was as dangerous or more so than over-exposure.[33] Another paper suggested that chronic vitamin D deficiency may have quite serious consequences for health, such as an increased risk of high blood pressure, MS, cancers of the colon, prostate, breast and ovary, and type 1 diabetes.[34] It is clear that there are great health benefits from ensuring adequate sun exposure, and hence adequate levels of vitamin D.

Primary prevention of MS with sun exposure

There is a striking geographical disparity in the incidence of MS from country to country. The Belgian School of Public Health study discussed earlier in relation to saturated fat intake examined latitude differences in MS incidence as well.[35] It found latitude was another independent predictor of the incidence of MS, quite separate from fat consumption. At first sight, this appears relatively meaningless. Why would there be virtually no MS at the equator, and why would the incidence rise in direct proportion to how far we go towards the poles? This study listed the countries studied in order of mortality rates from MS and compared this with latitude—that is, distance from the equator. With a few exceptions—these being where fish consumption is very high—it was very nearly a direct correlation (see Table 6). This has also been shown within countries[23, 36] and even north of the Arctic Circle.[37]

The explanation is exposure to sunlight. It is now widely accepted that adequate exposure to sunlight is one of the factors that may prevent the development of MS,[38, 39, 40] and there is a growing body of experimental work to support this. Sun exposure clearly plays a protective role in a number of other auto-immune diseases including MS, type 1 diabetes and rheumatoid arthritis.[24] The evidence in respect to preventing MS and diabetes in humans from epidemiological studies is convincing. There has also been some important work showing that MS can be prevented from developing in the animal model of MS (EAE) by pre-treatment with light, and that disease progression is slowed with regular light therapy.[41, 42] Recent evidence suggests that, at least in the mouse model of MS, ultraviolet light in the region of the 300–315 nm wavelength suppresses disease activity independent of vitamin D.[43] An important piece of evidence supporting this protective effect of sun exposure on the risk of developing MS came from a large US case-control study.[44] We have previously seen the value of case-control studies in evaluating the potential effects of different diets in MS. These researchers examined the effects of sunlight on MS using the death rate from MS in 24 US states as a measure. The study was substantial, with causes of death determined from all death certificates in these states over the period 1984–95. PwMS were matched against control patients of the same age dying of other diseases, and results were analysed allowing for age, sex, race and socio-economic status.

The more sun exposure people get, the less likely they are to develop MS.

Table 6: MS mortality rates (per million people) for men and women aged 45–74 by latitude, 1983–89

Country	Women	Men	Latitude (°)
Denmark	48.6	43.0	N55.7
United Kingdom	45.9	29.6	N51.2
Ireland	40.6	25.8	N53.4
Switzerland	39.7	29.6	N47.4
Poland	37.3	34.8	N52.5
Czechoslovakia	36.8	28.9	N50.1
Norway	32.8	29.7	N60.2
Netherlands	30.1	23.7	N52.1
West Germany	29.1	22.7	N52.5
Sweden	25.2	16.9	N59.4
Belgium	24.7	28.2	N49.6
New Zealand	24.5	14.6	S41.3
Austria	24.2	14.0	N48.3
Canada	22.6	16.9	N46.7
United States	19.6	13.5	N38.6
France	18.9	12.7	N49.0
Iceland	18.2	15.4	N64.1
Finland	15.6	17.7	N60.3
Australia	13.5	7.7	S33.9
Italy	13.2	9.8	N41.8
Bulgaria	11.1	11.0	N42.7
Greece	9.7	9.0	N38.0
Argentina	8.4	9.1	S34.6
Portugal	7.8	11.5	N38.8
Spain	7.1	7.4	N40.4
Japan	1.4	1.0	N35.7
South Korea	0.5	1.3	N37.5
Hong Kong	0.4	0.2	N22.3
Singapore	0.0	0.1	N1.4

(Modified from Esparza et al).[35]

The more sunlight people were exposed to in the course of their work, the less likely they were to die from MS. Further, people with high occupational exposure to sunlight who also had high sun exposure out of work had the lowest death rates by far, with an odds ratio of only 0.24—that is, they were only 24 per cent as likely to die from MS as those with low sun exposure. Swedish researchers provided further support, showing that those with high occupational exposure to sunlight had a 48 per cent chance of dying of MS compared to those with low exposure, and those with intermediate exposure had an 88 per cent chance compared with those with low exposure.[45, 46]

Researchers from Norway and Italy undertook a case-control study looking at people with and without MS who filled in questionnaires about their sun exposure while growing up.[46] They then compared the amount of sun exposure, measured in four categories, in those with MS to those without. Those with the least sun exposure in Norway had an 82 per cent higher risk of developing MS compared with those with the most sun exposure, and 49 per cent greater risk in Italy. Interestingly, it was also found that in Norway, frequent sunscreen use up to the age of six years old led to a 44 per cent greater risk of developing MS. It seems likely that the greater risk reduction from frequent sun exposure seen in Norway was because, in summer, it was much more common for people to get frequent sun exposure, and there was a much bigger difference between summer and winter in the amount of sun exposure. The greatest effect of infrequent sun exposure was seen in early childhood in Italy and in late adolescence in Norway. The paper reinforces the evidence showing that adequate sun exposure in those at high risk of MS—that is, close relatives of PwMS—is important for reducing that risk.

Another study from Oxford University on a very large database of people in the United Kingdom found that PwMS were only half as likely to get skin cancer.[47] They had similar rates of all other cancers, so it seemed likely that sun exposure was affording some protection against MS, in that people getting more skin cancer due to their sun exposure were much less likely to get MS.

An interesting study from the Menzies Centre for Population Health Research in Tasmania, the Australian state furthest from the equator, looked at the rates of MS and malignant melanoma in each of the major cities of the states of Australia and compared them with the amount of sunlight in the area.[48] The causative role of sunlight—specifically UV radiation—in the development of malignant melanoma, the most lethal of the skin cancers, is well accepted in medicine, and is the reason behind much of the public health message about avoiding sun exposure. The scientists conducting this study showed that the correlation between low UV radiation and MS was somewhat stronger than that between high UV and melanoma.

Other Australian researchers have studied MS incidence according to month of birth in Australia, in an attempt to determine whether sun exposure during pregnancy relates to MS risk. Their findings add further evidence that sun exposure plays a crucial role in determining whether MS develops. For the 1524 PwMS born in Australia from 1920 to 1950 out of a total population of 2,468,779, there were 34 per cent more cases of MS for people who were born at the end of winter rather than the end of summer.[49] MS incidence also varied according to latitude (and hence sun exposure), as these researchers have previously shown.

There has also been good experimental work from Tasmania showing that adequate sun exposure—particularly in winter and between the ages of six and fifteen especially—reduced the risk of developing MS in later life by about two-thirds.[50] This has been strongly supported by an interesting US study in 79 pairs of identical twins, comparing their sun exposure in childhood with whether they developed MS in later life.[51] Each of the nine sun exposure–related activities during childhood about which they asked conveyed strong protection against MS, ranging from 43 to 75 per cent reduction in risk. They concluded that the benefits of sun exposure were independent of genetic susceptibility to the disease. These and other studies provide very strong evidence supporting the role of adequate exposure to sunlight in preventing the development of MS.

Primary prevention of MS with vitamin D

So studies have shown that adequate sun exposure seems to prevent MS. Further studies have examined the levels of vitamin D in blood and the subsequent risk of developing MS. One examined the stored blood of over 7 million US army recruits from 1992 to 2004, and compared the vitamin D levels with their risk of developing MS.[52] It found 257 new cases of MS in the group. There was a significant decrease in risk with increasing vitamin D levels among Anglo-Americans, but not African Americans or Hispanics, who had lower vitamin D levels than Anglo-Americans because of their skin colour. Interestingly, when looking at the actual levels of vitamin D, levels of 100 nmol/L or more seemed to be protective, with almost a two-thirds reduction in risk for those with these higher levels. These levels were likely to represent an indication of sun exposure, as vitamin D supplementation—certainly at the sorts of doses used today—was not common at the time of that study.

Lower vitamin D levels have consistently been associated with higher risk of developing MS.

In a large prospective study of 332 children presenting to Canadian healthcare facilities with an episode of demyelination, researchers at the Toronto Hospital for Sick Children confirmed the strong associations of MS with genetic predisposition and low vitamin D status.[53] They showed that, as well as a little over double the risk of developing MS for children with the particular genetic make-up of having one or more HLA-DRB1*15 alleles (a genetic marker for increased MS risk), for every 10 nmol/L lower the vitamin D level was, there was an 11 per cent increase in risk of going on to develop MS. A further study showed that PwMS had significantly lower levels of vitamin D than people without MS.[54] The authors showed that 61 per cent of PwMS had low vitamin D levels, and that many even had osteoporosis and muscle pain due to the low vitamin D levels.

But apart from sun exposure and the level of vitamin D in the blood, researchers have also examined directly the issue of whether vitamin D supplements can prevent MS. The US Nurses Health Study assessed the risk of MS developing in those nurses who supplemented with vitamin D compared with those who didn't take vitamin D supplements. Vitamin D supplementation reduced the risk of developing MS by 40 per cent, and this was with very low dose supplementation of anything over 400 IU.[55] This is an extraordinarily low dose to have such a major effect, given that all-over sun in Perth on a summer's day at midday produces this amount of vitamin D in just twelve seconds!

More recent work from the University of Bergen examined 953 PwMS and compared them with about double the number of healthy controls in terms of their use of cod liver oil during their childhood and adolescence.[56] Cod liver oil, as we have seen, is a potent source of dietary vitamin D, although in the amounts usually taken it still only provides a fraction of what is an optimal preventive dose. For those who took cod liver oil during adolescence, specifically between the ages of thirteen and eighteen, the risk of developing MS was one-third lower than for those who didn't. Those taking higher doses, but only 600–800 IU a day on average, had half the risk. Both these studies reported very low levels of vitamin D supplementation; in the doses recommended in this book, there is every likelihood that the risk of developing MS would be reduced by much more than in these studies.

Public health researchers from Harvard have assessed the potential of widespread population supplementation with vitamin D to prevent a significant proportion of MS in the community.[57] The researchers suggest that, on the basis of current evidence, nearly three-quarters of cases of MS in Europe and the United States could be prevented by keeping people's vitamin D levels above 100 nmol/L, and that very large national or multinational controlled studies need to be done to prove this. They also suggest studies of vitamin D supplementation, of the order of 4000–10,000 IU daily, for people with a first demyelinating event, to prevent progression to definite MS, and for PwMS to slow disease progression. An editorial suggested that there may already be a case for widespread supplementation, especially in areas like Scotland, where vitamin D levels are known to be very low, and the incidence of MS very high.[58]

Secondary prevention of MS with vitamin D

Apart from preventing MS from developing in the first place—that is, primary prevention—researchers have examined the question of whether sun exposure and vitamin D supplementation can slow MS disease activity and progression once a person has the disease—that is, secondary prevention of MS. This was first proposed by Goldberg in 1974.[59] He initially suggested that getting insufficient sunlight to form vitamin D could be the trigger for MS in genetically susceptible people. On the basis of amount of sunshine in areas with little MS and the rate at which vitamin D is formed in the body, he calculated that it would take 3800 IU of vitamin D daily to prevent the onset of MS. Remarkably, exactly this dose has been calculated to be the amount of vitamin D required to maintain a steady, reasonable vitamin D level.[60] The theory has now been revisited and refined.[61]

In 1986, Goldberg suggested that vitamin D supplementation could have a role in preventing disease activity and progression once diagnosed, and performed the first study of vitamin D supplementation in PwMS.[62] Sixteen people were admitted to the study, in which Goldberg compared their relapse rates after supplementation with those before. Participants were given 5000 units of vitamin D per day, in the form of 20 g of cod liver oil a day. This meant he was also supplying substantial amounts of omega-3 fish oils. He also gave large doses of calcium and magnesium.

The results showed that there were 2.7 times as many relapses per year before the supplements than after—a highly significant reduction. Some previous studies had suggested that the relapse rate falls with time the longer patients have MS, so he corrected for that, but the result was still significantly better with supplementation. A number of the PwMS dropped out of the study, and the numbers were small. Nonetheless, none of those who stayed on the supplements for the study period failed to have a lower rate of relapsing than before the supplements. In the group of six people who dropped out—mostly because they didn't want to keep taking supplements—the relapse rate overall fell, with only two getting worse in terms of number of relapses per year. These two had been in the study only eight and four months respectively.

Another study compared monthly vitamin D blood levels in 415 people from a particular area in Germany with the number of lesions detected on MRI scanning in PwMS from the same area.[63] High levels of vitamin D correlated closely with low levels of disease activity and vice versa. A study from Finland added further support.[64] Researchers measured vitamin D levels during relapses and compared these with levels during remission. They found the levels to be lower during a relapse, and concluded that vitamin D may be involved in the regulation of disease activity in MS. They found that, although levels were lower during relapses, they were mostly still in what would currently be considered to be the 'normal' range, suggesting a requirement for a higher vitamin D level to optimally control the disease. A follow-up study by the same group demonstrated that relapses were more common the lower the vitamin D level was in PwMS.[65]

This evidence has been replicated elsewhere. Vitamin D levels were significantly lower in another study in PwMS than a control population of people without the illness; further, levels were again shown to be lower during relapses than when in remission.[66] Similarly, a US study of PwMS in a long-term care facility showed high levels of osteoporosis, suggesting vitamin D deficiency.[67] Many authorities now recommend that PwMS get adequate vitamin D both to control the illness itself, but also to minimise the risk of complications like osteoporosis, falls and fractures.[68]

Another US study examined 219 veterans with progressive MS in the MS Surveillance Registry.[69] They found that low sun exposure prior to MS diagnosis was associated with more than twice the rate of progression to disability. Further, taking cod liver oil (containing vitamin D and omega-3 fatty acids) at any time in childhood or adolescence more than halved the risk of progression. This adds to the data supporting the promotion of regular low-dose sun exposure and vitamin D supplementation to people with an increased risk of developing MS—that is, those who are related to PwMS, and those living further from the equator—and also suggests a protective secondary preventive effect of sun exposure and vitamin D supplementation, even before the diagnosis of MS is made.

Researchers at the Harvard School of Public Health analysed data from one of the interferon studies, looking at the level of vitamin D in the blood in people recently diagnosed and commencing either the interferon or placebo as part of the BENEFIT randomised controlled trial.[70] There were nearly 500 PwMS in the study, nearly 300 of them taking interferon and the remainder a placebo. Those with a low vitamin D at the outset had much worse disease activity and progression than those with higher vitamin D levels. For every 50 nmol/L increase in vitamin D level at baseline, there was a 57 per cent decrease in new MRI lesions and a 57 per cent lower relapse rate, with less brain shrinkage in those with higher levels. Those with higher vitamin D levels also had less disability progression over the subsequent four years. The authors suggested that identifying and correcting low vitamin D levels early in the disease had an important role to play in the early treatment of MS.

Further study of the Tasmanian population was undertaken by Canadian researchers who studied 142 people with relapsing-remitting MS.[71] The lowest relapse rate throughout the year of 0.5 per 1000 days occurred in February (mid- to late summer); this compared with a rate of 1.1 per 1000 days for the rest of the year, a 55 per cent reduction. This correlated with higher UV exposure and high vitamin D levels. Again, this supported the protective role of sun exposure against relapses. A Dutch study looked at 73 PwMS over 1.7 years, tracking their vitamin D levels and the number of relapses they had. For every doubling of vitamin D level, there was a 27 per cent reduction in relapse rate.[72]

Polish researchers have suggested another reason for PwMS to take vitamin D. They analysed the literature on vitamin D levels and how they influenced the effectiveness of a variety of medications for diseases such as MS, atopic dermatitis, infectious disease, kidney disease, osteo-porosis and epilepsy.[73] They noted that vitamin D deficiency in Poland is at epidemic proportions with 83 per cent of babies born there being vitamin D deficient due to their mothers' vitamin D deficiency. They analysed the results of studies showing that having such low levels of vitamin D actually makes medications much less effective. They showed that for every 10 nmol/L rise in vitamin D for PwMS taking first line disease-modifying therapies, there was a reduction in the relapse rate of nearly 14 per cent. Similar patterns were observed in the other diseases treated with standard medications.

Interestingly, recent research shows that vitamin D deficiency in newborn babies, while very common, can be prevented by the mother taking supplements during pregnancy. With as little supplementation as 2000–4000 IU daily, babies of mothers taking the supplements had on average normal vitamin D levels (81 nmol/L) versus deficient levels for those whose mothers were not taking the supplements (42 nmol/L).[74] This is critically important for mothers who have MS, as there is now ample evidence that MS can be prevented if babies are born with healthy vitamin D levels.[75] Taking larger doses in pregnancy would result in higher levels in the newborn baby, with the aim of a level over 100 nmol/L for optimal prevention.

Of course, taking the supplements is likely to be helpful to the pregnant mother as well as the baby. Unfortunately, there has been very little formal study of supplementation of pregnant women with MS in randomised controlled trials. In one small study reported in 2015, fifteen pregnant women were randomly allocated to receive 'high-dose' vitamin D3 (50,000 IU a week or around 7000 IU daily) or standard care—that is, no vitamin D—during pregnancy.[76] As expected, those women supplemented with vitamin D had a rise in their blood level of vitamin D, from 15.3 ng/mL (38 nmol/L) to 33.7 ng/mL (84 nmol/L), whereas those not being supplemented were noted to have a falling vitamin D level over the pregnancy. There were no safety concerns with the dose of vitamin D, with no reported side-effects. Of great interest, however, those in the vitamin D group had no relapses at all in the six months after delivery, while those not receiving vitamin D averaged 0.4 relapses over that period. Disability, as measured by EDSS, also worsened in the group not receiving vitamin D, whereas it was stable for those getting supplements. While small, this study was the first trial published on this critical issue of supplementation of pregnant women with adequate doses of vitamin D, and the results are extremely promising.

Australian researchers have provided important evidence about the value of maintaining a high vitamin D level for PwMS.[77] In a prospective study as part of the Southern Tasmanian Multiple Sclerosis Longitudinal Cohort Study, they followed 145 PwMS for an average of 2.3 years. Many of these people were taking vitamin D supplements, although surprisingly most were taking a tiny dose (below 400 IU/day), and therefore supplementation did not have any effect on vitamin D levels, as would be expected. The important findings were that for every 10 nmol/L higher in the vitamin D level in blood, there was a 12 per cent reduction in the risk of relapse. This effect was linear—that is, the benefit did not seem to reach a threshold level over which there was no additional benefit. Their graph showed essentially a straight-line relationship between risk reduction and increasing vitamin D levels. If the line was continued down to no risk, it intersected at a vitamin D level of around 150 nmol/L, suggesting that this is the important level of vitamin D in the blood for which PwMS should aim year round.

This is strong evidence supporting the value of PwMS maintaining a high vitamin D level. The study further showed that, for most people in Tasmania, the level was related to time outdoors and physical activity, and this is the ideal way to obtain vitamin D. The study did, however, show that on average, the whole group was vitamin D deficient during winter.

The study from the Belgian School of Public Health[35] showing the large variation in risk of developing MS related to latitude has now been replicated in relating the risk of relapse to latitude once a person has the disease. Australian researchers using the large MSBase databank showed recently for the first time that peak relapse rates occurred in both the Northern and Southern Hemispheres in early spring (when vitamin D levels are lowest immediately after the lack of sun in winter) and lowest in autumn (immediately after summer, when vitamin D levels are highest).[78] In the Northern Hemisphere, relapses for PwMS peaked on 7 March, and in the Southern Hemisphere, they peaked on 5 September. The further one got from the equator, the greater the difference was between the peak relapse rate in spring and the lowest relapse rate in autumn, and the shorter the time between the lowest level of UV radiation in winter and the subsequent peak in relapse rates. This suggests that the further from the equator one is, the lower the vitamin D, and therefore the earlier a person reaches a particular threshold level for immune system activation of the inflammation associated with a relapse.

This was a particularly strong study, as it involved prospective collection of data about relapse rates from the physicians of PwMS, and so was not affected by the kind of bias present when people try to recall when they had a relapse. It was also a very large study, including nearly 10,000 PwMS from twenty countries, with over 30,000 documented relapses—by far the largest study of its kind, and therefore very likely to provide accurate and reliable results.

The first observational study has been published showing decreasing relapse rates in PwMS taking vitamin D supplements, according to how much these supplements raised their vitamin D levels. As noted earlier, a number of observational studies of groups of PwMS have shown that the higher the blood vitamin D level, the lower the relapse rate. However, these studies were in people who were not systematically being supplemented with vitamin D. Many experts argued that it was actually the illness being active that stopped these people getting outdoors, and hence their vitamin D levels went down, rather than the vitamin D reducing the relapse rate. This phenomenon is called reverse causality, and is often mentioned in this type of population study.

This study, however, looked at 156 people with relapsing-remitting MS in Paris, France, divided into two groups—one that started on disease-modifying drugs before starting vitamin D supplements, and the other where the two treatments were started at the same time.[79] The dose of vitamin D used averaged out to be a little over 3000 IU a day, although it was given as a periodic megadose rather than a daily dose. The researchers noted that this level of supplementation with vitamin D should now reasonably be considered 'routine care' for PwMS. They also noted that their aim was to have participants reach a blood level of 75–200 nmol/L—that is, in the normal range. In this study, the average blood level of vitamin D went up from 49 nmol/L (indicating the group was deficient at the outset) to 110 nmol/L. It should be noted that the dose of supplementation was relatively small, and that the final blood level was also relatively low compared with what is recommended in this book. The results were highly statistically significant, with every 10 nmol/L rise in vitamin D level reducing the relapse rate by nearly 14 per cent. The researchers found no additional reduction in relapse rate above a blood level of 110 nmol/L. However, the methodology for this study was not ideal for determining the optimal blood level; the researchers only supplemented people with levels lower than 100 nmol/L. Determining the optimal level exactly will need to wait for randomised controlled trials of supplementation using different doses, achieving higher blood levels.

There is strong evidence that people with MS should maintain high levels of vitamin D in the blood.

This study provides strong support for regular vitamin D supplementation for PwMS, and confirms that vitamin D blood levels of around 50–75 nmol/L, commonly recommended as adequate by some doctors, are not optimal for PwMS. Higher levels than this are likely to result in significant reductions in relapse rates and disease activity.

A small Canadian study looking principally at the safety of vitamin D compared escalating doses of vitamin D (averaging 14,000 IU of vitamin D per day) in a small group of PwMS to a low dose (averaging 1000 IU per day).[80] There was a dramatic difference in health outcomes between those PwMS who took high doses versus the low dose recommended by many doctors. For those who took the higher dose, only 14 per cent had a relapse during the study, versus 40 per cent for those who took the lower dose. Measures of their immune system balance also showed a move away from an inflammatory profile towards at Th2 profile. People with vitamin D levels above 100 nmol/L did best. Although this study aimed to look at the safety of high-dose vitamin D supplements and was not primarily designed to detect outcomes in the medical condition of these PwMS, it is interesting to note that the mean number of new MS lesions more than halved over the short period of the study.

One small randomised controlled trial of vitamin D supplementation showed reduced disease activity in MS.[81] While too small (66 PwMS randomised to treatment or placebo) and too short (twelve months) to really show much clinical difference in the people in the trial, it did show a marked reduction in new MRI T1 contrast-enhancing brain lesions in the group with the vitamin D supplementation. Unfortunately, there were a few problems with the study. A very low dose of 20,000 IU a week, or under 3000 IU a day, was used. That only raised vitamin D levels in the blood to around 100 nmol/L. Additionally, they did not use a one-off megadose to get people's levels up quickly, so the participants spent several months at the beginning of the study with low vitamin D levels that were gradually coming up, so that at six months, three-quarters of the treated group had levels over 85 nmol/L, and by twelve months, 84 per cent had reached this level. This study, described as promising by the authors, demonstrated that brain inflammatory disease activity is reduced with the addition of relatively small doses of vitamin D to standard interferon therapy for MS.

People with MS should aim for a blood level of vitamin D above 150 nmol/L (60 ng/mL).

Further studies support the maintenance of a vitamin D level above 150 nmol/L for optimal secondary prevention of MS. The first was a small study from Ireland,[82] in which investigators looked at the effect of supplementing healthy volunteers with doses of 5000 and 10,000 IU of vitamin D. This was performed in preparation for a prospective study of vitamin D supplementation in people with a clinically isolated syndrome (CIS). As would be expected, given the location of the study, all subjects were low in vitamin D at the beginning of the study, with an average level of 38 nmol/L. The four participants took 5000 IU daily for ten weeks, then two participants increased their daily dose to 10,000 IU and the other two continued at 5000 IU for the following five weeks. Those on 5000 IU achieved maximum levels of 152 and 191 nmol/L, while those on 10,000 IU had peak levels of 152 and 223 nmol/L. Note that all these levels remained within the normal range for vitamin D (75–250 nmol/L).

To assess the effect on immune function, the investigators measured the production of the anti-inflammatory cytokine IL-10 and the activity of pro-inflammatory Th17 cells, a type of Th1 cell. Th17 cells have an important role in the animal model of MS and are associated with disease activity. They found that following supplementation with vitamin D there was a 'striking' increase in production of the anti-inflammatory IL-10 and a significant decrease in activity of the pro-inflammatory Th17 cells. These responses increased over the course of the study and were more pronounced in the higher-dose group. The study confirms that high-dose vitamin D modulates the immune response in PwMS so that inflammatory episodes are less likely. A recent review confirmed these findings in a number of other studies.[83]

HOLISM study findings on vitamin D, sun exposure and latitude

As with the other aspects of the HOLISM study, we sought to shed light on the associations between quality of life, relapse rate, disability and, in this case, sun exposure, vitamin D supplementation and latitude. We asked the participants about geographical location, intentional sun exposure for health and supplementation with vitamin D including dosage, among other lifestyle variables.

Of 2301 participants answering these questions, 82 per cent were women and the median age was 45 years, with a median time since diagnosis of six years. The majority (62 per cent) had relapsing-remitting MS. Nearly two-thirds lived in the Northern Hemisphere, mostly in developed countries. Two-thirds reported deliberate sun exposure to raise their vitamin D level, and the great majority (82 per cent) took vitamin D supplements, mostly 2000–5000 IU a day on average. We undertook sophisticated regression modelling incorporating deliberate sun exposure, latitude and vitamin D supplementation, controlling for gender, age, disability, physical activity and fish consumption. We couldn't detect any benefit of deliberate sun exposure, but felt that just asking such a simple question, without collecting any other reliable data about sun exposure, may have seriously limited our ability to find any associations. In contrast, associations between vitamin D supplementation and quality of life were strong, with a dose–response effect. This means that the higher the dose of vitamin D taken, the better the quality of life—a strong argument for vitamin D actually causing this improvement. We also detected a one-third lower rate of relapses annually in those PwMS in the sample who were taking any dose of vitamin D supplement, compared with those taking no vitamin D.

Of latitude, deliberate sun exposure and vitamin D supplementation, only latitude was significantly associated with disability, with an increase of latitude by one degree (further away from the equator) predicting 2 per cent increased odds of moderate disability and 3 per cent increased odds of high disability compared with no/mild disability. This means that in round figures, for every ten degrees one lives further from the equator, there is a 20 per cent greater likelihood of having moderate disability, and about a 30 per cent greater likelihood of high disability. Many PwMS would see this as a modifiable risk factor—that is, one could move further south if living in the United States, or further north in Australia, to a sunnier climate, to reduce the risk of disability progression—assuming the association we found was causal. So in the United States, this would mean moving from, say, New York to Florida. In Australia, it would mean moving from Melbourne to Brisbane. Many people might consider such a move—and, indeed, many people have moved to warmer climates for these and other health reasons.

Latitude was also associated with relapse rate, with a 1 per cent increase in the odds of having a relapse in the previous year for every degree of latitude further from the equator. This meant that, using the opposite of the above examples, moving from Brisbane to Melbourne is associated with a 10 per cent increase in the odds of having a relapse.

In summary

Sun exposure and vitamin D supplementation have significant protective effects in preventing the development of MS, and in preventing progression to disability for those people diagnosed with the disease. The further one lives from the equator, the higher the risk of the disease developing, and of having relapses and becoming disabled for people with the disease. The literature now is congruent and wide-ranging, across many different research formats. There is little doubt that this should be used in a preventive medicine approach to managing MS, in both primary and secondary prevention.

HOW

Introduction

There are several strategies related to sun exposure and vitamin D supplementation that PwMS can adopt to minimise the risk of their close relatives developing MS (primary prevention) and of themselves having relapses or progressing (secondary prevention). Sun exposure works partly through its effect of raising vitamin D levels, but also through a number of other mechanisms. So, ideally, sun exposure and vitamin D supplementation should both be adopted as prevention strategies. This, of course, is harder in some places than in others. The further one is from the equator, where the risk of developing MS and of it worsening is highest, the harder it is to get the very thing that can keep you well. So for those in places like Canada or Scandinavia or Tasmania, where it can be hard to get adequate sun exposure even in summer, vitamin D supplementation takes on an even more important role in MS prevention.

In a nutshell

- Increasing sun exposure and supplementing with vitamin D can prevent MS in those at risk.
- Regular low-dose sun exposure is important for those at risk and those with MS: around ten to fifteen minutes on most of the skin when the UV index is 7, and more sun when there is less UV.
- For primary prevention, a blood level of over 100 nmol/L (40 ng/mL) is recommended; for adults, this requires around 5000 IU a day, proportionately less for children.
- For secondary prevention, a blood level of over 150 nmol/L is recommended; for adults this may require up to 10,000 IU a day, the maximum safe amount of supplement.
- For those with low levels on first testing, a one-off megadose of vitamin D is recommended.

MS prevention with sun exposure

The evidence strongly suggests that the key issue for primary prevention of MS is adequate sun exposure during childhood and adolescence, around the ages of six to fifteen, particularly in winter. This fits with all the data presented. But getting adequate sun exposure during pregnancy is also clearly important for expectant mothers. For women with MS, the real potential here is to stop their children from developing MS, despite their markedly higher risk than the rest of the population, but also to reduce the risk of relapse for the mother after childbirth. Secondary prevention of MS through regular sun exposure is also important for everybody with MS.

For most people who have heard and adopted the messages about reducing skin cancer risk by avoiding sun, this takes quite a bit of attitude and habit changing. It is important to lose our fear of the sun; there is no doubt that it is safe in small regular doses. So, practically, this means that people in relatively sunny countries should encourage their children not only to play outdoors and go to the beach more often, but also to uncover somewhat when doing these activities, although not for long periods.

It is important to get regular sun exposure, taking care to limit exposure to short periods.

In summer in warmer climates, it is still important to avoid the midday sun for lengthy periods in order to reduce the risk of skin cancer, which remains quite real, although it is quite acceptable to have short periods in the sun during the middle of the day—preferably mostly uncovered. If going out into the sun to play, children should be encouraged to play with their shirts off. Hats are still a very good idea, as the face is more exposed to the harmful effects of UV radiation throughout life than any other part of the body. But getting the arms, chest and back, and legs exposed increases the skin area with which to manufacture vitamin D, and so means that more vitamin D is made from a shorter period in the sun. Similarly, it also allows the other more direct effects of sunlight on immune cells in the skin to occur over a larger area of the body, and so potentially to have greater effect.

In most countries, it is not difficult to find information on the UV Index on a particular day. In Australia, for example, the Bureau of Meteorology website, <www.bom.gov.au>, has information showing the UV Index on any given day for most parts of the country, and how this varies with time of day. Several mobile phone apps do this as well, even allowing for cloud cover on any given day. Willy Weather, <www.willyweather.com.au>, is a good one in Australia. In the United Kingdom, the Met Office website is <www.metoffice.gov.uk>; in the United States, go to <www2.epa.gov/sunwise/uv-index>.

How much sun?

On a UV Index day of, say, 14 in Perth in mid-summer, one needs to be in the midday sun for about five to seven minutes uncovered to get the full 15,000 IU of vitamin D, or proportionately less vitamin D for younger people with smaller body size and therefore skin area. Going out at 10.00 am means one can stay out about a third longer, or about ten minutes, to get this amount of vitamin D. When taking the children to the beach at this time of year, it is preferable to go earlier or later so as not to get too much sun, and to uncover as much as possible and get full sun for this amount of time, then to put on sunscreen for the rest of the time at the beach, or cover up or stay under an umbrella. This means that the children get their full dose of vitamin D, but don't run an increased risk of skin cancer in later life. The same applies to adults who themselves have MS and are aiming to get adequate sun exposure to prevent disease progression.

This amount of sun exposure is very safe, as evidenced by the report of the ANZ Bone and Mineral Society, Endocrine Society of Australia and Osteoporosis Australia, which recommend six to eight minutes of sun in summer and 25 minutes of sun in winter to prevent osteoporosis.[84] Unfortunately, their recommendation was just to get this exposure on the hands, face and arms. As noted previously, people who get this amount of exposure over the whole body get far more vitamin D, and the evidence suggests that more vitamin D is needed for MS than for osteoporosis prevention.

 Surprisingly small amounts of sun exposure in sunny climates make large amounts of vitamin D.

In spring or autumn, when the UV Index might be 5, using the yardstick of ten to fifteen minutes of uncovered exposure on a UV Index 7 day to make 15,000 IU of vitamin D, going out at midday would mean needing about fifteen to twenty minutes of uncovered exposure to make the same amount of vitamin D. In winter, when the UV Index might be 2, this amounts to 35–50 minutes of sun. This can obviously be quite difficult, especially in winter in most places, where it is simply too cold to stay outdoors for that long uncovered. One can, for instance, choose to do some exercise outdoors—like swimming in a heated pool for 35 minutes, or running or walking, largely uncovered—to get the full amount of vitamin D.

It can be quite hard for people to know exactly what the UV Index is at certain times of the day, and one doesn't want to be on the smartphone or computer looking these things up regularly. With practice, however, after looking it up a few times at different times of the year, it gets easier and easier to get a pretty close approximation to the UV Index. A useful rule of thumb is that if your shadow is longer than you are, then you will probably make negligible amounts of vitamin D from sun exposure because the UV Index is too low.

MS prevention with vitamin D

For most people and places, the alternative is to take a vitamin D supplement throughout winter, as mostly it will be difficult to get this sort of sun exposure. First, though, it is important to dispel a few myths about vitamin D. For many years, some members of the medical profession have been overly concerned with the potential for toxicity from supplementing with vitamin D. We have also quite significantly under-estimated the doses required for optimal health. As previously discussed, vitamin D levels in the body can be easily measured with a simple blood test. For many years, a level of less than 25 nmol/L was considered to represent moderate to severe deficiency and a level of 25–50 nmol/L mild deficiency, with anything over 50 nmol/L considered normal. There is quite a bit of evidence that we have set these levels too low, and that optimal levels are really quite a bit higher.[85] Even at these levels, 80 per cent of women and 70 per cent of men living in hostels in the Australian states of Victoria, New South Wales and Western Australia are deficient.[17] In women in the city of Geelong, for example, 30 per cent had deficiency in summer and 43 per cent in winter, and the rate of falls and fractures was higher in winter.[18, 86]

Contrary to some opinion, the evidence shows that vitamin D is a very safe supplement.

The recommended daily allowance (RDA) of vitamin D in Australia is 200 IU; this is acknowledged to be well out of date, being from a 2006 Australian government set of guidelines.[87] This amount of vitamin D is way too low. It is based on the amount required to prevent rickets, a disease where the bones bend because they don't have enough calcium in them, but is not nearly enough to prevent other diseases like MS, rheumatoid arthritis or type 1 diabetes. It is equivalent to the amount of vitamin D one's skin makes in six seconds of all-over sun at midday in

Perth on a summer's day. US authorities have recently revised their RDAs, setting a minimal amount of 600 IU a day for those under 70 years of age and 800 IU for those over.[87] Again, these are way too low.

Vitamin D levels and dosage

In sunny countries where auto-immune diseases are uncommon, vitamin D levels are at least 100–140 nmol/L, and often around 135–250 nmol/L, raising the likelihood that a level of 200 nmol/L may actually be optimal.[16] Others have suggested that a level as high as 250 nmol/L may be optimal.[88] Most laboratories some time ago changed their recommendations for the normal range of vitamin D levels, reporting the range of 75–250 nmol/L as being normal. PwMS should aim for at least the middle of that range, and the evidence presented earlier strongly suggests that a level of 150 nmol/L is the minimum level for which PwMS should aim year round. To achieve a level of 100 nmol/L requires a daily intake of about 4000–5000 IU of vitamin D for people who are not getting any sun. To get to 150 nmol/L needs about 10,000 IU a day in the absence of sunlight. It has been shown that average healthy men's bodies use about 3000 to 5000 IU a day.[60]

Because vitamin D is fat soluble, and is stored in the body in fat tissue, the dosing can be spread out so that intermittent higher doses will maintain levels just as well as daily doses. This is particularly important for children, where it may be much more convenient to administer, say, a weekly dose if the child doesn't like taking medicine. If someone aims to be taking 7000 IU a day, for example, based on what dosage keeps their blood level stable at a particular reading, then that can be given as, say, 50,000 IU once a week. This can really simplify the process, given that many online providers now sell 50,000 IU capsules. It is probably best not to take the dose less frequently than weekly, though. One Australian study looking at bone fractures contradicted much previous research showing that vitamin D prevented bone fractures and raised some concerns among vitamin D researchers.[89] But it appeared that the issue was that they used an annual megadose of vitamin D. Interestingly, they also showed that this single annual megadose had no effect on mental well-being or depression,[90] contradicting other research. Given that we would optimally get our vitamin D from the sun, and that under normal circumstances we wouldn't get intermittent megadoses from sun exposure, it is probably best to mimic this natural process by not having long periods of no vitamin D intake. Annual megadoses of vitamin D clearly don't work as well as regular smaller doses. Megadoses should be reserved for bringing one's levels up quickly.

Vitamin D toxicity

It is important to note that vitamin D toxicity is not possible if it all comes from the sun. Only supplements have the potential to produce toxic levels. The only published toxicity is from supplements of 40,000 IU a day or higher.[91] The dose escalation study discussed earlier showed that increasing doses of vitamin D in twelve people over 28 weeks, increasing the dose from 4000 IU per day up to 40,000 IU per day, produced levels of vitamin D in the blood that were extraordinarily high. These levels were much higher than was previously regarded as toxic, with average levels increasing to around 400 nmol/L and the highest measured level at 800 nmol/L. Despite these very high levels, no patient developed high calcium levels or any side-effects. It is clear now that supplementation with vitamin D at quite high doses is very safe, and the way is clear to use these larger doses in research situations to examine the effect on relapse rates and disease progression.

A very sound research study applied the risk assessment methodology used by the Food and Nutrition Board in the United States to derive a revised safe tolerable upper intake level (UL) for vitamin D.[92] The risk assessment, based on relevant, well-designed human clinical trials of vitamin D, concluded that the UL is 10,000 IU of vitamin D per day— in other words, it is safe to take up to 10,000 IU of vitamin D per day. Even with plenty of sun exposure, supplementing even up to this dose appears to be quite safe. It may give rise to levels above the upper limit of what most laboratories regard as normal (250 nmol/L)—even as high as 350 nmol/L—but there do not appear to be any associated toxic effects if the daily dose does not exceed 10,000 IU. For those who get regular sun, it is sensible not to take such a high level of supplementation in summer, only in winter. The best check on supplementation doses is always the blood level of vitamin D, and it is safest to keep that between 150 and 250 nmol/L if possible.

Unfortunately, many of the societies and institutes that produce guidelines about vitamin D supplementation are very out of date with these research findings. For instance, the US-based Institute of Medicine (IOM) sets guidelines for vitamin D supplementation. Its most recent guidelines in 2010 recommended an upper safe limit of vitamin D supplementation of only 4000 IU. A report on this published in the *New York Times* in November 2010 created some alarm among people taking vitamin D supplements.[93] The report alluded to the deliberations of the fourteen-person expert committee assembled by the IOM. This group attempted to frame dietary reference intakes (DRIs) for vitamin D and calcium—in other words, they were looking at coming up with the estimated average requirement, which is the amount estimated to satisfy the needs of 50 per cent of people in the American population. A press release from the IOM stated that, 'Most Americans and Canadians up to age 70 need no more than 600 international units (IUs) of vitamin D per day to maintain health.' They subsequently suggested an upper safe limit of supplementation of 4000 IU per day.

Most people reading this report would be very surprised about these findings. Haven't we been reading paper after paper about the worldwide epidemic of vitamin D deficiency due to sun avoidance? But the findings can be explained partly by the purpose of the committee, which was to update long-standing and out-of-date dietary reference values for vitamin D and calcium. DRIs were introduced in 1997 to broaden existing guidelines around Recommended Dietary Allowances (RDAs) that were used in the United States, Canada and Australia to provide nutrition advice with a substantial margin of safety. The RDA was essentially the minimum intake required to meet the requirements of 97–98 per cent of *healthy* individuals.

The problems with the IOM report were that it was not their brief to examine what supplement amount would be best for people with serious illness—just to look at an average requirement for healthy people. And this was just an average amount needed for maintenance, not even for the prevention of serious illness, let alone its treatment. New data are appearing all the time on the potential of vitamin D to prevent a variety of cancers in addition to heart disease, depression, hypertension, diabetes and so on, as well as osteoporosis. The IOM focused completely on bone health. But higher doses and higher blood levels of vitamin D are required for management of auto-immune illness than for maintenance of bone health.

 Doses of vitamin D up to 10,000 IU daily are perfectly safe.

It is important for PwMS trying to do the best for their health not to be deterred by such reports. In this case, it is about balancing risks: the risk of what will happen to people with a serious progressive neurological disorder like MS waiting until such groups decide that vitamin D supplementation is proven beyond doubt to prevent and improve the outcome from MS far outweighs the remote potential risk of toxicity from supplementation at the doses recommended here.

Fortunately, the Endocrine Society has published Clinical Practice Guidelines for the evaluation, treatment and prevention of vitamin D deficiency, providing a sensible, evidence-based rebuttal of the IOM's recommendations.[94] Led by internationally renowned expert in vitamin D Dr Michael Holick, the Taskforce concluded that substantially higher levels of supplementation than those recommended by the IOM were appropriate. It is important to note that this group was not examining the requirements for people with various diseases using vitamin D as a potentially helpful supplement, but the levels of vitamin D that could be regarded as normal and deficient, and the sort of level of supplementation needed to avoid deficiency. Their recommendations, as might be expected, are very conservative, and will not go any further than robust available evidence allows, although they note the paucity of research on higher doses of vitamin D supplementation.

Given the concerns raised by some people about their doctors' responses to the level of vitamin D supplementation they are using, it is important to note their recommendations which they compare, based on the best available evidence, with those of the IOM. They recommend an upper limit of vitamin D supplementation for adult males and females of 10,000 IU a day, as recommended here, and for pregnant and breast-feeding women also 10,000 IU a day.

To illustrate the safety limits of supplementation, Kimball and Vieth reported the case of a man who had been supplementing with very large doses of vitamin D.[95] This 39-year-old man with MS had steadily been increasing his self-prescribed dose of vitamin D over four years, from 8000 IU per day to a whopping 88,000 IU per day. This latter level would be expected to produce some toxic effects. In fact, the amount of calcium in his urine started to rise, and then blood calcium levels started to go up, with a vitamin D level in his blood of 1126 nmol/L. He displayed no symptoms, though. At that point, he stopped taking vitamin D, and within two months all his blood tests were normal, although vitamin D levels remained high at 656 nmol/L. While not recommended, this at least shows that it takes very large doses of vitamin D to produce any increase in calcium levels and toxicity.

A very large study in Minnesota examined over 20,000 vitamin D measurements over ten years.[96] The researchers found that around 8 per cent of people tested had values over 50 ng/mL (125 nmol/L), 0.6 per cent over 80 ng/mL (200 nmol/L) and 0.2 per cent over 100 ng/mL (250 nmol/L), but only one had any problem with toxicity. This was a person who had been taking 50,000 IU a day for three months, with a level of 364 ng/mL, or 910 nmol/L, as well as calcium supplements, and understandably the calcium level was elevated, indicating vitamin D toxicity. This level of supplementation is five times the maximum recommended in this book, and is not a safe level of supplementation.

What kind of vitamin D?

The correct form of vitamin D to take is cholecalciferol or vitamin D3. In this form, vitamin D is extremely safe. As it is the pro-hormone from which calcitriol is made—and it is calcitriol that is primarily responsible for increasing the uptake of calcium from food in the intestines—toxicity is not seen with even very large doses of vitamin D3. In a pilot study of a high dose of the end-hormone calcitriol in PwMS, for example,[97] a number of patients developed side-effects and high calcium levels, in contrast to the studies of those taking high doses of vitamin D3. They did, however, find some benefit from treatment, and that is an encouraging step in the continuing development of vitamin D as a treatment for MS.

Vitamin D as a supplement should be taken in the form of vitamin D3, or cholecalciferol.

Vitamin D3 or cholecalciferol is the natural form that is made in the body in response to sunlight. Because Australia is such a sunny country, regulators have in the past not allowed vitamin D to be sold in high dose supplement form. Until recently, the only form available in Australia was vitamin D2 or ergocalciferol. This is produced by UV irradiation of the plant sterol ergosterol, available by prescription only, and is not the optimal form to take. There is also evidence concluding that it doesn't work as well as vitamin D3,[98] with one Australian study showing that it doesn't work at all in MS.[99] It is also expensive. Vitamin D3, on the other hand, is cheap, and because it is naturally occurring, it cannot be patented by drug companies.

The easiest way to obtain supplies at a reasonable strength is on the internet. There are many reputable suppliers of vitamin D3 on the web, at a variety of doses. Sites like <www.iherb.com> and <www.prohealth. com> offer a range of strengths, including 1000 IU, 2500 IU, 5000 IU, 10,000 IU and 50,000 IU, and a range of formulations, some in gel capsules containing olive oil, others in capsules containing dry powder. Both are fine for children, as the capsules can be broken apart and the powder sprinkled on food such as cereal, and the soft-gel capsule in olive oil can be squeezed onto food or into drinks.

What to do about vitamin D at diagnosis

When first diagnosed, people should ask to be tested for their vitamin D level immediately. It is very common for this first level to be low, and often this is why the attack happened. Australian researchers are now calling for 'active detection of vitamin D insufficiency among PwMS and intervention to restore vitamin D status to adequate levels . . . as part of the clinical management of MS'.[100] Most neurologists are now doing this routinely at diagnosis. If the level is very low, it can be brought up very quickly with a one-off megadose of vitamin D followed by regular capsules.[3] After a one-off dose around 500,000 IU if the initial level is low, a regular supplement of around 5,000–10,000 IU a day in winter should keep the level above 150 nmol/L. MS Australia has published guidelines for vitamin D supplementation for PwMS developed by the respected Menzies Research Institute. It concurs with the advice here that it requires about 4000 IU of vitamin D a day to reach a level of 100 nmol/L, and that if levels are low, a single dose of 500,000 IU can be taken.[101]

The level should be checked at the end of each winter of supplementation to make sure it is not being overdone. It may, in fact, be more important for men to keep their vitamin D levels high and check their levels frequently as it has been shown that women with MS have considerably higher levels than men with MS.[102] Holick, a world authority on vitamin D, suggests annually checking one's vitamin D level as a routine.[12]

When to start vitamin D

In terms of MS primary prevention, the best age to start supplementing children with vitamin D is minus nine months! Many authorities are now saying that the majority of cases of MS in the world could be prevented if women took vitamin D supplements during pregnancy. So what is the ideal dose for a woman planning to get pregnant? As noted above, adults should be taking enough to stay above 150 nmol/L year round, and for most that means supplementing with 10,000 IU a day for much of the year. It would be ideal if this dose didn't have to change because of pregnancy, and the good news is that it doesn't. While there is some lack of knowledge about safe dosage of vitamin D during pregnancy among doctors, the evidence is quite clear that high doses are required because of the additional needs of the growing foetus.

 Vitamin D supplementation should be started during pregnancy.

The important thing about this is the risk of the child developing MS as an adult, and much less about the mother's health, as pregnancy is very protective for the mother. It is critical to lower the roughly 40 times higher risk that children of PwMS have of getting MS than others in the population. The evidence base around supplementation in utero is growing rapidly. There has been much published about the risks of developing MS related to season of birth, and hence sun exposure. The most recent paper highlighting the lower risk of MS in babies born in the months just after summer finished by noting, 'The findings here provide the first population based evidence beyond month of birth patterns to indicate that vitamin D supplementation for the prevention of multiple sclerosis might also need to be considered during in utero development.'[49] Chaudhuri, a Glasgow neurologist, advocated this early in this century: 'Prevention of MS by modifying an important environmental factor (sunlight exposure and vitamin D level) offers a practical and cost-effective way to reduce the burden of the disease in the future generations.'[75]

The only real question is the optimal dose of vitamin D. Many neurologists are not really familiar with dosages for vitamin D supplementation, as they do not use this in any of the other neurological diseases they manage. There is also a widespread irrational fear in medicine about over-dosage of this naturally occurring hormone. Consider that if you step outside in, say, Perth or Brisbane in summer with only a bathing suit on for around five minutes at midday, you will make 15,000 IU of vitamin D immediately. Why would you be told not to take 1000 IU then? How could that be toxic? Hollis says that around 6000 IU a day during pregnancy probably reflects actual requirements.[103] But of course, to prevent MS, that dose should be higher.

So ideally, women with MS planning to fall pregnant should aim for a stable high-normal blood level of vitamin D of around 150–250 nmol/L in the months before trying. As noted, this usually requires around 5000–10,000 IU of vitamin D throughout winter and less in summer. Once pregnant, vitamin D requirements actually go up, as the vitamin D is for two now, rather than one. There is no safety issue about taking the maximal dose of 10,000 IU a day throughout pregnancy—and, indeed, that is ideal for primary prevention of the baby developing MS in later life, and keeping the mother well through and after pregnancy, when the risk of relapse goes up. Incidentally, it is important that mothers continue to breastfeed for as long as possible after the birth to minimise this risk of relapse.[104, 105]

Is there any controversy about vitamin D for MS prevention?

For secondary prevention of MS—that is, reducing disease activity and progression in people with established MS—vitamin D supplementation is critically important. It is now uncommon for doctors treating PwMS to be unaware of all this literature in favour of vitamin D supplementation in MS, but for those whose doctors don't support such supplementation or give incorrect advice about dosage, the following publication should help. In 2013, the editor of the *Multiple Sclerosis Journal*, the world's biggest journal devoted solely to MS, convened a debate in the journal about whether neurologists themselves would take a supplement of 10,000 IU of vitamin D a day if they had a CIS and an MRI scan suggestive of MS, or a family member did.[106] The conclusion was that yes they would, which should reassure those worried about whether to take the supplement and at what dose. The author identified that a supplement of 10,000 IU of vitamin D a day is safe, achieves levels of vitamin D in the band 150–225 nmol/L, the level at which vitamin D has its optimal effect on the immune system (and is safe up to levels of 380 nmol/L), and reduces disease activity and relapse rate.

The really surprising part, though, was that despite stating that this was the course of action neurologists would take themselves or recommend to relatives, the accompanying editorial noted that they would not prescribe the same supplement to their patients with MS, as there wasn't yet conclusive evidence. By conclusive they meant that there were no large-scale randomised controlled trials. This is a really surprising position, and makes one reflect on what evidence-based medicine has done to doctors to have made us so pedantic that we would not prescribe a naturally occurring vitamin, taken at physiological doses at which there are no known side-effects, that has been shown to reduce the incidence of cancers and other auto-immune diseases as well as reduce the risk of relapse of MS, despite being enthusiastic about taking the same supplement ourselves. As recipients of healthcare, it also makes one wonder about our medical advisers, who would do one thing for themselves and quite another for their patients, despite being convinced enough of the value and safety of the supplement to take it themselves.

While neurologists wait for conclusive trials before prescribing vitamin D for their patients, PwMS should follow the advice neurologists would follow themselves or give to their own relatives. PwMS should take vitamin D in doses of 5000 IU to 10,000 IU a day, aiming at a blood level above 150 nmol/L. Their relatives should also take vitamin D supplements, aiming at levels above 100 nmol/L, as primary prevention against developing MS. This is supported by 2014 Consensus Guidelines from the Brazilian Academy of Neurology.[107] In a wide-ranging review of vitamin D supplementation conducted by its Scientific Department of Neuroimmunology, expert neurologists and researchers examined the vast literature on vitamin D supplementation in MS. Noting that doses up to 10,000 IU are safe and might be needed, they recommended 'individualized doses until reaching serum levels between 40 ng/ml and 100 ng/ml' (in Australia, New Zealand and the United Kingdom, 100–250 nmol/L).

> The dose of vitamin D should be lowered appropriately for children.

For children, these doses need to be lowered according to body weight. So, using a 50 kg person as the standard adult for the purposes of calculating dosages, a 25 kg child—say, an eight-year-old—would need half the usual adult dose. As a good preventive dose for an adult is around 5,000 IU a day, aiming at a blood level of 100 nmol/L, this child would get 2500 IU a day. For, say, a 10 kg child—perhaps a two- or three-year-old—the dose would be one-fifth of the adult dose, so 1000 IU a day. I deliberately recommend using 5000 IU a day as the comparative adult dose, rather than the 10,000 IU a day dose proven safe by Hathcock and colleagues, because for primary prevention it is not necessary to reach the recommended blood level of 150 nmol/L, but rather 100 nmol/L. If one is keeping to this recommendation for children of a reduced dosage based on weight and using the 5000 IU dose as the baseline, this has the advantage of allowing for an appreciable margin of safety. In turn, this means that checking children's blood levels is not necessary, in contrast to secondary prevention, when a higher level is needed. I recommend this approach for primary prevention as it is best to be cautious about not raising vitamin D levels too high for children who are essentially healthy.

Should we take calcium as well as vitamin D?

Most Western societies have overdone their public health messages about sun avoidance to the extent where a very large proportion of the population is low in vitamin D or frankly deficient. As the main effect of vitamin D in the body is to extract calcium from the food we eat and incorporate it into bone, this has resulted in a virtual epidemic of osteoporosis in Western countries. Rather than modify the messages to promote modest sun exposure, which as we have seen has a range of health benefits, the response has been to recommend calcium supplementation. As a result, we have a huge food industry growing up around adding calcium to foods and encouraging substantial dairy consumption.

The evidence, however, is that this is not having an impact on osteoporosis and bone fractures. In fact, there is evidence that populations that eat mainly vegetarian or vegan diets have lower rates of osteoporosis and fractures, and that high milk intake is associated with more rather than fewer fractures.[108] A US study showed that the incidence of forearm and hip fractures in men was no lower in those with high calcium intakes than those with low intakes.[109] Likewise, a very large prospective study from Boston of over 77,000 women showed there was no difference in fracture rates in women with high calcium intakes compared with those with low intakes.[110] Indeed, there was a trend to higher fracture rates in those with high calcium intakes. A detailed review of the literature shows that there is no evidence that increasing cow's milk consumption has any beneficial effect on children's bone health.[111] The Centre for Nutrition and Food Safety at the University of Surrey recommended that a 'fruit and vegetable' approach to osteoporosis may provide a very sensible alternative therapy for osteoporosis, and is likely to have many other health benefits.[112]

The problem with widespread calcium supplementation for populations of people with low vitamin D levels is that most of the calcium that is added to food is not absorbed into the body because of the low vitamin D. It has been shown, for example, that people with a blood level of vitamin D of 86.5 nmol/L absorb two-thirds more calcium than those with blood levels of 50 nmol/L, yet both levels have until recently been considered normal.[113] For people with osteoporosis, the best thing to do is get out in the sun regularly as recommended by the guidelines in this book, not to consume more calcium. Of course, it is also easier to exercise more when outside, further strengthening bones. MS and osteoporosis often go hand in hand, especially for people with advanced disease, because they don't exercise much and don't get outside much. PwMS must get out in the sun.

As consumers, we now face constant advertisements about whether we are getting enough calcium, designed to get us to take calcium supplements. The dairy industry has seen an opening here to market its products as high in calcium and therefore healthy, obscuring the very real health risks associated with dairy products, particularly for PwMS. It has actually taken a long time for researchers to begin to investigate whether this widespread calcium supplementation is doing any good or, more particularly, whether it is possibly doing harm. After all, many of our elderly are on drugs called calcium channel blockers, particularly those with heart and vascular disease, and intuitively it seems problematic to be giving them the very mineral the effects of which we are trying to block in the body.

As previously discussed under dietary supplements, there is now substantial evidence to suggest that calcium supplementation is not only unhelpful, but also probably harmful, and this is likely to be particularly true for people supplementing with vitamin D. As a result, I do not recommend calcium supplementation unless there is a compelling reason to do so.

OVERVIEW

The vitamin D issue can be a source of great frustration for PwMS. Studies confirming benefits for PwMS keep coming, with very little evidence contradicting these important findings. Yet our medical advisors continue to demand more evidence before making any recommendations. The evidence for sun exposure and vitamin D supplementation is now vast and congruent, all pointing to reducing risk of getting the disease and of its activity. My recommendation of regular low-dose sun exposure is not only highly protective for PwMS but also effective in prevention of a range of internal cancers, and a variety of auto-immune diseases.

Professor Bruce Taylor, a highly respected expert in MS, particularly in the research around sunlight and vitamin D, has finally started a serious conversation at a high level among neurologists about whether our sun-avoidance public health policies based on skin cancer risk have gone too far, and whether we should be promoting judicious exposure to UV light (in sunlight) to promote a healthy immune system.[114] Slowly, the experts are starting to discuss this. In the meantime, PwMS should continue to be highly proactive and look to get regular sun exposure and take vitamin D in the amounts suggested here. The risk for PwMS, and those susceptible to MS, of waiting for more research far outweighs any perceived risks.

STEP 3

EXERCISE REGULARLY

Those who think they have not time for bodily exercise will sooner or later have to find time for illness.

Edward Stanley
Address at Liverpool College, 20 December 1873

INTRODUCTION

A key part of the OMS Recovery Program is exercise. For a range of diseases, there is overwhelming evidence that exercise improves not only outcome from the disease, but also quality of life. People who exercise regularly live longer, healthier and happier lives. They have less depression and better cognitive function. The situation is no different for PwMS, despite the obvious limitations many have with physical ability. Making the change to regular exercise—of any sort—is an important habit for PwMS to develop.

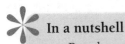

In a nutshell
- Regular exercise improves the health of PwMS.
- Both aerobic (endurance) exercise and progressive resistance (strength) training are beneficial.
- Preliminary evidence suggests that regular exercise slows disease progression.
- The HOLISM study found better quality of life for people with MS who exercised more, regardless of level of disability; the biggest benefits were between those who did little exercise and those who exercised moderately.

WHY

Exercise has wide-ranging benefits for physical and emotional well-being.[1, 2] Studies have shown that regular physical exercise is important in the primary and secondary prevention of a range of diseases, particularly heart disease, type 2 diabetes, cancer and osteoporosis.[3] Indeed, researchers have shown that regular exercise provides around as much benefit for a range of diseases as currently prescribed medications.[4] Exercise is medicine!

Regular exercise also reduces the risk of premature death. One study showed a three- to five-times higher risk of premature death from any cause for people in the lowest exercise category compared to the highest, with a higher rate for women than men.[2] Physically inactive middle-aged women had a roughly 50 per cent increase in death rate from all causes, twice the cardiovascular-related mortality and about a 30 per cent increase in cancer-related mortality compared with physically active women.[2] These risks are fairly similar to the risks caused by high blood pressure, high cholesterol and obesity, and not much short of those associated with smoking, but are not well known by most people. Exercise is an important risk factor in chronic illness, and for most people relatively easy to do something about.

How much exercise?

While generally the rule is the more exercise the better, even small improvements in physical fitness significantly reduce the risk of early death.[5, 6] Quite modest changes to increase physical fitness in inactive people have major effects in improving health overall, particularly for people with many chronic illnesses.[7-12] And it doesn't have to be a sudden change—indeed, it is probably safer to increase physical activity slowly but surely. One study showed that people who became fit over a five-year period nearly halved their risk of death compared with those who remained inactive.[13]

Two large-scale studies published in 2015 showed that, in general, the more exercise we undertake, the lower our risk of dying. The bigger of the two studies examined 661,000 people. Importantly, it showed that even by doing a small amount of exercise compared with none at all, there was a major 20 per cent decrease in death rate.[14] There was additional benefit for those who complied with current guidelines and did 150 minutes of moderate exercise a week, with an additional 11 per cent reduction, and for those who exercised on average more than an hour a day every day, there was an additional 8 per cent reduction. But it is important to note that the major benefit comes with just doing something versus doing nothing.

The other study looked at over 200,000 Australian adults and reached similar conclusions.[15] Additionally, it showed that occasional vigorous exercise provided some extra benefit in terms of reduced death rate. The findings of these two studies, while looking at a general population, and using death rates as the measure of benefit, can nevertheless be extrapolated to PwMS, in that the health benefits are likely to be similar. Of course, there may be less scope for vigorous exercise for many PwMS who are significantly disabled, or even moderate exercise for some.

Regardless of age or level of disability, exercise can be recommended as a preventive therapy. Regular exercise eventually leads to a state of physical fitness, which means a state of well-being that allows a person to physically meet the demands of daily living. Of course, for those who are active sports people, regular exercise results in physical fitness that allows optimal performance of their sports. For general health, physical fitness improves health status, including cardiovascular fitness, muscular fitness, body composition and metabolism, and also improves quality of life and well-being.

Not exercising, or physical inactivity, is a risk factor for the development of many chronic illnesses, including heart disease, high blood pressure, diabetes, cancer—particularly of the breast and bowel—osteoporosis, obesity and depression.[2] So exercise is an important measure for the primary prevention of these diseases. One meta-analysis showed marked improvement in depressive symptoms for people with neurological diseases, including MS, who exercised—particularly those who met current physical activity guidelines.[16] Increasing physical activity also improves outcomes from established heart disease and high blood pressure, diabetes, certain cancers[17, 18] and osteoporosis.[19] So exercise has an important secondary prevention role as well.

Regular exercise, even in small amounts, prevents disease, but also makes a big difference to health and physical abilities in those who already have illness.

Sadly, physical inactivity is surprisingly common. But one doesn't have to get physically fit to derive benefits from exercise. Just increasing physical activity, even without any change in level of fitness—particularly in the elderly and the disabled—leads to better health outcomes. Regular low-level exercise leads to reductions in risk factors for chronic disease and disability without necessarily affecting fitness.[20] Just increasing the strength and endurance of muscles, without necessarily making any difference to cardiovascular fitness, improves health and reduces the risk of chronic disease and disability.[21] This is particularly important for elderly and disabled people, as a little more muscle strength can mean the difference between being able to do simple tasks of daily living and not being able to do them.

Just a small change in strength or endurance can also help those with established disease—for instance, it can mean being able to get out of a chair without help. Without the added strength derived from some exercise of the muscles, a vicious cycle can start, with reduced muscle fitness leading to more inactivity and growing dependence on others for help. This is particularly relevant for PwMS. People with higher levels of muscle strength are able to do more and have less risk of developing other chronic diseases like heart disease, diabetes and stroke.[22] Systematic reviews of published studies in the area show that better muscle fitness improves functional independence, mobility, bone health, well-being and overall quality of life;[20, 21] people with lower levels of muscle strength and fitness have a higher risk of falls and illness. So things like resistance training and flexibility exercises at least twice a week can really help to maintain functional independence and improve overall quality of life.[23]

Exercise in MS

As long ago as 1974, Professor Ritchie Russell, Professor of Clinical Neurology in Oxford, published a book entitled *Multiple Sclerosis: Control of the Disease*, in which he detailed a specific exercise program that he felt arrested disease progression in MS.[24] It was called the Rest–Exercise Program (REP). The program involved PwMS doing short bursts of vigorous exercise, preferably in a prone (lying down) position, such as press-ups or weight-lifting exercises, followed by periods of rest. Russell thought this would help by protecting the blood–brain barrier, which we know is intimately involved in the development of MS. He reported in his book the details of 21 PwMS of various ages and the good results they achieved with this therapy.

There is now a wealth of evidence about the benefits of exercise specifically for PwMS. One study using meta-analysis to examine the overall effect of exercise training interventions on quality of life in PwMS looked at thirteen studies with 484 MS participants, and found a significant improvement in quality of life for those exercising, particularly for fatigue-related measures.[25] A 2015 Cochrane review, examining 72 studies overall, found that exercise is safe and moderately effective in reducing fatigue for PwMS without increasing the risk of relapse.[26] Unfortunately, increasing disability can lead to decreasing levels of exercise for PwMS,[27, 28] as pain, weakness and problems with balance may limit a person's exercise ability. While exercise appears to improve fatigue, many PwMS find that fatigue acts as a major disincentive to exercise. Indeed, many are told that they need to conserve energy. Inactivity can also contribute to an increased risk of other illnesses like heart disease or obesity, which are known to increase disease progression in MS[29] and may also lead to deconditioning and muscle weakness.[30]

In the 1970s, there was quite a strong prevailing medical opinion that PwMS should avoid exercise—that it could somehow be detrimental. There is now good evidence that exercise improves fitness and function in mild MS and maintains function for people with moderate to severe disability.[31] Randomised controlled trials have also shown that moderate aerobic exercise does not worsen symptoms of MS.[32] There is strong evidence that exercise therapy, including aerobic exercise and resistance training, improves muscle power, exercise tolerance and mobility-related activities such as walking in people with significant disability.[33–40] Exercise also improves mood,[41] general well-being,[35, 42, 43] fatigue[44, 45, 46] and quality of life.[25, 47, 48] Walking distance has been shown to be increased with regular treadmill training.[49] Interestingly, some of the benefits of exercise in MS seems to be more pronounced in women.[50] Exercise has been shown to be superior to neurological rehabilitation in improving exercise tolerance and walking ability in people with mild to moderate MS.[51] Several studies have also reported beneficial effects of exercise on quality of life in PwMS[52, 53, 54] and in significantly reducing the chances of depression.[43]

Progressive resistance training

Progressive resistance training (PRT), or strength training, uses external resistance (or body weight) to progressively increase the force of muscle contraction through step-by-step weight increases working on different groups of muscles. PRT is very good at building up muscle strength.

Researchers at La Trobe University in Victoria, Australia, studied the effects of PRT using a tailored gym program with weight training for the lower limbs for PwMS. They showed that the exercise improved muscle performance and fast walking speed, but also quality of life, as well as reducing fatigue. Importantly, the benefits for quality of life and fatigue disappeared once the training stopped. Participants noted that the perceived impact of MS on their physical function was reduced.[55] They also found that using encouraging leaders with a good knowledge of exercise, and exercising in a group, contributed to the success of the program.[56]

A Danish study analysed all the well-conducted published studies in the area of PRT.[57] They summarised evidence that PRT helps functional capacity, such as walking distance and gait, and balance, including reducing the fear of falling. Importantly, as in other studies, they confirmed that PRT is also of benefit in improving fatigue, quality of life and mood. One small study showed that treadmill training was superior to PRT in improving walking for those with mild to moderate disability.[58] While studies exploring how these benefits occurred were scarce, there was some suggestion that exercise tended to shift the immune profile towards an anti-inflammatory state, and that risk factors for heart disease—which we know are similar to those for MS—were reduced.

Strength training improves health even if only twice a week, has no significant side-effects and is preferred by many people to endurance training.

None of the studies on PRT reported any adverse events or any serious symptom exacerbations. Further, almost everybody adhered to the program and there were very low drop-out rates from the PRT groups. One important advantage of PRT for PwMS is that PRT is a time-efficient way to exercise; studies have shown major improvements with just two one-hour sessions a week. PRT is also easily done in a community setting, in groups. Another advantage is that PwMS who are sensitive to heat tolerate PRT better than endurance training.[59] A two-year study showed that PwMS can stick with this form of exercise for long periods; it also showed marked benefits to functional capacity over that period—that is, PwMS were able to recover lost function. Importantly, when the group training stopped and the participants took over their own training, they maintained these benefits at six months after group cessation.[60] This research group argued:

Physical activity is a basic prerequisite for optimal body functioning and health in humans, and even more so in MS patients with known reductions in physical activity. As such it can be argued that the goal is to increase the physical activity level of MS patients by promoting all types of exercise that will induce this. This is an important consideration given that long-term adherence to a more physical active lifestyle may depend strongly on motivation and enjoyment of exercise. However, given that exercise therapy, and PRT in particular, is probably the most well-documented non-pharmacological symptomatic treatment in MS, this exercise modality is highly recommendable. Moreover, PRT is a safe intervention without known side-effects, showing excellent short-term adherence and low drop-out rates, and has beneficial effects on numerous common MS symptoms and deficits . . . Not many symptomatic treatments, even pharmacological ones, have such a profile![59]

It is difficult to argue with this comment—and why would we? Drawing a favourable comparison with drug therapies is unusual for a lifestyle-based intervention.

Aerobic exercise

Of course, many PwMS—particularly those with earlier stage disease and less disability—prefer aerobic exercise such as running or swimming. Aerobic exercise is likely to have some advantages as well, if PwMS are able to do it. One literature review concluded that 'evidence exists for recommending participation in endurance training at low to moderate intensity, as the existing literature demonstrates that MS patients can both tolerate and benefit from this training modality'.[61] It seems there is a complex interplay between lack of exercise causing depression and fatigue, and fatigue causing depression.[62] Aerobic exercise is very helpful in breaking this cycle, but needs to be regular to maintain the benefits.[30] Certainly, any aerobic exercise is better than none. As we have seen from studies in other conditions, physical inactivity is a key risk factor. Getting physically fit is not necessary; just getting active brings numerous health benefits—particularly to quality of life, mood and well-being.

One Iranian study of 90 PwMS randomly allocated them to three groups, one doing aerobic exercise, another yoga and a control group not doing exercise. The aerobic exercise group did a half hour of walking three times a week after a warm-up, and the yoga group a half hour of yoga three times a week. After twelve weeks, the researchers found that in both active groups, fatigue, emotional role, social function and energy had improved, and that pain was somewhat better compared with those not doing the exercise.[63] So yoga may also be beneficial.

Exercise and cognitive function

Many PwMS have memory problems—up to half in some studies. To date, no treatment has been shown to improve that memory loss in clinical trials. US researchers have investigated the potential for aerobic exercise to affect memory after other trials showed some benefit in the elderly and in people with schizophrenia.[64] They used an array of detailed tests to check memory status, and used functional MRI to look at potential changes in the size of the hippocampus—the part of the brain responsible for memory formation, organisation and storage. This was a small pilot study of just two people—both women—one of whom undertook aerobic exercise (exercise that raises the heart rate and works out the cardiovascular system) and one who did non-aerobic exercise (such as lifting weights).

The results were very encouraging, with the woman undertaking aerobic exercise showing an increase in her memory scores of over 50 per cent, and her hippocampus increasing in size by 16.5 per cent, whereas the woman undertaking non-aerobic exercise had negligible increase in hippocampal size and no change in memory. The authors stated that this may be the first effective memory treatment for PwMS. Importantly, they noted that it is cost-effective, widely available and has no adverse effects. Another recent randomised controlled trial in older women also showed that aerobic exercise increased the size of the hippocampus, again suggesting a likely beneficial effect on memory of this sort of exercise.[65] This is a key reason for PwMS to undertake regular vigorous aerobic exercise to the extent they are able.

Another important benefit of exercise is likely to be an improvement in other aspects of cognitive function. One study by Australian scientists examined the effects on cognitive function of two sessions of weight training a week in the gym for elderly people with mild cognitive impairment (early dementia).[66] The researchers from the University of Sydney randomly allocated 100 elderly people with early dementia to a group who did PRT and a control group who did seated calisthenics. The training involved chest press, leg press, seated rowing, standing hip abduction and knee-extension exercises, all designed to improve strength.

They found that the group with the resistance training had marked improvements in cognitive function; by six months of training, about half the resistance training group had normal cognitive function compared with only a quarter of the control group. It is interesting to note that the control group who did the calisthenics also experienced an improvement, but the resistance training had a much more marked improvement. Importantly, when tested a year after the end of the study, the benefits in improved cognitive function persisted.

 Exercise can improve cognitive function.

There had been some previous work on aerobic exercise in people with mild cognitive impairment that showed some improvement in higher executive functions, but only in women, and with no real benefit for memory.[67] So both aerobic exercise and PRT are likely to be helpful in preventing cognitive decline and even improving memory—a key issue for PwMS (Figure 10).

How might exercise work?

Two proteins, brain-derived neurotrophic factor (BDNF) and nerve growth factor (NGF), have been shown to have some protective effects for nerve cells in PwMS, helping them to repair. Exercise has been shown in one study to significantly increase the levels of these proteins in PwMS.[68] In summarising the literature on exercise playing a role in preventing cognitive decline, German researchers have also shown increased levels of neurotrophic factors in PwMS who undergo exercise training.[69]

Not only does exercise improve symptoms in MS and prevent depression, but it has also been suggested that it may have a neuroprotective effect, and that this could modify the course of the illness.[70, 71] Other

Figure 10: Exercise is good for the brain

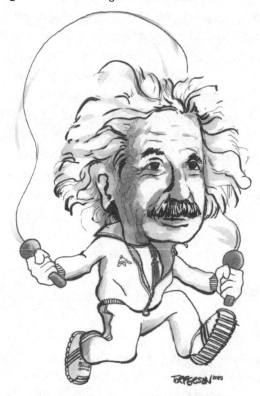

researchers have suggested that regular exercise promotes neuroprotection, neuroregeneration and neuroplasticity through the production of nerve growth factors,[72] and by inducing immune modulation through alteration in cytokines and stress hormones, and that this could reduce long-term disability.[73] It is likely that exercise has an anti-inflammatory effect, and we have seen the importance of shifting the balance in MS away from inflammation.[74]

Does exercise affect disease progression?

But while the literature on exercise in MS strongly suggests that it improves quality of life, fitness and function, muscle power and exercise tolerance, as well as mood, fatigue and general well-being, what is not clear from the evidence base is the answer to the obvious question: does exercise slow the progression of the illness? Danish researchers have attempted to examine this question through a systematic review of all the studies on exercise that have addressed this.[70] Naturally there is less evidence here than about drug therapies in MS due to a lack of funding for suitable studies. Nevertheless, the authors found considerable evidence in the animal model of MS, EAE, as well as in clinical studies of PwMS, to suggest that exercise may well have a disease-modifying effect. In experimental animals the onset of disease was delayed and the illness was less severe for those animals that exercised; in humans, there was considerable evidence of a benefit for exercise in disease progression, symptoms, cognitive function and walking impairment.

A longitudinal study of PwMS showed that those doing more exercise at the beginning of the study had less functional decline over time than those doing less exercise, suggesting that exercise may prevent disease progression.[75] Importantly, there is no evidence that exercise is in any way harmful for PwMS,[32, 76] and does not seem to trigger relapses.[77]

 Exercise, like diet, prevents inflammation and degeneration.

It appears likely that exercise, like diet, is effective against both the major ways in which MS causes its damage, immune activation and degeneration. This is very likely in MS, just as it has been seen in modifying the progression of many other immune-mediated and degenerative diseases. One study of 611 PwMS provided some confirmation, showing that exercise had a positive impact on the progression of disability, as well as quality of life.[78] Unfortunately, recent studies have shown that PwMS do less exercise than those in the general population.[79, 80] It is important to consider the benefits of this lifestyle change, not only for general health, but specifically also for MS.

HOLISM study findings on exercise

As outlined above, previous evidence about exercise for PwMS has been extensive and largely congruent, showing beneficial effects for PwMS in terms of quality of life, fatigue and depression, with a suggestion of benefit for disease progression. The HOLISM study investigators were very interested to see, in the real-world setting, what sort of levels of exercise were being undertaken by the two and a half thousand PwMS in our study sample, and whether the benefits seen in previous studies were substantiated.

Our study used the International Physical Activity Questionnaire (IPAQ) scoring system to categorise the amount of exercise PwMS were doing. This score was filled in by PwMS themselves, but has been shown to correlate reasonably well with other external measures of the amount of exercise people do. It is categorised from the amount of physical activity undertaken in the last week into low active, where no or little activity is reported; moderately active, where the amount of exercise meets any one of a number of criteria (three or more days of vigorous activity of at least 20 minutes per day, five or more days of moderate-intensity activity or walking of at least 30 minutes per day, or five or more days of any combination of walking, moderate-intensity or vigorous intensity activities); and high active, where participants satisfied any one of the following criteria—vigorous-intensity activity on at least three days or seven days of any combination of walking, moderate-intensity or vigorous intensity activities.

Of the 2519 PwMS completing this section of the HOLISM study, about 41 per cent were low active, about 32 per cent moderately active and about 27 per cent high active. These data again confirm the fact that the HOLISM sample of PwMS comprised a large number who were very proactive about their health; to have nearly three in every five PwMS in the sample doing moderate amounts of exercise or more compares more than favourably with most other populations previously studied. PwMS, even those with mild disability,[81] have in other studies been shown to generally do less exercise than the general population,[27, 82] although exercise has benefits for PwMS no matter how disabled they are.[83, 84]

As expected, the more disabled people were, the less they exercised, although there may have been some contribution here from less exercise leading to more disability, given the evidence previously presented that exercise has a disease-modifying effect in MS.[70] Our results, however, showed that exercise was associated with better quality of life outcomes, regardless of disability level. Increasing levels of exercise were associated with increased levels of energy, social function, physical, mental and

Figure 11: Quality of life by level of physical activity

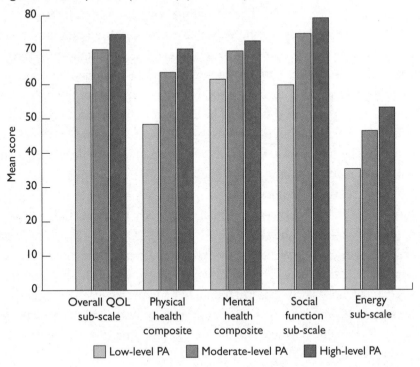

overall quality of life, as measured by the MSQOL-54 while controlling for age, gender and disability level (see Figure 11).

A very important finding was that the increases in quality of life between low and moderate levels of exercise were bigger than those between moderate and high levels of exercise. This means that PwMS who currently do little exercise may benefit more in terms of improved quality of life from increasing exercise levels than those with moderate levels increasing to a high level of exercise. In other words, you don't have to do a lot of exercise, but it is important to do some. How exercise improves quality of life has been the subject of some debate. Some argue that it works through better social participation; others suggest it reduces fatigue, improves mood, increases a sense of empowerment or improves functions of the body in general.[48, 75, 85–88]

Another important finding was that those who exercised more had a 40 per cent higher energy sub-scale of quality of life. Fatigue is one of the most debilitating symptoms for many PwMS, so the association of increasing exercise with having more energy is an important one for PwMS to note. A review has previously strongly suggested this apparently beneficial effect of increasing amounts of exercise on fatigue and energy levels for most PwMS.[89] Other important findings included increases of more than 25 per cent on the physical health composite, and increases of around 15 per cent on the mental health composite, social function sub-scale and overall quality of life sub-scale between high and low levels of exercise. The size of these effects of exercise on quality of life is consistent with most studies looking at this question.[53, 54, 90–94]

Most of these studies have included only people with mild to moderate disability. However, a small pilot study which included PwMS with high disability showed increases on MSQOL subscales of energy (60 per cent), physical health composite (30 per cent), mental health composite (22 per cent) and social function sub-scale (13 per cent) after a relatively modest exercise program involving twelve weeks of treadmill training.[84] In line with this, our study too showed that, even in those with more major disability, the more exercise one did, the better the quality of life became.

In terms of relapse rate, our initial analysis showed that PwMS with relapsing-remitting MS who were exercising more had lower relapse rates. However, when we applied more advanced statistical techniques, controlling for age, gender and disability level, we found no significant association. This is probably because those having relapses more frequently were less likely to exercise rather than the other way around. Our data also showed that for PwMS with low to moderate disability, more exercise was related to a healthier body-mass index (BMI), which is associated with better physical health overall.[29]

HOW

Introduction

While there are guidelines about how much exercise is optimal for the general population, guidelines for PwMS are harder to find. Such guidelines need to take into account the many factors that affect the capacity and motivation of PwMS, particularly for different forms of MS and for different stages in the disease process. It would be very unhelpful to be recommending vigorous aerobic exercise for people with major disability; for such people, gradual introduction of strength training, starting with very small amounts of resistance and progressing very gradually to increasing resistance levels and more frequent training, would be more sensible. So one size does not fit all.

In a nutshell
- When starting out, a qualified fitness trainer can help, especially for those with significant disability.
- Start by aiming for half to three-quarters of one's maximal predicted heart rate for age, doing about half an hour of exercise two to three times a week.
- Start low and increase slowly.
- Try aqua exercise, aerobics, weight training, yoga and balance programs, or more vigorous exercise with walking, jogging, swimming, cycling or a sport.
- Consider strategies for staying cool, including swimming in a pool or wearing an ice vest.
- Try setting goals and using devices that measure activities.

Exercise recommendations from MS organisations

There are some good guidelines for exercise produced by the major MS organisations. MS Australia, for example, produces a series of brochures entitled *MS Practice for Health Professionals*; its brochure on strength and cardiorespiratory exercise for PwMS has guidelines for both PRT (strength training) and aerobic exercise (cardiorespiratory training).[95]

The strength training suggestions are that the weight to begin with should be around two-thirds of the maximal weight that one can handle initially. So if one can move, say, 60 kg with a knee-curl machine at the gym, then training should begin with 40 kg or so, depending on how comfortably one can lift that. Between one and three sets of around eight to fifteen repetitions of that knee curl should then be done about three to five times a week. The weight should be increased by 2–5 per cent—say, 1 kg—once twelve to fifteen repetitions can be done without problems over two training sessions. Of course, that exercise would gradually increase the strength of the muscle group used—in this case, the quads. Other exercises would need to be used to develop other muscles—say, the calf muscles. Some gym equipment may not offer such small increments in weight, so a specialised training area at one of the MS societies might be more helpful.

People starting out with an exercise program can benefit from the assistance of a qualified trainer.

Such formulae can be useful for people beginning a program. By signing up with a gym, or using the local MS society gym, and getting help from a qualified fitness trainer or physiotherapist, it is possible to develop a program targeting the key muscle groups that are most important for that individual. If walking is a major problem, then targeting the particular leg muscles used in walking is key. An experienced trainer can be very helpful—for instance, in starting the resistance at the appropriate level, and in recommending the best technique for the various exercises. Being flexible about the training routine is very important, rather than rigidly sticking to a pre-determined exercise program.

If starting out on an aerobic exercise program, depending on age and other possible illnesses, it can be important to have an initial health and fitness check with a doctor or experienced gym instructor. The sudden introduction of too high-intensity exercise can potentially be very damaging for those with other diseases, such as heart disease. A variety of machines and programs is available in most gyms to enable this form of exercise. These might include treadmills, stationary cycles or even cycles where one can lie down, aqua aerobic programs and, for wheelchair users, arm-crank machines. Alternatively, PwMS—particularly those who have been newly diagnosed—may wish to simply start a walking, running or swimming program.

MS Australia recommends aiming at around half to three-quarters of the maximum predicted heart rate for the person's age, doing around half an hour of exercise—possibly broken into two sessions—two or three times a week, progressing in intensity and effort to maintain that target heart rate.

Most of the major MS organisations have similar guidelines. The National Multiple Sclerosis Society in the United States has a particularly helpful one, written in very plain language, with sensible recommendations.[96] This reflects the fact that it was written by a person with MS, Mary Harmon, who has lived with the disease since 1988. She clearly exercises regularly, and is able to offer many of the insights she has gained throughout those years. The guidelines offer many alternatives for aerobic exercise, such as aqua exercise, weight training, yoga or other stretching exercises, balance programs such as with a Swiss ball, gentle martial arts and aerobics. The guidelines also advise on the availability of a range of adaptive sports, particularly for people with disabilities, such as modified basketball, handball, tennis or golf, in addition to a range of aquatic sports. Importantly, they offer useful advice on starting out, setting realistic goals and being mindful of safety concerns. Warming-up and cooling-down are emphasised, as are tips to deal with fatigue and for keeping cool. The brochure concludes, 'Take it slowly. Exercise is not a battle with the body to overcome spasticity, weakness or any other MS symptom. Instead, it's an opportunity to do everything possible for good health. And to have fun!'

For many years, Canada has had very authoritative guidelines for physical activity. Its most recent 2011 guidelines for healthy adults[97] have now highlighted the importance of combining both aerobic and strengthening exercises, with about two days of each per week. They encourage people to participate in a variety of activities that are enjoyable and safe, through planned exercise sessions, getting from place to place, recreation, sports, or occupation over and above the incidental physical activities of daily living. They note the importance of starting with small amounts of activity and gradually increasing how long, often and hard they are done.

They suggest a total of at least two and a half hours of moderate to vigorous aerobic activity a week (so, for most people, say five days of half an hour of exercise each), of at least 10 minutes' duration in each session, but also to have at least two days of muscle- and bone-strengthening activities. It is important to note that these guidelines are designed for healthy people; PwMS, depending on their health status, might need to adopt considerably less rigorous exercise programs, at least until their aerobic capacity improves.

These guidelines were developed with assistance from the Canadian Society for Exercise Physiology (CSEP), the principal body for physical activity, health and fitness research and personal training in Canada. This group has published specific guidelines for physical activity for PwMS with mild to moderate disability, based on the national Canadian guidelines.[98] The Toolkit notes that, in the past, PwMS were told they shouldn't be physically active, but that in fact meeting the guidelines may reduce fatigue, improve mobility and enhance overall well-being. They suggest finding a mix of moderate-intensity activities that suits a person's situation and lifestyle.

For those with minor or no disability, they suggest walking, cycling, dancing, swimming or an aqua fitness class, a team sport or an active game with family or friends for aerobic activity. For strength training, they suggest weight training using free weights or machines, resistance bands, using body weight or doing adapted push-ups or squats. For those with moderate disability who are in a wheelchair, they suggest cycling with a hand cycle or on a stationary bike, wheeling, swimming or an aqua fitness class, or playing a sport or an active video game (for example, using the Wii). For strength training, they suggest weights (free weights or machines) or resistance bands. They also suggest tai chi, yoga, Pilates and stretching in addition to these physical activities to build flexibility, balance and body awareness. They reinforce that it is important to start slowly, rest afterwards and believe that you can do it.

Some of these guidelines appear to aim very high and possibly to be out of reach for many PwMS, particularly those with significant disability. Canadian researchers have previously noted that low-intensity exercise is generally better accepted by people who are new to exercise training, those who are out of shape and older people,[3] and this also applies to many PwMS. As previously noted, low-intensity exercise can improve health status without any real change in physical fitness. In effect, any exercise—indeed, any physical activity—is better than none, and any activity will improve health. So this could be light gardening or walking for around an hour a day on most days of the week.

But ideally, PwMS who are out of shape or older would start with such low-intensity exercise and add some strength training over time. More moderate-intensity exercise might be, say, brisk walking or dancing for around a half an hour or more, three to five days a week. Others who are in better shape or have gradually moved through low- and moderate-intensity exercise levels and can now do them without difficulty might add running, cycling or swimming, again for half an hour a day or more, three to five days a week. Adding strength training in a gym might involve one or two sets of about ten repetitions of a range of weight-training exercises of moderate intensity using the large muscle groups, particularly of the arms and legs, twice or more per week. Again, using a weight about two-thirds of the maximum that can be lifted or pushed is ideal, but for those who are older or weaker, using lesser weights, but doing more repetitions—say, 15—may achieve similar goals.

Gentle stretching exercises, such as in a yoga or Pilates program, are also very helpful and suit many PwMS. Holding the stretches for 15–20 seconds, and doing these twice weekly or more, provides optimal benefit. Many PwMS will choose to do some light-intensity, some moderate-intensity and some high-intensity exercise, and some weight training, along with yoga or Pilates, mixing and matching to ensure that the activities are enjoyable. The aim really is to enjoy the exercise as well as reap the health rewards. An important additional benefit is that maintaining an active lifestyle or taking up light or moderate physical activity like walking or moderately heavy gardening significantly reduces the risk of cardiovascular disease and death.

How much exercise is enough?

It seems that good health is very closely related to how much exercise we do, and how intense it is, with the most benefit gained by those exercising the most and the most vigorously. However, any exercise is better than none, and even regular light physical activity brings health benefits. As noted earlier, the biggest benefit seems to be in moving from no or little exercise to regular moderate exercise. It doesn't have to be vigorous to get marked health benefits.

Any exercise is better than none.

PwMS who use pedometers or swimming watches will be familiar with the calorie count on these devices, which shows the number of kilojoules used in the exercise. For instance, a half-hour run at around six minutes per kilometre pace will use up around 1700 kilojoules (400 calories) of energy. Most authorities recommend a minimum of around 4000 kilojoules (1000 calories) a week for significant health benefits, but even half this amount used up in just a couple of brisk hour long walks weekly produces health benefits. This sort of weekly energy expenditure is associated with around a 20–30 per cent lower death rate from all causes;[2] double this expenditure to around 2000 kilojoules (500 calories) a week, and people have been shown to gain around two extra years of life.[2] There does seem to be a consistent increase in health benefits for a range of conditions, not just MS, with increasing levels of exercise and increasing intensity, so for PwMS it is important to develop healthy new habits that incorporate generous amounts of exercise, tailored to the degree of disability if present.

Pedometers and other devices like swimming watches and cycle computer devices are being used increasingly. One can monitor not only calorie expenditure, but also number of steps, distance swum or cycled, and times. This makes them really useful for setting training goals. For instance, increasing the number of steps taken by 3000–4000 per day during walking brings that person up to current public health requirements for healthy exercise levels. One could, for example, start a pedometer-based walking program by adding 500 steps a day each week until reaching the goal of 3000–4000 additional steps per day. Many people find that such devices that give instant feedback on how they are progressing provide additional motivation to keep going and to get healthy.

The fitter one is to begin with, the more exercise and the higher intensity needed to improve the level of fitness. This is good news for the elderly and those in poor condition, as even just adding a little regular exercise will result in marked improvements in fitness levels. But the health and quality of life benefits continue to accrue as more exercise is added, so a progressive training program is ideal for those who are out of condition, so that eventually they will be doing exercise on most days of the week. Such a program needs to be prescribed and overseen by a health professional for those who are significantly disabled or have other chronic health conditions. But for most of us, exercise is something that we prescribe for ourselves, and also manage ourselves.

 Regular strength training can result in surprising improvements in apparent disability.

What type of exercise?
Most authorities recommend aerobic exercise that lifts the heart rate and makes you sweat, like walking at a good pace, jogging, swimming, cycling, rowing and aerobics. But they also recommend some strength training, usually added after someone has started to build up some fitness and endurance.[99] We all start to lose muscle in adulthood, but most noticeably after the age of 60 or so. This is especially true for people who don't use their muscles. For PwMS, the cycle of disability and fatigue leading to failure to exercise, leading to muscle deconditioning and loss of muscle mass, then leading to more disability and fatigue, can become a vicious one. Many PwMS who have been disabled for some time and have lost a lot of capacity to do things for themselves are surprised to find that when they enter a strength training program and gradually build back up the muscle strength of big muscle groups like those in their legs, tasks that were previously beyond them become possible again, quite independently of any neurological recovery or reduction in the number of lesions in the brain or spinal cord.

Some find that they can start walking again, even after a considerable time of not being able to walk, and believing that they were disabled due to the MS disease process itself. For people in this position, it is often best to start with gentle stretching exercises, as muscles have tightened up and there may be considerable spasticity, moving on to some gradually increasing weight training to redevelop strength in the affected muscles, and then light aerobic exercise. For some, moderate-intensity exercise like swimming or brisk walking may even become a possibility, but that needs to be developed slowly. Many people will find that these activities are easier in a group setting where motivation may be easier to find, and some will find it easier doing short, sharp bursts of, say, ten minutes at a time, with adequate recovery in between, some of them with a group, and others on their own.

So, while aerobic exercise is great for fitness, it is important to add some strength training, as aerobic exercise on its own doesn't make a lot of difference to the amount of muscle we have, or its strength. This can make a great difference to how much one can engage with the ordinary activities of daily living, like doing the shopping or climbing stairs. While most people associate this sort of training with gyms and fitness studios, it is actually not difficult or expensive to do this at home, using simple things like stretching bands or heavy objects from around the house. Sometimes, the help of a partner or other family member can be required; it is also a good way to spend time together. Others might want to invest in some equipment to keep in a spare room; a lot of gym equipment is available these days at reasonable prices, sometimes as an all-in-one machine. Alternatively, many MS societies offer just these facilities for their members, often with some experienced instructors on hand to guide the program.

Ideally, this strength training should be done two or three times a week, in addition to the aerobic exercise. In any one session, it is impor-tant not to overdo things, particularly at the beginning, exerting oneself at around 50–70 per cent of what would be considered maximal exertion, and repeating the movement twelve to fifteen times, with a break of at least a minute between these repetitions. At the beginning, it is best just to do one round of these repetitions for each major muscle group, doing both lower and upper body if possible. With time and increasing strength, one can add more rounds.

Other exercise issues

For those who struggle with the heat, and find that exercise worsens their symptoms because they heat up, there are a number of options. I prefer to swim in an outdoor pool at around 26–28°C, getting my exercise and sun in the one session and avoiding the problems that many people get with the MS symptoms worsening when they get hot. This would also fit nicely into Professor Russell's notion that exercise in the lying down position is the best form.[24]

Others may find that tailoring the particular exercise to the weather helps. For instance, on very cool days one might choose to go running or walking. On warmer days, one might choose swimming in a pool or walking on a treadmill in an air-conditioned gym. Others have found that ice vests are helpful for keeping cool when doing vigorous aerobic exercise, particularly on hot days.

One thing that has helped my exercise program is to set exercise goals. Not long after being diagnosed with MS, I set myself the goal of running the Perth City to Surf annually. This is a 12-kilometre run from Perth city to the coast. Many thousands of people do it each year, including many people with disabilities. Having the goal four months away at that stage was a great motivator. It also got my son, now in his twenties but twelve years old at the time, involved in his first ever City to Surf.

Setting goals can help with the motivation to exercise regularly.

OVERVIEW

Overall, exercise forms an important part of the OMS Recovery Program. There is clear evidence that regular, vigorous exercise has many beneficial effects on health in general, including better quality of life and mood, improved memory and cognitive function, and reduced depression, and the evidence suggests that it has similar benefits specifically for PwMS, with less fatigue and potentially some benefit in delaying disease progression. It also has physical benefits in enabling more endurance, and even overcoming some apparent disability.

STEP 4

MEDITATE AND USE THE MIND–BODY CONNECTION

The gift of learning to meditate is the greatest gift you can give yourself in this lifetime.

Sogyal Rinpoche

INTRODUCTION

There is a vast literature on the interaction of the mind and the body, and how this interaction can result in good or poor health. The evidence is scattered through the medical literature, and not easily found or summarised. The literature strongly supports the hypothesis that our mental lives and our physical lives are inextricably linked, for better or for worse. The wonderful film *The Connection* (see <www.theconnection.tv>),

216

by filmmaker Shannon Harvey, has popularised many of these ideas. Central to this mind–body connection are the harmful effects of certain types of stress for most people, particularly PwMS, and the beneficial effects of a sense of empowerment and the practice of meditation.

WHY

In a nutshell

- Stress triggers MS relapses, so managing stress is very important for preventing MS disease activity.
- Being proactive and empowered to be the captain of your own health ship is a key ingredient in recovering from MS.
- A vital first step to empowerment is finding hope.
- Meditation helps recovery by reducing negative reactions to stress and shifting the immune balance to a Th2 response.
- HOLISM data show that people with MS who meditate have a better quality of life than those who don't.

Stress

Our bodies are programmed to respond to stressful stimuli in our lives in a particular way. In response to a sudden dangerous event, like a vicious dog running towards us, our bodies activate the so-called fight or flight response (see Figure 12). Through secretion of chemicals like adrenaline and direct nervous system effects, this response activates our

Figure 12: Triggering the fight or flight response

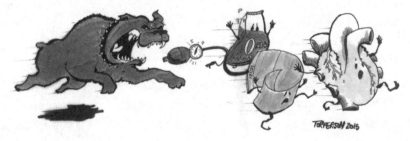

sympathetic nervous system so that our heart rate speeds up, our blood pressure rises, the blood vessels to our muscles open up and blood starts pumping through our bodies much faster, getting us ready to fight, or to run away. The chemicals secreted in this response make us more alert, so that we can appreciate the danger and calculate our possible responses more quickly, and trigger an immune response, resulting in activation of inflammation and thickening of our blood, so that if we are injured we can stop bleeding and heal more quickly.

This is a very useful response in the context of a clear danger, such as a vicious dog. Unfortunately, in today's world this response is triggered many, many times a day in situations where there is no vicious dog, and no reason to fight or flee. Someone pulls out in front of us in traffic, a friend or relative gets angry with us, or any of a wide range of other stimuli can equally trigger the fight or flight response, and do so on a regular basis, throughout the days and weeks of our lives. Now this constantly triggered fight or flight response is no longer useful—in fact, it is highly counter-productive. If we are sitting in our cars with adrenaline flowing through our bodies, with our immune systems activated, our blood sticky and so on, over and over again, it is obvious that our bodies will increasingly be damaged by this response that was once so useful to us. Worse still, there is evidence that even when we get out of the traffic, arrive home and try to relax, our bodies don't resume their baseline relaxed state so easily. We usually assign the term 'stress' to this build-up of stimuli that continually trigger this fight or flight response. In fact, over 40 years ago, scientists discovered a contrary response—the relaxation response—that needs to be practised and cultivated in order to balance out the harmful effects of the fight or flight response.[1]

Stress and MS

In terms of primary prevention, there has long been speculation that stress can trigger the development of MS in susceptible people—that is, those with a genetic background predisposing them to the illness. One population-based case-control study from the Karolinska Institute examined many thousands of PwMS and compared their patterns of shiftwork while young to those of people without MS.[2] They found a

30–60 per cent increased risk of MS for those who undertook shift-work at a young age; for those doing significant amounts of shiftwork before age twenty, there was roughly a doubling of risk. The authors hypothesised that this may be due to sleep disruption causing changes in melatonin secretion and a shift towards a pro-inflammatory state.

With respect to secondary prevention, there has also long been a view that stress may precipitate relapses in MS. It is well known that major life events like marriage breakdown, moving house, losing or changing jobs, and losing close friends or loved ones may have a profound effect on our general well-being. Good research now confirms that, for PwMS, major stressful life events—or, more particularly, our reaction to them—often trigger MS relapses. Scientists have summarised basic molecular and animal experimental research, as well as human clinical and epidemiological studies, showing that stress can precipitate relapses and worsening disability through a variety of mechanisms, including an 'overshooting' of the inflammatory response, and through worsening degeneration.[3]

There is clear evidence that major stressful life events trigger relapses in MS.

In the context of the immune system balance of Th1 versus Th2 cytokines that is intimately involved in the development of relapses in PwMS, it has been shown that stressful events like students' final examinations can significantly increase one of the known Th1 cytokines, tumour necrosis factor alpha (TNF-alpha) levels.[4] Literature reviews on the effects of stress for PwMS have concluded that stressful life events are associated with relapses and the subsequent development of brain lesions.[5] It has been noted that acute short-term stressors generally cause no problems. In contrast, longer term stressors such as interpersonal conflicts, loss and complicated grief, poor social support, anxiety and depression are risk factors for MS relapses.[6]

One study followed 50 women with MS on a weekly basis, looking at the occurrence of major life events such as those listed above, and their MS disease activity.[7] Nearly half of all major life events were followed within six weeks by a relapse. Relapses were, however, more common in those people who were more clearly affected by the events, as demonstrated by a higher resting heart rate and blood pressure. Another study of 73 PwMS from an MS clinic showed that, during the study period, 70 experienced major stressful events. Stress resulted in a more than doubling of the relapse rate over the following four weeks.[8]

A unique study from Israel looked at the development of relapses in PwMS who were exposed to rocket attacks on civilian centres in northern Israel during the 2006 war between Hezbollah and Israel.[9] The researchers clearly showed that there was a major increase in the number of relapses for these people during the 33 days of the war compared with the periods both before and after it. Another study looked at women with MS for over a year, noting the number and type of stressful life events they had and their subsequent risk of relapses.[10] Experiencing three or more stresses during a four-week period caused a five-fold increase in the MS relapse rate. Having at least one stressful event associated with psychological effects lasting over two weeks was associated with three times the rate of MS relapses during the following four weeks. This study is strong evidence of the association between stress and relapses in MS because it was studied prospectively, not in hindsight.

Another study correlated the development of new MRI lesions in PwMS with stressful life events. After major life stresses, people were roughly 60 per cent more likely to develop a new lesion in the next eight weeks.[11] This study noted that those with good coping mechanisms could reduce this risk.[12] Another study asked participants about stressful life events, categorising them as negative or positive.[13] This was in recognition of the fact that many stresses are perceived by the individual as positive, particularly where the person has some control over the event and it is meaningful.

For instance, breaking up with a partner can be seen as positive or negative, depending on the type of relationship and who instigated the break-up; a court case can be seen as positive or negative depending on the outcome, and so on. The researchers found that major negative stressful life events resulted in nearly 80 per cent more new MRI lesions over the subsequent four to nine weeks, and around 60 per cent more new or enlarging T2 lesions (the so-called black holes that are closely associated with worsening disability). Perhaps the surprising part of the study was that positive stressful life events had a protective effect; those who experienced a positive event had about half the number of new contrast-enhancing lesions on MRI.

Stressful life events can be negative, with harmful effects, but also positive, with some protective effect.

This study is important not only because it reinforces the causative effect of negative stressful life events on worsening MS disease activity, but also because it highlights the fact that stressful events can be both positive and negative, with positive stressful events actually providing some protection. This is critical information, as one of the goals of the OMS Recovery Program is to get healthy and to be able to fully engage with life again, with all its ups and downs. The term 'stress' is often thrown around indiscriminately, but this study reminds us that we can live life to the fullest extent, and go through significant personal crises, but that the quality of the stress and its meaning to us are the important factors in determining whether the stress is helpful or harmful to our health. It reinforces the notion that, for people overcoming MS, it is important to change jobs, relationships and circumstances if these are proving negative in our lives. While changing these things can be perceived as stressful, and cause concern about possible health consequences, in fact these changes can be very helpful and improve our chances of staying well or recovering.

So, given the pivotal damaging role of stress in MS, it is critical that PwMS find ways to better manage stress. Possibilities include a more proactive approach, using meditation to develop a less reactive response to stress—effectively using it as a form of stress prevention. They also include finding better ways of coping with stress once it has been experienced, such as keeping a diary, using counselling or group work to better understand and integrate stressful events into our lives, and developing a stronger social support network to help buffer the effects of stress on our lives.

Empowerment

The concept of empowerment is an important one to explore for PwMS aiming to do as much as they can to get control of the illness, and ultimately to start on the road to recovery. Empowerment goes by many names in the medical literature, such as self-efficacy, locus of control and patient activation. In a health context, it essentially means a process whereby people gain control over their own health. In the literature on patient empowerment, it has been described as both a process and an outcome: 'a process to increase one's ability to think critically and act autonomously . . . an outcome when an enhanced sense of self-efficacy occurs as a result of the process'.[14] This is distinguished from a person simply becoming more compliant with the directions of their healthcare provider, although greater adherence to physician recommendations is also a likely outcome of greater empowerment.

In simple terms, empowerment really means becoming the captain of one's own ship. It means that, through our own efforts, actions and changes, we not only get back a sense of controlling our own health destiny, but also see tangible improvements in our health as a result of our own actions. The whole notion of empowerment fits very neatly into the area of preventive medicine, which is also about modifying health and lifestyle behaviours to change health outcomes.

One aim of the OMS Recovery Program is to become captain of your own health ship.

A critical point here is the attitudinal shift that happens for people when they start to become more proactive in their pursuit of health and control over the illness, as opposed to being simply the passive recipients of healthcare. Some people call this positivity, or a positive outlook, but it is much more than that. By becoming the captain of one's own ship, and making decisions for oneself about all aspects of health, including what to eat, how much exercise to do, how much sun exposure to get, how to eliminate risky behaviours like smoking, and being actively involved in stress reduction, but also deciding on whether to take medications and which medications to take, the whole situation changes for a person with MS.

In recent years, there has been a paradigm shift in the management of chronic diseases towards a patient-centred approach to self-management and prevention. People who are proactive in their health achieve better outcomes than those taking a more passive approach. Studies measuring empowerment have found positive associations with a range of benefits, including healthy lifestyle behaviours, better quality of life and functional status, fewer health visits and decreased depressive symptoms, among others.[15, 16, 17] For PwMS, increasing empowerment predicts improvements in walking ability and physical and psychological impact of MS.[18] Higher levels of empowerment are also associated with lower depression scores and better quality of life.[19] Recent research has shown that empowerment positively affects cognitive function in PwMS, and that preventing disease activity helps preserve this sense of empowerment.[20] These benefits can be critical not only to how people with MS or any other disease perceive their lives, but also to the actual progress of the physical illness—given that we know that depression, for example, not only worsens quality of life, but also exacerbates the level of physical illness, with a more rapid rate of progression for PwMS who are depressed.

People with a greater sense of control over the illness, representing the sense of empowerment that proactive patients experience, have better understanding of their condition, often a more balanced and better relationship with their health provider, and better outcomes. So not only do people who become more empowered feel better about themselves and their futures, and are therefore less likely to develop depression and fatigue, but they are also more likely to make the necessary lifestyle modifications to influence the course of the illness, and thus get the physical benefits of the OMS Recovery Program as well.

Gaining a sense of empowerment also makes active engagement with other like-minded people in similar situations and with similar outlooks more likely, resulting in empowered people finding the social and emotional support they need from interacting with other PwMS with whom they can relate their health experiences. It has been shown that social support is a significant predictor of quality of life,[21] and having more positive experiences, including those that promote physical and mental health or involve social interaction, is associated with better quality of life and fewer depressive symptoms.[22] This reinforces a person's hope for the future, and having greater hope is thought to improve one's ability to adjust to or cope with MS.[23]

There is considerable literature on the positive effects of people having a feeling of control over their illness. Dr Bernie Siegel, a US cancer surgeon, has written a number of books that are rich with stories about people he has seen who have transformed themselves and overcome serious illness because they were active, positive participants in the process. Bernie describes the survivors of serious illness as people who, on learning of the diagnosis, actively seek out information, look for people to talk to who have overcome such illness, question their doctors about alternatives and generally become what doctors think of as 'difficult' patients. This is one of the reasons I am so keen on a preventive medicine approach to the management of MS and other chronic Western diseases. People have to be actively involved in their own health and empowered to make the healthy lifestyle choices that form the core of this approach.

Sadly, empowerment is often somewhat overlooked in many traditional healthcare settings. Many PwMS attending their doctors for advice and assistance often feel like patients, passive and uninvolved in their own care. This makes for much worse health outcomes. Finding a good doctor who understands the importance of a more balanced relationship, with the person with MS at the centre of the interaction, can be crucial in ensuring the best possible health outcome. In Australia and New Zealand, the Australasian College of Nutritional and Environmental Medicine (ACNEM, see <www.acnem.org>) is an organisation of doctors trained in integrative medicine. Under their Find a Practitioner directory, one can find doctors who understand the importance of particularly nutrition, but also exercise, meditation and so on to health outcomes. Many people find this a useful site to visit to find a local doctor with the right background to enter into a useful partnership to give themselves the best chance of having an empowering relationship with their healthcare provider, and hence the best possible health outcome. There are likely to be similar organisations in other parts of the world.

But the first step to gaining some control over the illness, to becoming empowered, is to find hope—hope that it is possible to influence the course of the illness.

Hope

In a number of media interviews I have done about the OMS Recovery Program, interviewers have asked questions about whether the whole notion of recovery from MS is giving people 'false hope'. Dr Bernie Siegel, a cancer surgeon who works in New Haven, Connecticut, has written much about this. I recommend his books to those looking for hope. Bernie has convinced me that there is no such thing as false hope. There is only 'false no hope'. While statistics help us describe the outcome for a particular group of patients, they are quite useless for any individual patient. There are always those who do better and those who do worse than the statistics. There are always extraordinary survivors, no matter how bleak the outcome or how advanced the disease. We can always have real hope that we will have a similar course. This is especially true for MS, which is such a variable disease. We know that there is a group of people who do very well—those with so-called benign MS. At the very least, why shouldn't we hope that we will be one of these people? How much better is it for someone to live positively in hope than negatively in depression, when there is a real possibility that they won't deteriorate.

Much more than that, though, in reality the evidence presented in this book and elsewhere clearly indicates that lifestyle modification has a profound effect on disease course in MS. Making the necessary changes acts in its own right to improve quality of life and reduce depression through the sense of empowerment it brings; it not only positively affects MS disease course, but also reduces the risk of other chronic Western diseases like high blood pressure, diabetes and heart disease. It is more than a win–win situation; it is a win–win–win situation! This provides more than enough reason for PwMS to have real genuine hope for their futures.

Researchers have shown one of the principal reasons for chronic sorrow in PwMS is their loss of hope.[24] The problem with telling someone that the usual outcome in MS is significant disability is that it may then become a self-fulfilling prophecy. The doctor's relationship with the patient is charged with such authority that patients usually do their best to please their doctors; patients will often live out exactly the prescription they have been given. This 'false no hope' takes away our genuine hope, weakens our resolve and literally takes away some of our power to heal the illness. It defeats the human spirit to take this away from people, in turn leading to loss of empowerment, depression and worsening physical illness.

Hope has, however, been poorly studied in the medical literature. Sadly, the bias against undertaking such research is strong, given the lack of commercial benefit derived from such studies, and the distorting influence of commercialisation on the research agenda in medicine.[25] One important study from psychologists in Queensland, Australia, recruited 296 members of the MS Society of Queensland.[23] The participants completed questionnaires at baseline and again twelve months later. The researchers were interested in how much hope they had, and whether there was a difference in response to stress, and in anxiety, depression and state of mind, between those with high hope and those with low hope. They used established scales to measure these variables.

 Hope has an important protective effect for the health of PwMS.

PwMS with high hope had a more positive state of mind, greater life satisfaction and less depression; hope buffered the effects of high stress, so that under high stress there was an even greater difference in favour of those with high hope, and they were considerably less anxious. The researchers concluded that hope is a potent protective resource for PwMS. Interestingly, they undertook the same study of the caregivers of the participants in this research and found a similar relationship, with hope buffering stress.[26] Importantly, in terms of clinical practice for clinicians managing PwMS, the authors suggested that there are benefits in promoting hope in PwMS. The science is clear: not only is hope important, but it is also important for our doctors to promote hope.

Faith

Faith is a very misunderstood concept. Faith and belief are somewhat different things. Faith doesn't necessarily mean believing in something. Faith is living life as if something is true, as if a desired outcome is actually going to be the outcome. Faith and belief actually form part of a continuum. My friend Siegfried Gutbrodt, Therapeutic Director of the Gawler Foundation, specialises in laughter therapy. Siegfried always tells his audience about the positive effect of laughter on our bodies, about the good chemicals that are released during laughter. But, importantly, he points out that it can be faked. That even if you are not feeling too good but make the effort and have a big laugh, the same chemicals are released. It works too! Try it yourself if you don't believe it. It's amazing how much better you feel after a good laugh, even if you fake it. I use that analogy a little for the concept of faith becoming belief. Faith is a bit like faking it: living life as if something is true but not necessarily believing it to be true. But if you live that way for long enough, you gradually start to believe it, and it gradually starts to happen.

Personally, when I started this regimen of diet, sunlight, meditation and so on to gain control over MS, even though I had seen all the evidence and collated it carefully, I still had to find faith and live as if it was going to work. The sceptical approach of some medical authorities can be very powerful, especially for a traditionally trained doctor. Years of seeing PwMS coming into hospital emergency departments with serious disability and illness can have a profoundly negative effect on one's view of the disease. But as the years of good health have gone on, faith has given way to a growing belief. And, more and more, my belief is reinforced as I see evidence of other PwMS who show faith in their ability to overcome this illness.

One of the ways in which the energy we need to take control over our health can be wasted is when we are consumed with fear. In many respects, fear is the opposite of faith. MS is a frightening disease, particularly when first diagnosed. Most of us want to live a long, healthy life. So often we hear people say, 'I hope I drop dead with a heart attack' or, 'I hope I die in my sleep after a healthy life'. The fear of incapacity and a long, drawn-out demise is very distressing for most people. Yet that is precisely what comes to mind when given a diagnosis of MS. Suddenly the wheelchair comes into view, and being fed, and catheters. But most people, when told, are comparatively well. It makes no sense to spend some of the precious time we have now, when we are well, consumed with worry about what might be if and when we are not well. Worse, using that energy worrying robs us of the energy we need to make the necessary changes in our lives, to become empowered. Similarly, for those of us who have significant disability, it is important to live life as if we can make a difference to the course of the disease, to have faith that we can stabilise the illness and even recover some of our lost function. That is not wishful thinking; the evidence presented in this book strongly supports it.

 The antidote to fear is faith.

My great mentor, Dr Ian Hislop, captured it perfectly when he said, 'The principle is straightforward. You have to replace fear with faith. Faith in yourself, your future, and perhaps in something which transcends both.' It is interesting how often people facing serious illness or death come to similar conclusions.

Using the mind–body connection

The mind–body connection is one of the most interesting but least understood areas in medicine. In six years of medical school, I learnt all about disease, micro-organisms and the treatments we, as doctors, could give to patients to help them get better. To a much lesser extent, I learnt about how patient factors could predispose them to illness, and how various lifestyles and behaviours put people at risk of acquiring certain diseases. What was conspicuously absent was any discussion or study of the complex interplay between people's emotions, personalities and lives and the diseases to which they are predisposed, and what patients themselves can do about disease once they have developed it. In effect, there was a lot of discussion about cures, but little about healing.

Yet for most of the history of medicine, this has not been so. For previous generations of doctors, who had few effective resources with which to treat disease, there was a strong emphasis on patient factors in disease. Great medical minds of prior times were convinced that patients held the key to their recovery from illness. But today's doctors, surrounded by a vast array of technological wonders and marvellous drug therapies, have lost sight of just how important the patient is in determining recovery from illness.

The patient's influence on illness

Emotions play a very significant role in the development of illness. Dr Bernie Siegel describes the years he spent trying to keep a detached, impersonal relationship with his surgical patients, before realising this was doing neither the patients nor himself any good. He then began ECaP, a group for exceptional cancer patients. Unlike 'traditional' cancer surgeons, he actively encouraged his patients to look everywhere for ways to heal, to explore every possibility, to become 'active' participants in their healing. In his book, *Love, Medicine and Miracles*, which every doctor should read, he describes what it is that sets apart these people who recover from serious illness.[27] In general, they find the illness both a challenge and an opportunity for personal growth. They tackle the illness actively, rather than being passive recipients of doctors' treatments. They go to every source for information, are open-minded about possibilities, try everything that has a reasonable chance of success. They feel empowered by the discoveries they make to take control of their illnesses—and, indeed, their lives.

These are difficult ways for a conventionally trained doctor to respond to illness. To illustrate this, as Bernie says, imagine the different responses to this situation. A woman comes into a lecture theatre full of medical students. She describes how she was diagnosed with terminal cancer with secondaries everywhere just a few months ago, but says the latest scans show she is better, that there are no more lesions. The students will be filled with awe, and ask how the patient did it, what she tried and so on. Imagine the room is full of doctors, particularly those who have been qualified for some time. The responses will be very different. They will suggest that the original pathology reports must have been mixed up with someone else's, that the scans must have been switched, that the tumour must have been benign. They will do almost anything rather than remain open to the possibility that this illness has been healed. What makes us become so closed-minded? Where do we lose our openness to such ideas?

There is a significant movement in medicine away from the conventional parentalistic view of impersonal doctors treating passive recipients of their care: patients who don't argue or say what they want and who are therefore not empowered to tackle the changes they must make to improve their outcome from disease. Visionary physicians like Deepak Chopra and Bernie Siegel lead this revolution. They understand what potential we have within us for modifying the course of disease, if only we choose to and are encouraged to use it.

Illness as a challenge

Serious illness is viewed by many who survive it as a challenge. Yet many come to regard it as a gift. Like other challenges in life, out of the kernel of the problem may come wonderful insights and answers that transform our lives. For those of us with MS and cancer and many other serious diseases, it is worth remembering that the illness is part of us. In many ways, the analogy that is often used of a fight or a battle against an invader just doesn't fit with this basic tenet. It doesn't make sense to fight yourself: it just empowers the illness. It is more useful to see MS as representing a complex system that is out of balance, and to understand that our lifestyle changes will tip the balance away from inflammation to a more calm, anti-inflammatory setting.

> Our reaction to illness is very important in determining the outcome of the illness; the outcome is not arbitrary or a matter of chance.

We have extraordinary power over how our bodily cells behave. If we get anxious and our blood pressure rises, we lower our heart rate to compensate. We don't have to do it consciously—indeed most of us can't do it consciously. If we get too cold, we start our muscles shivering to generate heat. Similarly, if we are infected with a virus, we mobilise our immune system to fight the invader and almost always win. When we break a bone, we don't have to tell our body how to heal itself. Built into the DNA in every cell in our bodies is the blueprint for fixing itself when things go wrong, for developing into an adult, for producing children.

But our bodies need help. Our mind is actually the key player here. Our mind both sets the intention for the actions we undertake in making changes to our unhealthy lifestyle behaviours and holds the key to the attitude we have, to our reaction to stressful life situations, to our sense of control. The body has a tremendously effective ability to heal when it is in balance. The difficulty is to overcome the normal tendency of our minds to chatter aimlessly, to ruminate over the past, to be fearful and project and fantasise about the future, and instead use the mind–body connection to allow the normal state of balance in our bodies to be facilitated. This is where meditation and mindfulness come in.

Freeing the mind from its usual preoccupations is important. A variety of tools can help, with meditation at the forefront. Other techniques, such as expressing our difficult emotions through counselling, keeping a diary or attending a group, can help to free up our very powerful subconscious mind from its frequent preoccupation with unresolved conflicts and suppressed anger and grief in order to enable it to help deal with disease. The key to understanding this is realising that, apart from setting the intention to change habits and behaviours, the conscious mind does not have the power to heal us.

The late Dr Wayne Dyer has written much about the conscious mind actually being insane, because it believes it is something it is not.[28] It believes it is the body, the accomplishments of a person, the history of a person. The conscious mind deals in thoughts. Every minute of every day, we have a never-ending stream of thoughts passing through our minds. If we are focused on a particular problem, the thoughts may be centred around finding a solution, perhaps working through alternatives. More often than not, if we stop to actively listen to the thoughts, they are nonsense. There may be a strain of some song we have recently heard, playing along in front of an imaginary conversation with someone we have seen earlier or are about to see later.

These constant thoughts rob us of the energy we need for healing. We waste that energy dealing in the abstract with countless unimportant matters we think about over and over again. Serious illness demands that we focus our available energy in the present, on healing ourselves. Most of what is happening in the conscious mind distracts us from actually being present in the now, in the present moment. Being centred in the present moment actually requires some effort and some commitment. It is all about being mindful of the distractions that constantly pull us away from the moment.

Living in the moment

The present moment is all we have. Many people are locked into a lifetime of thoughts and inner struggles about things that have long since passed, or will never happen. As Mark Twain said, 'I've lived through some terrible things in my life, some of which actually happened.' Yet those constant thoughts and preoccupations would have no existence, except for the fact that they are being thought by the thinker. If the thinker wasn't present right now, none of it would exist. This is very powerful stuff to consider for those people who feel that the past controls their lives. Many people feel that they would be better people, or far better able to cope, or less anxious, if only certain things in the past hadn't happened. For instance, some blame their parents for not loving them sufficiently, or for always criticising them. This is often still the case many years after the parents are gone. But the only reason the parents' actions still exist in any sense is because of the thoughts that person is thinking *in the present moment*.

> The present moment is all we will ever have; it is important to live in that moment.

Wayne Dyer has a useful metaphor for those who see themselves as slaves of their past. See yourself as a ship on the ocean, looking down from above. Behind the boat stretches the wake. Is it possible for the wake to be driving the ship? No, it is just the history being left behind. The power to drive the ship lies within the ship itself.

On reflection, time is an illusion. Over the years, humans have become more and more sophisticated at measuring time exactly. The concept of what a person would be doing at 3.00 pm on a given day next week would have meant absolutely nothing to Stone Age people. Now, with superannuation and booking ahead for holidays and diaries full of appointments, we have come to believe in time as a very real thing—so much so that we spend much of the present moment either in the future or the past, or both, planning or worrying about what is going to happen or analysing or trying to work out what we should have done in situations that have already happened. We have precious little time left to be experiencing the present.

But in reality, now is all we will ever have. Even at the moment we lie on our deathbeds preparing to depart this life, we will still be in the present moment. How much of it will we have wasted before then by not being centred and present in the moment as we live? Excessive thinking gradually removes us from the present moment by dulling our senses to what is really going on in our lives. The antidote to excessive thinking is to concentrate on feeling and sensing our physical bodies again in the present moment—to literally come to our senses. This is where the technique of progressive muscle relaxation (PMR) is of great benefit. As an introduction to meditation, it is really good for relaxation but more importantly, because the focus of concentration is on how the physical body is feeling, it helps to centre us again in our bodies, and hence helps us to live in the present moment. It has been shown to be of value for PwMS in a UK study.[29]

Very early on, after being diagnosed with MS, when I was battling mentally to come to terms with it, I started focusing on where I wanted to get to with all the changes I was making. Diet, meditation, exercise, sunlight, visualisation—what was the aim of all of these things? The aim, I realised, was to keep myself the same as I am now. That is, my end-point was identical to the process I was going through every day. What I was aiming at was not some distant future goal: I had my aim already. I was already fit, active and had essentially no disability, and I was living life in a healthy, balanced way after many years of poor balance in my life. That was the very outcome I was after. I was already there.

This was a revelation in many respects. The whole trick was to ensure that I was living life to the full every day and enjoying the present moment, not concentrating on some far-distant goal. If I did things right, that would take care of itself. I realised that every day is an end in itself. The process is the outcome. I hung these two messages on my study wall, 'Every day is an end in itself' and 'The process is the outcome'.

They remind me, when I forget as we all do, to stay centred in the present moment.

Subconscious issues

Sometimes the continuous mind babble that we all have keeps returning to a theme. It might be how we have been harshly treated by a friend, or how we were hurt in a particular relationship. This indicates that, at a deeper level in the subconscious, we have not resolved an important issue in our lives. The subconscious mind is very powerful. Until we satisfactorily resolve such issues, it will keep returning to the problem. This may not happen consciously—although it often does—but may take the form of dreams around a certain theme. Worse, it may manifest as illness. To have the necessary energy to heal the illness, we have to heal the underlying problem in our subconscious. To marshal all our energies to deal with the illness, we have to resolve those underlying issues so that the energy is ours again to deal with the illness.

Carolyn Myss shows in *Anatomy of the Spirit* how these destructive patterns develop, and how we can resolve some of these issues. Just by being aware of these mechanisms, we may liberate enough energy to begin dealing with the problems. Mainstream researchers are starting to explore this area too. A major review of the brain–immune function connection in MS noted that psychological factors like mood and cognition exert a modulating effect on the immune system in MS.[30]

My great mentor, Dr Ian Hislop, started me off on the process of understanding the importance of unresolved issues when he mentored me as a young medical intern. Then, when I was diagnosed with MS, he helped me to start tackling issues that I had left unresolved. The first part of the process is to quiet the conscious mind enough to begin to get in touch with the subconscious. This is one value of meditation. Some prefer other methods of quieting the mind: yoga, tai chi, playing music, gardening—all may be helpful, depending on personal preferences. Until the mind slows down, though, and leaves enough gaps in the constant stream of mental chatter, the issues bubbling up from our subconscious remain elusive. While music or gardening may be helpful for quieting the mind, they are only really capable of slowing it a little.

Often, there is a background of chatter going on in the mind when one is doing these things. Meditation is the most helpful way of slowing the mind.

An important part of using the mind–body connection to facilitate healing is to trust instincts and feelings. Many people who take the time to quieten the mind and reflect after a serious diagnosis realise that they need to attend to important unfinished business. It is important to listen carefully to the immediate gut-level reactions that occur when first hit with the shock of serious illness. Later, when things have settled down, it may be much easier and more comfortable not to confront the things that were instinctively felt to be in need of sorting out. But they have to be confronted.

Another important ingredient is to learn to let go. Part of the development of faith is to learn to relinquish control, and just go with what is happening and what you are feeling and trust that things will work out. In the words of Bill Harris of Centerpoint Technology, 'Let whatever's happening be okay.' Part of this is to learn to let go of past resentments, removing their ability to still have power over you. Forgiveness is an interesting virtue. While, at face value, it may seem that the act of forgiving has a lot of benefit in it for the person being forgiven, the forgiver benefits greatly from forgiving. In many respects, it is a win–win situation. Forgiveness may not just be about working out grievances from the past and working actively to seek reconciliation; rather, it is something to be practised as a daily exercise. Just as we get back energy from forgiving those against whom we harbour negative feelings from the past, so we lose energy beginning the process anew every day.

Meditation

Meditation is a key part of healing from any disease. To heal, the body needs to be in a state of balance to allow its natural healing mechanisms to operate. Stress—most particularly our negative reactions and responses to stress—upsets this balance, and has been shown in many studies to worsen MS. Meditation can help us to achieve that balance. One review of published studies on meditation in MS found that positive effects of meditation included improved quality of life and coping skills,[31] but there seems little doubt that it can also affect the progression of the disease through its modulating effect on stress.

Slowing the mind is the correct physiological term for what actually happens in meditation. Normal brainwave recordings show many low-amplitude waves of a frequency of greater than twelve cycles per second, termed beta waves, together with waves of eight to twelve cycles per second, termed alpha waves. As meditation proceeds, or as we get into reflective states while listening to music or gardening, the frequency slows (see Figure 13). This is the state we reach early in meditation, or when we are in that focused attention state—like when we are watching a movie, and other things are blocked out. For most people, this is where most meditation happens. In deeper alpha states, we reach a twilight state—like just drifting off to sleep—and the frequency drops further. This state is good for learning, and people feel very relaxed.

As meditation deepens, the brainwave frequency slows further to between four and eight cycles per second, becoming theta waves. This

Figure 13: Meditation slows brain waves

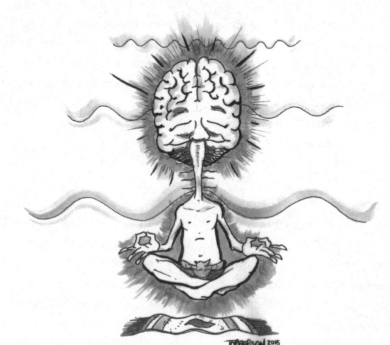

is the brainwave pattern associated with dreaming during rapid eye movement (REM) sleep. It is also associated with visionary experiences, enhanced creativity and sudden breakthroughs. Some experienced meditators get down to this level without difficulty.

As the brain quiets even further, the wave pattern continues to slow and grow in amplitude until we are experiencing waves that are large, but below four cycles per second. This is the delta wave pattern, and it represents the subconscious mind. By now, the brainwaves are very large and slow. This is the state of deep dreamless sleep, but if it is experienced with awareness, as during meditation, there is an intense feeling of oneness and connection with the underlying energy of life. Mystics and very experienced meditators describe this state in detail, and clearly have experienced it. Getting into this awareness of the subconscious mind can throw up all sorts of emotional difficulties, as long-buried issues surface into conscious awareness. But, as a result, it also has the potential to be very healing.

 Meditation has many beneficial effects for those with chronic illness, particularly auto-immune disease.

Meditation is particularly important for those with chronic illness. The evidence for the benefits of meditation on health is enormous and growing rapidly. One review showed that there was clear evidence of benefit for epilepsy, premenstrual syndrome, menopausal symptoms, mood and anxiety disorders, auto-immune illness and emotional disturbance in cancer patients.[32] Given the difficulties associated with proof in medicine, it is likely that meditation is helpful for considerably more conditions. Others find alternatives to meditation that may be just as effective. Researchers have shown, for instance, that music therapy improves acceptance and reduces anxiety and depression in PwMS.[33]

One study found that people who meditate regularly find it easier to cope with pain because their brains anticipate the pain less.[34] Comparing non-meditators with meditators with varying levels of experience, brain scans showed that the most advanced meditators were the least likely to anticipate pain produced by a laser, making the experience more bearable. The meditators had unusual activity in the brain region that controls attention and thought processes when potential threats are perceived. The lead researcher, Dr Chris Brown, said, 'Meditation trains the brain to be more present-focused and therefore to spend less time anticipating future negative events.' This fits neatly with the previous comments on the process being the outcome, and learning to stay grounded in the present moment rather than in future imaginings.

An important study on PwMS from Switzerland showed that an eight-week course of mindfulness training improved quality of life and reduced depression compared with a control group receiving usual care.[35] Mindfulness training is one of the most common forms of meditation practised, incorporating non-judgemental awareness of moment-to-moment experience. The trial clearly showed a benefit for all measures studied, including quality of life, depression, fatigue and anxiety. Mindfulness training was especially helpful for those who had problems with depression, fatigue and anxiety before the trial, suggesting that for those PwMS who are experiencing these problems, this is a very worthwhile treatment to try. The paper also discussed the important concepts of acceptance and courage, reinforcing the importance of the mind–body connection in healing.

Another important study from London examined the effects of mindfulness training in 40 people with primary or secondary MS.[36] To date, as we have seen, many authorities contend that there are few effective therapies for this group. The researchers randomly allocated them to an eight-week course in mindfulness training, or remaining on the waiting list for such training—that is, with no mindfulness training. The mindfulness training was actually delivered via Skype, not even face to face. The study showed a strong effect of mindfulness training in reducing distress, but also in reducing fatigue, pain, depression, anxiety and the impact of MS on the lives of the people in the treatment group. The effect persisted and actually increased at the three-month follow up. The authors concluded that such treatment improved outcome and was highly likely to reduce healthcare costs for these people.

A systematic review of the research evidence underpinning specific health interventions used to make a difference to quality of life for

PwMS found that self-management produces a definite improvement in quality of life.[37] These self-management approaches included health promotion education and chronic disease self-management courses. The medications tested in these studies were those intended to treat specific MS symptoms, not disease-modifying drugs like the interferons. The study showed that these medications also have a small but significant benefit on quality of life, particularly levetiracetam for control of neuropathic pain. Cognitive training had a moderate effect on quality of life, particularly memory and attention training, as did exercise, with resistance and aerobic training having the biggest effects. To the surprise of many clinicians, however, psychological interventions had the biggest and most significant effect on quality of life. The interventions included cognitive behaviour therapy and mindfulness meditation. Interestingly, the biggest effect of all the interventions overall was from mindfulness meditation.

Another review paper summarised the medical literature on mind–body medical interventions for PwMS.[38] The researchers examined the results of well-conducted clinical studies in various mind–body modalities for treating PwMS. They found that mindfulness-based meditation had a positive effect on quality of life, fatigue, anxiety and depression. In particular, meditation was associated with stress reduction, a lower rate of poor coping strategies and increased resilience for those with MS. Yoga was helpful for fatigue, and relaxation techniques were shown in good-quality research to improve quality of life. Biofeedback was helpful with bladder incontinence.

Mind–body medicine can be a difficult area to study, as it is impossible to blind participants to the technique when they are required to actively participate; randomised double-blind, placebo-controlled studies are much more applicable to drug therapies, and harder to conduct for these types of interventions. There is also little commercial imperative to conduct such studies, and most research funding in MS still comes from the pharmaceutical or device industries. Nevertheless, it is heartening to see doctors and researchers exploring this important area, and it reinforces the broad-based OMS approach of using mind–body medicine to assist in MS recovery.

HOLISM study findings on meditation

Our HOLISM study also examined the associations of meditation with health in our large international cohort of PwMS.[39] Of around two and a half thousand PwMS doing our study, 2244 completed the questions about meditation. Around half had meditated at least once in the previous year. But over 1000 PwMS in our sample had never meditated—a surprisingly high number given the well-documented benefits in MS of this simple, free therapy. Women, those with higher educational status, those working part-time and older participants were all more likely to have meditated.

Those who meditated at least once a week had considerably better quality of life in terms of mental health (9 per cent better), better cognitive function (10 per cent) and better perception of their own health (13 per cent). Health distress (11 per cent) and emotional well-being (8 per cent) were also significantly better for the meditators. Physical health was significantly better too, but not by as much (6 per cent). Those meditating at least once a week were also around half as likely to screen positive for depression. This is a very important consideration for PwMS, given that half will be diagnosed with depression at some stage during the illness. At any one time, around a quarter of PwMS have depression.[40] Meditation appears to be a really simple way of reducing that risk. The study showed no significant associations of meditation with fatigue or with relapse rate.

Overall, the study added considerable weight to previous randomised controlled studies showing the benefits of meditation for PwMS. Given that it is not an expensive treatment modality, and that it has countless other health benefits, why wouldn't one meditate?

Writing down feelings

There has been little formal study of the benefits of keeping a diary or written expression of feelings on health. The Department of Psychiatry at New York State University published a unique study of 112 patients with chronic asthma or rheumatoid arthritis (RA).[41] Like MS, RA is an auto-immune disease, but the target of the immune system is the joints rather than the nervous system. Asthma is also a disease mediated by the immune system. This was a formal randomised controlled trial where the 'treatment' group was asked to write on just one occasion about the most stressful event of their lives. The 'control' group was asked to write about a neutral topic.

With this simple intervention—that is, getting people to express feelings that may not completely have been released before—the 'treated' patients got better and the others did not. This should not surprise us, but to a sceptical medical community this scientific 'proof' was something of a shock. The magnitude and duration of the effect of this simple one-off expression of feelings was stunning. The RA patients had a 28 per cent reduction in disease severity (this is about the same benefit as derived from interferon and glatiramer in MS), and the asthma patients a 19 per cent improvement in lung function. And this effect persisted for four months after the 'treatment'. Effects of this size and duration are difficult to achieve with drug therapies without producing side-effects. Yet all this was achieved with only one session. Imagine if these people had regularly expressed their feelings.

JAMA (the journal of the American Medical Association) carried a powerful editorial by David Spiegel, a psychiatrist from Stanford University, commenting on the article.[42] Perhaps the most surprising thing about the editorial is that he sounds surprised. Yet there is abundant scientific evidence of the effects of the mind and spirit on illness. Most of us know these things to be so resonant with truth that they require no proof. But the medical community has become sceptical in these days of miraculous drug therapy. This is despite evidence that people are more likely to die after than before their birthdays and holidays, for example.[43] Or evidence that patients with psoriasis (a chronic skin condition) heal faster with meditation training tapes played during treatment than without.[44] Or the abundant literature showing that patients who express their negative feelings[45] or develop a fighting spirit[46] do better in their recovery from cancer. These things have been known for a long time. Spiegel concluded with an interesting point:

Were the authors to have provided similar outcome evidence about a new drug, it is likely that it would be in widespread use within a short time. Why? We would think we understood the mechanism (whether we did or we did not) and there would be a mediating industry to promote its use. Manufacturers of paper and pencils are not likely to push journaling as a treatment addition for the management of asthma and rheumatoid arthritis.

Spiegel finished his editorial by saying, 'In this, and a growing number of studies, it is not simply mind over matter, but it is clear that mind matters.'

Bernie Siegel recommends—not only to people with serious disease but also to everyone—that they start keeping a journal or diary. On the three-month 'anniversary' of being diagnosed with MS, I started mine. We were just coming back from holiday in the south-west of Western Australia, around the well-known Margaret River winery area. I chose the day to start because of the special significance I attached to three months without a relapse. I picked out a nice diary from our favourite general store in Dunsborough. It was purple and had an opening sunflower on the cover. A good symbol, I thought. For some time, I made it a daily ritual to sit down in the evening and write my thoughts about the day. I now do it when I get the feeling that something is going wrong or something major has happened. It helps me to become more in tune with how I am feeling.

The diary has been really helpful to me. I can look back from time to time and see how I was feeling at certain times, see what things helped me stay positive, and so on. Some time ago, I re-read an entry I made about eight months after the diagnosis of MS. I had only just begun regular injections of medication, having made the decision that I should use every avenue open to me to control the illness even though I was not keen on injections. Within weeks of commencing, I started to feel really low. It is clear now, on looking back through the entries I made at the time, that once I started injecting I began feeling like 'a sick patient'. To that point, I had been positive and full of faith and confidence but, paradoxically, the addition of injections to my regime was a powerful psychological blow to my confidence and made me see myself as sick.

The diary really helped, though. I sat down to write one night, and resolved as I was writing that I would let myself get no lower. I drew a little signpost with the date on it (31 December 1999), and a message that this day marked the lowest point of my mood and that from here I would recover. Sure enough, that is what happened.

Depression

One of the potential consequences of stress and lack of empowerment is the development of depression. Depression is very common, being diagnosed in over 50 per cent of PwMS at some time during the course of the disease.[47] One Italian study found that 46 per cent of PwMS in the study had major depressive disorder,[48] and a Norwegian study revealed that 59 per cent of PwMS assessed had depression.[49] An Australian study found higher rates, with two-thirds of surveyed PwMS being depressed.[50] Further, it has also been found in quite a large study that one in four PwMS has unrecognised and undiagnosed symptoms of depression.[51] It has been shown that PwMS who experience depression mostly do not seek medical help or treatment,[52] although in a large Canadian study, 40 per cent of PwMS had been treated with anti-depressants during the study period.[53] In any one year, about one in five PwMS will be diagnosed with depression.[54]

Depression worsens the physical disease in MS.

Researchers have shown that the single most important factor in determining the quality of life of PwMS is not disability or fatigue or work, but the presence or absence of depression.[55] This is supported by a US study that showed depression was the best predictor of quality of life for PwMS, and that cognitive function was the best predictor of ability to work.[56] A major US consensus statement on depression in MS reported that depression was common in MS, had a major negative impact on quality of life, and was under-recognised and under-treated.[57] US researchers have suggested that the key issues influencing depression in MS are social support, coping ability, how people feel about themselves and the illness, and stress.[58]

An important point to note about depression in MS is that the development of depression almost certainly worsens the physical disease by shifting the immune balance towards a Th1 response.[59] Further, it has been shown that treatment of depression corrects this immune disturbance,[59, 60, 61] and so probably slows disease progression. Along with fatigue, depression worsens not only the psychological but also the physical impact of the disease on PwMS.[62]

Researchers have looked at depression in MS and compared it with the incidence of depression in other chronic diseases.[63] They found that depression is a specific feature of MS. That is, while having MS can cause one to get depressed—as can non-specific factors in having a chronic disease in general—there is something very specific about the disease process in MS that makes PwMS much more likely to get depressed. Further, it is not only the physical progression of the illness that increases the distress of PwMS about their health. In fact, the 'invisible' features of MS—such as pain and depression—are much more likely to precipitate health distress than the more visible features.[64]

So avoiding depression takes on a much more important role in the management of this illness than is generally recognised. A Cochrane review of pharmaceutical treatment of depression in MS, however, failed to find any anti-depressant medication that was significantly effective in treating depression for PwMS.[65] While this is of concern, it is important to note that medications are by no means the only treatment option for depression.

 Modifying lifestyle risk factors can help avoid or alleviate depression.

There is clear evidence that lifestyle factors are linked to the development of mood disorders.[66] Yet there is often little consideration of this treatment strategy, and pharmacological and psychological therapies seem to be the treatments most often offered to PwMS.[66] One important randomised controlled trial showed that modification of diet, sun exposure, exercise and sleep patterns was effective in treating depression.[67] Meditation is also a proven treatment for depression in PwMS.[35] Similarly, smoking[68] and lack of social support are risk factors for depression that can potentially be modified.[69, 70] This evidence really suggests that a secondary preventive approach to MS management not only is important for preventing disease progression, but also should become a routine part of prevention and treatment for depression. It is, of course, associated with additional benefits for general health—particularly in reducing the likelihood of other chronic Western diseases such as cardiovascular disease and diabetes.[66, 68, 71] Hope and empowerment are also important factors in avoiding depression.

The omega-3 fatty acids are effective in ensuring optimal cell membrane function and improving the immune system, but they also prevent depression.[72, 73, 74] This is probably also due to a membrane effect on the nerve cells in the brain. Both animal and human work has now shown that fish oil supplementation improves learning. But there is also evidence that low levels of eicosapentanoic acid found in fish and fish oil correlate with depression.[75] There are also data from large population studies that show countries where fish forms a major part of the diet have much lower rates of depression than those where fish is not eaten much. Japan and Taiwan, for example—where fish consumption is the highest in the world—report rates of depression below 1 per cent of the population. West Germany, Canada and New Zealand, where fish-consumption is very low, report rates of 5 per cent or over. One large meta-analysis of 26 studies involving 150,278 participants showed a 17 per cent reduction in depression risk for those in the highest fish-consumption group versus the lowest.[76] There is also evidence from small uncontrolled studies that omega-3 supplements can improve depression. And there is now randomised controlled trial evidence that omega-3 supplements improve depression in people with Parkinson's disease.[77]

As previously discussed, there is good evidence that regular exercise prevents depression. Given its other health benefits, exercise should form part of the health program of everybody who is able to undertake it. There is also long-standing evidence that low vitamin D levels are likely to precipitate or exacerbate depression and poor cognitive function.[78–81] This is a further reason to ensure that PwMS get adequate sun exposure, or take vitamin D supplements if that is not possible. Overall, this evidence strongly supports the secondary preventive approach to the management of depression in PwMS.

HOLISM study results on depression and fatigue

Our HOLISM study sought to clarify these lifestyle associations with depression in PwMS. This was the first major study in the world to examine lifestyle behaviours of PwMS potentially related to depression in detail. We used the Patient Health Questionnaire depression module short version (PHQ-2) to screen for depression risk in our large international sample of PwMS. The PHQ-2 is a shortened form of the PHQ-9 that has shown good validity in studies of PwMS.[82] The PHQ-2 is quite good at predicting major depression with a score $\geq$ 3.[83] This cut-off was used in our analysis as a positive screen for depression risk. Participants were also asked to indicate whether they had a diagnosis of depression, whether they were receiving treatment for it and whether depression limited their daily activities.

We had 2225 participants complete the PHQ-2 in our study, the majority from the United States, Australia and the United Kingdom, with participants overall representing 54 different countries.[84] Around one in five PwMS screened positive for depression. Overall, 19 per cent reported little interest or pleasure in doing things and 15 per cent reported feeling down, depressed or hopeless on more than half of all days or nearly every day—these being the two questions that made up the PHQ-2. Nearly one-third reported depression as a current diagnosis and, of those, 71 per cent reported receiving treatment for it and 39 per cent reported depression limiting their activities. Of the whole sample, 22 per cent were taking a prescription medication for depression. Almost everyone (93 per cent) who had this positive screening test for depression showed up as being significantly fatigued on our Fatigue Severity Scale.

PwMS who had never smoked had the lowest depression risk, with increasing risk for former smokers and greatest risk for current smokers. Those with moderate alcohol intake had significantly lower depression risk than those with low alcohol intake. Increasing levels of exercise were associated with decreasing depression risk. Taking a vitamin D supplement was associated with reduced depression risk; taking 5000 IU or more daily was associated with the least risk. PwMS who took omega-3s had a significantly lower depression risk, with those taking flaxseed oil having greater reduction than those supplementing with fish oil. More frequent fish consumption was associated with decreasing depression risk. Meditation was associated with lower depression risk, but only for those who meditated once or more per week.

Depression risk increased with increasing social isolation, but was only significant for those with very marked social isolation (no or one support person). Obese people had significantly greater risk of depression than those with a normal BMI. An increasingly poor diet was associated with increasing depression risk. Interestingly, those taking interferon had roughly 60 per cent higher risk of depression than those not taking a disease-modifying drug, whereas there was no increased risk of depression with the other medications.

This study demonstrated strong associations between the lifestyle factors in the OMS Recovery Program and the risk of depression. Diet, smoking, exercise, omega-3 supplementation (particularly flaxseed oil), fish consumption, social support, vitamin D supplementation, BMI, alcohol intake, meditation and choice of medication are important modifiable factors in depression risk for PwMS, and also strongly affect physical health and disease progression. There were no surprises in this study. All of the factors I have advocated for over fifteen years in the OMS Recovery Program were again shown to be important factors for preventing depression. It is important for clinicians and PwMS to be aware of the wide range of modifiable lifestyle factors that may reduce depression risk as part of a comprehensive secondary preventive medical approach to managing MS.

This was ground-breaking research. The study, led by psychiatrist Dr Keryn Taylor who also facilitates OMS retreats in Australia and the United Kingdom, will influence the management of PwMS globally. It has been common practice to accept that PwMS are at much higher risk of depression than other people, and to begin treatment with anti-depressants should a person with MS get depressed. This research opens up the important avenue of prevention; attending to these modifiable lifestyle risk factors raises the possibility of avoiding depression in the first place. Fortunately, in other parts of the HOLISM study, the very same risk factors have been shown to also be associated with better quality of life and reduced disease activity. The paper was the 'Editor's Pick' of the papers published in BMC Psychiatry in the week of publication! The MS Society of the United Kingdom, in a blog on the BMC Journal website, described the research as 'crucial'.

This led to important work on the commonly associated symptom of which most PwMS—around 85 per cent in clinical studies—complain:

fatigue. For many, this is the most disabling symptom they have. People often ask on forums and social media, 'What can I do about my fatigue?' Prior to this HOLISM research, there had been little to offer PwMS to counter fatigue—including no effective medications, although many had been tried. Our major international study of over two thousand PwMS, published in the world's biggest medical journal, *PLOS One*, changed all that.[85]

We found that around two-thirds of our sample (66 per cent) had clinically significant fatigue. This was considerably lower than in other big studies, probably because so many of those in our HOLISM sample were following the OMS approach, and therefore had fewer of the adverse lifestyle factors that we later identified as predicting fatigue in our study. We found people with progressive types of MS complained of significant fatigue two to three times more commonly than those with relapsing-remitting disease. To nobody's surprise, we showed that fatigue was markedly lower in those PwMS who adopted healthy lifestyles. We found increased fatigue in PwMS who ate a poor diet that was high in saturated fats (95 per cent more likely to be fatigued), were obese (84 per cent more likely) or took commonly used disease-modifying medications (83 per cent more likely), and reduced fatigue for those who exercised more (66 per cent reduction), supplemented with vitamin D (38 per cent reduction) and omega-3 fatty acids (37 per cent reduction for flaxseed oil, no reduction for fish oil), consumed fish frequently (34 per cent reduction) or drank alcohol in moderation (24 per cent reduction).

We considered these findings to be simply extraordinary. Many PwMS attending OMS retreats have reported that their fatigue lifted after they embraced the OMS Recovery Program. We found that the very lifestyle changes taught at the retreats, aimed at stabilising the illness and reducing relapse rates and disease progression, were exactly those that were associated with less fatigue. It is no wonder that people going to the retreats started to feel better, as their fatigue lifted. The HOLISM results fitted perfectly with the OMS preventive medicine approach. Given that the other HOLISM papers show that these healthy lifestyle behaviours are also associated with a better quality of life and reduced risk of MS relapses and depression, adopting the OMS Recovery

Program is a win–win situation all round! Doctors and PwMS everywhere will be heartened to know that fatigue need no longer be such a disabling problem.

HOW

Introduction

Given the enormously influential role of the mind when it comes to how the body functions and how we feel, it makes perfect sense to use that relationship to maximise our chances of a good health outcome after a diagnosis of MS, utilising the best available evidence and techniques. There is really no downside to this approach; it is not difficult or expensive, and it does not require any special equipment or drugs—just attitude and motivation. Nor is it in any way alternative; the science strongly supports using the mind–body connection to optimise health.

In a nutshell
- Meditate.
- Remember that any meditation is better than none; health benefits start from the very first practice.
- Try a few different techniques until you find one that suits.
- Use any technique that helps to resolve conflict and de-stresses: counselling, keeping a diary, imagery, visualisation—anything that helps to promote inner peace.

Meditation

There are many types of meditation; it is important to choose one that suits. This may involve a bit of trial and error. It is best not to get hung up about any particular technique; whatever works for you is best. But most people have trouble knowing where to start. Well-known meditation teacher, Tibetan monk and author of *The Tibetan Book of Living and Dying*, Sogyal Rinpoche, provides a really good description at

<www.buddhanet.net/e-learning/advicemed.htm>. Others who provide very useful guidance are Jon Kabat-Zinn, who popularised mindfulness meditation and mindfulness-based stress reduction (MBSR), based on Buddhist traditions, and Australian expert in mind–body medicine, Associate Professor Craig Hassed, coordinator of mindfulness programs at Monash University in Melbourne, where mindfulness has been part of the core medical curriculum since 1989.[86] Most of the published research on meditation is on this form of meditation, so it makes sense to outline how to do this in some detail. MBSR is now one of the most widely used mainstream psychological therapies in hospitals, psychiatry practices, schools and even prisons. Our website, at <www.overcomingms.org>, also has a range of very useful meditations to try online.

Essentially, mindfulness means paying attention on purpose, in the present moment and non-judgementally, bringing the attention back to a particular focus—usually some aspect of bodily sensation—whenever it wanders. Rinpoche points out that, particularly in the West, we are used to making a lot of effort to achieve things—often with considerable struggle—but meditation is just the opposite: it is fundamentally effortless. He describes meditation as simply being, like a melting piece of butter in the sun. Each session of meditation practice should be treated as something fresh, as if you were experiencing it for the first time. Rinpoche advises people to just sit quietly, with a still body, and their mind at ease, allowing thoughts to come and go, without getting involved with them, commenting on them or judging them. Essentially, it is like noticing a train coming through without getting on, or like watching clouds in a blue sky, coming and going when they are ready.

For most of us in Western countries, that is easier said than done, given the feverish pace at which most of us live our lives. So most forms of meditation employ a focus for the attention. In progressive muscle relaxation (PMR), for example, there is a systematic scanning through the different muscles in the body, usually beginning with the feet, progressing through the various body parts to the face and head. In most forms of PMR, that involves initially tensing those muscles, and then letting them go, noticing both the sensations of the tension and of the letting go. In other forms, one simply scans through the body parts slowly and systematically, noticing how they are feeling.

Generally, both processes result in deep relaxation of the body, which facilitates relaxation of the mind and the gradual calming of thoughts. Because the attention is focused on the body, there is less interaction with the stream of thoughts; when you notice that you have become distracted by a thought, you simply notice that, and then bring the attention back to the object of attention—usually the feelings in a particular body part—without commentary or criticism, non-judgementally. The gradual reduction in stirring up the thoughts means that the thoughts gradually lessen—a bit like the tealeaves settling in a cup of tea once you stop stirring it.

Other techniques use the breath as the focus of attention. Sogyal Rinpoche describes this as a very simple process. When breathing out, he says, know that you are breathing out. When breathing in, know that you are breathing in, without any extra commentary or mental gossip— just identifying with the breath. He notes that meditation in Tibetan means 'getting used to', and is really a process of getting used to our-selves by investigating our own nature and that of our minds through self-observation. Monash University uses the working definition of mindfulness as 'making a commitment to being fully present moment-to-moment, with an attitude of openness and acceptance (that is, without any judgment, labeling, or elaboration)'.[82]

 Try a few different techniques of meditation to find one that suits you best.

Most people in our Western culture, though, need more instruction than a direction to simply be. To that end, there are an endless number and variety of meditation packages these days, online, in books or on CDs, or through a variety of organisations that offer meditation classes. Many people seem to find that an introduction to meditation works well in a group setting, with the reinforcement and support of the others attending. It helps to start with a reputable source that is not aligned to any particular religion. Prof Craig Hassed has a number of online mind-fulness resources; some good ones can be downloaded free of charge from the University of Auckland's Computer Assisted Learning for the Mind website,[87] and others are on our website, at <www.overcomingms.org>.

Deepak Chopra, among many others, also offers meditation sessions at no charge, and several other commercial groups provide meditation lessons both online and in groups for a fee. Given how easily available many of the free sessions are, it doesn't make much sense to spend a lot of money accessing such resources.

One of Prof Hassed's most important principles is that mindfulness becomes a way of life—that it is not just something to be done every day in a meditation chair and then forgotten about. The goal of non-judgemental acceptance is an important one for daily life, not just meditation practice. The Monash mindfulness site offers a number of tips to enable this, like bringing the attention to the breathing at intervals throughout the day, noticing sounds and using them to remind you to be mindful, paying careful attention when eating to the colours, flavours and sensations of the food being eaten, noticing the sensation of our feet on the ground and the air on our faces, noticing if we are rushing, paying careful attention in conversations to what is actually being said without the need to be thinking ahead about potential responses, noticing bodily feelings whenever waiting and noticing any feelings of impatience, and focusing closely on activities that are usually thought of as chores, like brushing teeth, washing dishes or putting on shoes.

Rinpoche notes that perseverance is really important. Like everything else in life, meditation can be good one day and not so good the next, but persevering despite this is important. He likens good and bad meditation to good or bad weather, with an unchanging blue sky behind it. Like that sky, unperturbed by the weather, we can gradually be less perturbed by emotions, outside influences and experiences, potentially developing some stability. With perseverance, gradually our attitude starts to change, and grasping on to things and holding on to them tends to be less of a problem, with lightheartedness developing slowly.

When setting up the process of meditation, having sourced one of the many resources that are available to guide one through the process, many people find it helpful to set up a particular place where they meditate, and to commit to a regular practice of meditation. The evidence of the benefits of meditation for PwMS and for people in general is very clear but, like diet, it only works if you do it! It helps to find a comfortable chair, but not one that is so reclining or comfortable as to induce sleep. That is not the aim, although it is not a major problem. A lot of people also find that setting up a routine around when to meditate helps them to actually do it. The Buddhists have long recommended meditation when you feel inspired; they say that the morning is often the best time because, for many of us, that is when we are most inspired. Others find that it is good to just slot meditation in when they get a chance without too much routine about it.

For people who ask how they can find the time to meditate when they have such a busy job and a full home life, the Buddhist proverb goes that if you can't find the time to meditate for half an hour each day, then you should meditate for an hour. This is very wise, like many Buddhist proverbs. It is important to come to regard it as a priority to make time for meditation each day. How long and how frequently are somewhat individual choices. Rinpoche advises against allocating any particular amount of time; many other experts say that a minimum of twenty minutes a day is ideal. There is no doubt that you can get health benefits from less than this, but doing it for longer is more beneficial. Half an hour a day is a reasonable aim for most people. Many experts recommend meditation twice a day, but really, any time spent meditating is time well spent.

Imagery and visualisation

One way of harnessing some of the power of the mind–body connection is through imagery and visualisation, which are to some extent offshoots of meditation. This has become much more mainstream in recent years, particularly with the growth in sports psychology. It is not at all unusual now to hear about athletes who spend time visualising prior to an event succeeding in what they are about to do: they see themselves hitting the ball cleanly or putting long shots into the basket. Cricketers like great Australian opening batsman Matthew Hayden have described how they would sit on the wicket prior to the start of the day's play and visualise the bowler running in, and playing clean, powerful strokes to the bowling.

There is a growing science to back these techniques up—with stroke survivors, for example, visualising moving their legs for hours or weeks prior to being actually able to move them, and being shown to move them earlier using such techniques. The growing knowledge base around neuroplasticity provides a rationale for why this might work—with connections that are necessary for certain movements, for example, being made in the nervous system in response to such visualisations. It makes sense to use all the possible tools at our disposal in aiming to recover from MS. Using imagery and visualisation forms part of the toolkit for many PwMS.

Dr Bernie Siegel, for example, encourages his cancer patients to pay attention to their dreams. He says that the more open they are to this, and the more they pay attention to their dreams, the more they will see the signposts and messages their subconscious minds have for them. As he notes, many cancer patients have been able to effectively influence their disease by visualisation techniques, such as seeing their white cells as armed warriors shooting the cancer cells. This unfortunately isn't a very helpful image for PwMS, as the lesions of MS are part of our bodies and not outside invaders. But by paying attention to dreams, one can sometimes find symbols that are much more useful to use as the basis of visualisation.

There are a number of good accounts of how to develop a regular practice of visualisation. Both Carolyn Myss's *Why People Don't Heal, and How They Can* and Bernie Siegel's *Peace, Love and Healing* are excellent. The critical step is finding an image that is suitable. For MS, images of fighting or attacking are not of much use for most people. Because MS represents a system out of balance, some image related to balance may be of help. By paying careful attention to dreams, an image may arise that is unique and personal. Images thrown up spontaneously by the subconscious are likely to be of more benefit than those actively developed using the conscious mind. Whatever the image, finding something suitable and using it regularly—especially something related to balance—is very likely to assist the body in returning to a state of balance.

There are also many commercial CDs and online resources around imagery techniques. The Gawler Foundation offers some imagery CDs. One they use is a white light image, where one imagines a pure white light gradually passing through the body, cleansing the body of disease on the way through. PwMS might want to imagine such a white light passing through their brain and spinal cord, washing away disease and activating damaged nerve cells.

Counselling

An important part of dealing with any serious illness is through counselling. Knowing how important mental state and positivity are to successfully tackling disease, getting professional help to deal with the inevitable psychological response to serious illness makes very good sense. Everyone newly diagnosed with a major illness should consider some psychological counselling. We need every bit of our energy to tackle the illness. If we are wasting any energy dealing with things we don't need, or if we are tackling things in unproductive ways, it is usually easy for trained professionals to spot this. Of course, ongoing counselling may also be important. The journey on which MS starts people can be extremely difficult at times, and can lead to the exploration of unexpected issues. It is worth 'shopping around' a bit to find someone who really suits. An ongoing professional relationship with someone who really knows you, and whom you can trust, can be enormously helpful when the inevitable difficulties crop up in life.

This can be of great benefit, particularly when initially diagnosed, and also later if the disease progresses. Some people find this pretty confronting—and probably it needs to be if anything is really to be achieved. The focus should initially be on practical tips to help develop positivity, resolve conflict and unfinished business, and enjoy life. Finding someone you relate to well may be quite difficult. Often personal recommendation is the best strategy. As time goes on, if the right counsellor is found, the sessions can help with spiritual life. It is wise to shop around, though. Like all professionals, some are good and some are not so good. Some people find that close friends or relatives who feel comfortable talking about difficult issues can be a great source of support in a similar way.

 Counselling can be an important part of the OMS healing package.

It is important not to avoid tackling the unfinished business thrown up by these sessions. Avoidance seems the easier option at times, but it is important to remember that disease is often a manifestation of unresolved conflict. Resolving these issues may be the harder choice, but it is certainly the healthier one. MS is actually a great excuse to deal with issues of the past that still trouble us. Paradoxically, MS can provide a convenient excuse to contact someone with whom there have been difficulties in the past. Avoiding dealing with past issues makes it harder to heal. There is often a great sense of relief when these past issues are confronted; otherwise, they remain buried in the subconscious but continue to affect our daily lives. Biography becomes biology; if we live our lives in this way, our bodies will change. The most important skill to learn is that of forgiveness. Forgiving others and ourselves for past mistakes helps healing.

Positivity

Remaining positive in the face of a chronic progressive disease is difficult, although it gets easier when there is a commitment to significant life-style change, and the whole process becomes a challenge and a journey. Of course, if this results in continuing health—as it will for many people—positivity can continue to grow. Focusing on positive aspects of what has come out of having the disease is important. It is often difficult for people to see anything positive at all about having MS. But spending some time talking to someone close about the advantages and disadvantages of having MS can be quite illuminating. Not everyone will be able to see the disease as a gift. Staying focused on the lessons that can be learnt from conflicts and difficulties can help prevent bitterness and negativity. In the end, even if it appears that there are no choices, there is always a choice about how to react to the disease. Reacting positively will almost certainly bring physical as well as mental benefits.

One helpful way of developing positivity is to be surrounded by positive, strong people and environments. Most PwMS find that when they begin to confront the illness and change their way of life, many of their friendships change. Some people find it difficult to accept the changes, and want people to stay the way they were. Others relish the opportunity to assist and to change with the person. That is natural, and it is helpful to just accept it and let this reordering of friendships happen. A lot of people find it helpful to avoid people who always make them feel negative or down.

It can also be helpful to surround oneself with good stories. Reading about people who have recovered from serious illness or hardship, for example, can really provide some optimism in the face of all the difficulty. Books by Bernie Siegel, Ian Gawler, Nelson Mandela and so on can be really uplifting. So can the book *Recovering from Multiple Sclerosis: Real Life Stories of Hope and Inspiration*, by myself and Karen Law. Karen is a writer, musician, teacher and mother of three who is recovering from MS. The book represents the recovery stories of a dozen ordinary PwMS who have adopted a secondary preventive approach to MS management and are recovering. Some have had MRIs that have completely cleared of lesions! Surrounding oneself with good stories, rather than the negativity that we so often see from the mainstream media, and indeed many MS organisations, can provide the spark of hope that recovery is possible, and the faith to stay on the preventive path.

Keeping a diary

With the remarkable benefits shown in randomised controlled trials of just a single session of writing down difficult feelings, the potential that keeping a regular diary has for improving health is enormous. It is extremely helpful to keep a diary, particularly when going through difficult times. Expressing difficult emotions helps to free the subconscious mind from distractions and allows it to get on with the work of healing. It also helps to keep one in touch with feelings, and to provide some history against which to gauge one's progress. At first, when things are very difficult, many people find it helpful to write nearly every day. Later, it may suffice to write only when there is something major causing difficulty. And, of course, it is also good to write when things are going really well. The evidence is pretty clear that writing about difficult experiences can make a big difference to the physical expression of chronic illness. It is a simple strategy, but one that can be very liberating.

Keeping a diary can have significant health benefits.

How we view ourselves and the illness

The language we use around an illness is actually more important than many people think. Language can become a self-fulfilling prophecy. I suggest that it is important to avoid using the phrases 'MS sufferer' and 'MS patient'. The way we feel about the illness and refer to it has a big bearing on our outcome in my view. To use Carolyn Myss's terminology, 'biography becomes biology'. Like many others, she has seen that if people don't express their grief, they end up radiating grief. They get depressed. If people can't say what they want, repress their real wants and desires and feel powerless, then something like cancer may literally start eating them away. If people see themselves as 'suffering' with MS, they will probably end up suffering and get more attacks. People who take a positive approach to this illness, take an active stance and make the necessary lifestyle changes will do much better than if they allow it to dominate them and become sufferers. And people with advanced MS who are reading this may also get something out of reconsidering the attitude they have towards the illness.

Taking ownership of the illness, by referring to MS as 'my illness' or 'my MS', can also be problematic. Once people get on overly cosy terms with this illness, they may just end up adopting it and needing it to get on with the rest of their lives. Thinking of MS as an illness about which you are actively doing something, but that you expect won't be there in an active form for most of the time, allows you to focus on other, more important and productive areas of life. Similarly, there are good reasons not to talk about 'fighting' MS. MS is a manifestation of an imbalance in the body. It is not some outside invader like malaria or a virus. All the cells involved in MS are your cells and part of you. It makes no sense for you to fight yourself: it only empowers the illness.

We are trying to tip the balance back to a more favourable one, where the immune system is not over-active and nerves are in harmony with it. This can be done successfully with diet, meditation, sunlight and using the mind productively. It is not about fighting; it is about healing, which is multifaceted. Nor is it just physical healing: it is becoming clear that being sick spiritually impairs physical healing. Many of the ancient tribal healers knew this, but we are only now rediscovering it in a 'scientific' sense.

OVERVIEW

In the age of technological marvels and sophisticated medical equipment and pharmaceuticals, it is tempting to discount the health benefits of an active approach to illness, of empowerment, of being the captain of one's own ship. Taking such a positive and proactive stance has been shown to make a real difference to the outcome—both mental and physical. Using the mind–body connection is a critical part of getting well, of recovering after a diagnosis of MS.

STEP 5

TAKE MEDICATION
IF NEEDED

Some people have such mild symptoms that no treatment (with medication) is necessary.

Mayo Clinic

INTRODUCTION

The last two decades have seen an explosion of medical therapies for MS. Many authorities now recommend commencing one of these disease-modifying drugs (DMDs) licensed for use in MS as soon as possible after diagnosis to minimise disease progression. While these drugs are somewhat effective in reducing relapses, and may help slow the progression to disability for many people, their use needs to be balanced with a careful assessment of the potential for side-effects, some of them serious. Importantly, none of the research studies on these drugs has included groups of people adopting secondary or tertiary prevention strategies that are likely to offer considerable additional benefit. The best approach is a holistic one, modifying lifestyle risk factors in all cases and utilising the most appropriate drug therapies where needed; that approach offers the most realistic hope for a good outcome for people with MS, although some will find the lifestyle changes so effective that they don't require medication.

In a nutshell
- Steroids cut short relapses, but should not be used in the long term.
- The disease-modifying drugs can reduce the number of relapses, some quite significantly.
- There is some evidence that disease-modifying drugs can slow disease progression.
- Side-effects can be a serious issue with some of the drugs, and need to be carefully weighed up against potential benefits.
- Industry sponsorship raises questions about some of the clinical trial findings.
- HOLISM found only a small decrease in relapse rate for those on the disease-modifying drugs for longer than twelve months, but without any better quality of life.
- Overall, comprehensive lifestyle changes are an essential part of management, and disease-modifying drugs should be considered where needed.

WHY

Drugs to treat relapses
Steroids
While most of the advances in the pharmaceutical management of MS have occurred in the last twenty years, the role of steroids in managing relapses has been accepted for much longer. Most neurologists now prescribe steroids for acute relapses for people with relapsing-remitting MS. The evidence seems clear that they shorten recovery time from individual

relapses. This contrasts with any of the other disease-modifying agents currently available, none of which appears to have any effect on improving the recovery from an acute relapse. Not so clear about steroids are whether the actual degree of recovery is improved, the optimal doses, appropriate routes of administration and long-term benefits, if any.

'Steroids' is the accepted shortening of the word 'corticosteroids'. Steroids are found naturally in plants and animals, but corticosteroids are those particular steroids secreted into the bloodstream by the adrenal gland. Many are now also made in the laboratory. Typically, the synthetic corticosteroids are many, many times more potent than those that occur naturally. Some people will be familiar with the term anabolic steroids. These are the steroids used as performance-enhancing drugs by some sportspeople. Although the steroids used to treat MS are related to these drugs, and share some of their properties, they are different drugs. The term 'steroids' here means corticosteroids.

Steroids have widespread effects in the human body, but those for which they are used in MS are related to suppression of the immune system and changing the balance of the immune system chemicals, the cytokines, that affect inflammation. As relapses in MS are caused by inflammatory demyelinating lesions due to inappropriate immune system activation, this dampening effect on the immune system by steroids is a logical therapy. Some will be familiar with the use of steroid creams and lotions in inflammatory conditions of the skin, such as dermatitis. Steroids are also administered by mouth or injection for inflammatory conditions such as rheumatoid arthritis, asthma and systemic lupus erythematosus (SLE), and for certain lymph tissue and other cancers. Here again, they work through immune suppression.

 A course of steroids usually improves recovery from a relapse.

Studies of PwMS relapses being treated with steroids show that the steroids work by decreasing the levels of the 'bad' cytokines and eicosanoids and by making the cell membranes of the white cells more pliable and less sticky.[1] It is interesting to note how similar this is to the longer-term mechanism by which diet and essential fatty acid supplements work, but without the negative side-effects of steroids. Other evidence suggests that steroids also have an effect on the way the brain interprets the messages coming to it from the body's nerves.[2] MRI studies also show that steroids significantly decrease the amount of swelling around individual MS lesions, causing better nerve transmission through these affected areas. These effects are seen on MRI within hours of taking the first dose.

Fortunately, steroids are relatively safe when used in short bursts of up to seven days. A few rare cases of bone problems have been reported, as well as pancreatitis, but these are exceedingly uncommon. When used continually in the long-term, however, they are very toxic, causing weight gain, fluid retention, an increased risk of infection, stomach ulcers, muscle weakness, changes in behaviour including depression or psychosis, cataracts and osteoporosis. Long-term use is not a good idea in any condition, unless there is no real alternative. But used as a short, sharp burst for an acute relapse, these drugs are very safe and there should be no hesitation in using them.

Trials of steroids in MS

Studies over many years have shown a beneficial effect in recovery from acute relapses in MS when the relapses are treated with intravenous steroids. In 1987, one study randomised 50 PwMS to receive either methylprednisolone (MP) 500 mg intravenously (IV) for five days or an inactive placebo.[3] Assessments were carried out at one and four weeks after the treatment by a 'blinded' neurologist who didn't know what the patients were taking; 73 per cent of MP-treated patients improved compared with 29 per cent of those on placebo. The treated group contained people with classic relapsing-remitting MS but also people with chronic progressive MS, and both categories benefited from MP. This study caused most neurologists around the world to subsequently offer IV MP to people with MS for relapses.

Although most inflammatory diseases for which steroids have been used have shown similar benefit for IV and oral routes of administration, most neurologists have used steroids for MS only by the IV route. This seems to have stemmed from the results of a study in the early 1990s that studied steroids in the condition optic neuritis.[4] As discussed earlier, this is where the nerves to the eyes become inflamed, causing visual disturbance. It has long been known that people who develop this condition are at risk of going on to get MS. In this particular study, IV MP seemed to delay the development of MS in these people for longer than oral MP. While this may have just been a quirk in the way the results fell in that particular study, it was very influential in its effect on the prescribing habits of neurologists. Most tended to give only IV steroids after the results of the study were published, even for people who had typical MS relapses and not optic neuritis.

This was first challenged by the results of a small study of 35 people with MS that showed equivalent benefit for oral and IV steroids.[5] Because of the size of the study, most doctors did not change their prescribing practice to favour oral steroids, despite the advantages of this route. A later study of 80 PwMS comparing oral prednisolone versus intravenous MP found that oral was just as good as intravenous.[6] There was no difference between the groups in terms of degree of neurological improvement at one, four, twelve or 24 weeks after therapy. Indeed, there was a slight trend to better results for the orally treated group.

Another study randomised 51 PwMS with an acute relapse lasting less than four weeks to receive either placebo orally or oral prednisolone 500 mg per day for five days, then a tapering-off dose.[7] After one, three and eight weeks, 4 per cent, 24 per cent and 32 per cent in the placebo group and 31 per cent, 54 per cent and 65 per cent in the prednisolone group improved one point on the Kurtzke Scale score. Study participants also rated their symptoms as having improved much more with the steroids at three weeks and eight weeks. As expected, no significant side-effects were noted.

The definitive study on oral versus intravenous steroids was published by French researchers in *The Lancet* in 2015.[8] This study enrolled 199 PwMS to either oral or IV methylprednisolone 1000 mg daily for three days. At one month, they had comparable disability scores, indicating that both modes of drug delivery were equally effective. There was no significant difference in side-effects. The researchers indicated that clinicians should consider oral treatment with respect to access to treatment, comfort and cost.

Some doctors now offer oral steroid therapy for a relapse. But if only IV steroids are offered, it is worth mentioning the evidence that oral steroids are just as good. From the patient's point of view, oral is really much better. For a start, no special expertise is needed to administer the drug, which means no day hospitals and inconvenience. Second, there is no discomfort, bruising and so on. It's worth pressing this issue.

 Oral steroids work just as well as intravenous steroids for MS relapses, and are much more convenient.

There is still, however, considerable debate about the optimal dosage of steroids and the duration of the course. Indeed, there are still neurologists who never prescribe steroids, believing that they confer no benefit despite the evidence. In the United Kingdom, this is about 5 per cent of neurologists. Most use them for selected relapses but not all, and about 50 per cent use them for all relapses. Similarly there is a lot of variation in whether oral or IV steroids are usually used. UK neurologists in the past overwhelmingly favoured IV, despite the evidence that oral is just as effective. In the late 1990s, over 90 per cent used IV steroids, and only about 5 per cent routinely used oral steroids.[9] The current situation is unknown.

The most common dosage schedules for steroids in acute relapses are oral prednisone or prednisolone 500 mg a day for five days, or IV methyl-prednisolone 500 mg or 1000 mg a day for three days. The oral and intravenous doses have been shown to be roughly equivalent in terms of biological availability.[10] The 2014 UK National Institute for Health and Care Excellence (NICE) guidelines now unequivocally recommend 500 mg of oral methylprednisolone for five days.[11] They do recommend, however, considering IV methylprednisolone 1 g daily for three to five days as an alternative where oral steroids have failed or not been tolerated previously, or for those who need to be admitted to hospital for a severe relapse. Further, the guidelines suggest that steroids shouldn't be used more than three times a year, or for more than three weeks at a time in any given episode. It is also important to note that tapering doses are not needed after the initial course, despite commonly being prescribed. One study showed that there was no difference in outcome with or without a tapering dose,[12] and the shorter the course, the safer the drug.

Another possibility is that the course of steroids may be more effective if it is given at night.[13] Because there is a natural rhythm of steroid secretion in the body, varying between day and night, Israeli researchers compared outcomes and side-effects of steroid therapy for relapses between one group of PwMS given the treatment during the day and the other at night.[13] The outcome was better for those receiving the treatment at night, side-effects were fewer and patients expressed a clear preference for night-time treatment.

Most neurologists treat only some relapses. They argue that only attacks that are severe and likely to leave some disability should be treated. The NICE guidelines disagree. From the point of view of a patient, all relapses can leave lasting symptoms that can be quite distressing, even if they are 'just' disturbances in sensation, and some of these sensory lesions may result in quite a bit of pain in the long run. Therefore, most relapses should be treated with steroids. A relapse is also a sign that maintenance disease-modifying medication might be considered. That said, most neurologists would not treat a relapse until symptoms had been present at least 48 hours and were progressing; many apparent relapses resolve more quickly than that, and require no treatment. The previous NICE guidelines from 2003 recommended treating 'an acute episode sufficient to cause distressing symptoms or an increased limitation on activities'. So what constitutes 'distressing' is clearly up to the person with the illness.

It is a good idea to discuss with your doctor the possibility of keeping a prescription for steroids at home in case of a relapse, and what sort of symptoms might warrant taking the course. Interestingly, the 2014 NICE guidelines specifically say that doctors should not provide a supply of steroids for people to keep at home for management of future relapses.[11] Providing a prescription that can be quickly filled after a phone discussion with one's doctor is obviously different, however. Sometimes it can take quite a while to get an appointment with a neurologist, and the earlier these drugs are started in a relapse the more effective they are likely to be. Many patients and their neurologists will be comfortable with this sort of approach, although clearly it is not for all those with MS. Not everyone—even neurologists—feels confident enough about what exactly constitutes a relapse. It can be easy to be confused between a true relapse and a phenomenon called Uhthoff's syndrome or sign, when neurological symptoms get worse due to over-heating, either with exercise or with fever due to infection; in the latter case, this can cause symptoms to be quite persistent until the fever reduces, and can sometimes be confused with a relapse.

If steroids are so effective when given in short, sharp courses for relapses, some have investigated whether they might be of benefit in preventing relapses if given in the longer term. When steroids are given for a first attack, there is a longer delay before the second attack than if they are not given, suggesting that if used continually, there might be fewer attacks. The problem with this approach is the side-effects of long-term use of steroids. In short, intermittent courses, steroids are remarkably well tolerated, considering what powerful drugs they are. In long-term use, however, they have unpleasant side-effects, some of which are probably more unpleasant than the disease they are being used to treat.

Long-term continual treatment of MS with steroids was shown over 40 years ago to be unhelpful.[14] However, there still remains the possibility that intermittent so-called pulses of steroids, which have minimal side-effects, can be beneficial in slowing the rate of progression to disability. One study looked at monthly IV doses of methylprednisolone 500 mg in a group of nine people with MS who were getting monthly MRIs.[15] After six months on treatment, there was a 44 per cent reduction in the number of new lesions compared with the baseline six months on no therapy. This clearly warrants further study.

Another study compared two different dosages of MP given every other month for two years to people with secondary progressive MS.[16] The investigators studied 108 PwMS and found that the group with higher dose MP took longer to go into a sustained progression of disability than those with the lower dose. This suggests there may be significant benefit from intermittent pulsed steroid therapy in progressive forms of MS. Another interesting piece of research has studied a novel way of giving the steroids. After repeatedly administering a long-acting steroid directly into the spinal fluid, essentially by the same technique as lumbar puncture, patients with progressive MS experienced substantial improvements in walking distance and speed.[17, 18] Larger studies may help determine whether this has a place in the management of people with progressive MS.

Overall, there is convincing evidence that steroids are useful for improving recovery after a relapse of MS. It is probable that steroids delay the onset of the next episode as well. The oral route is as effective as the IV route. There is also likely to be a role for long-term, intermittent, high-dose steroids, but more work is needed before this will become clear. For the time being, for most relapses, there should be no delay in starting a short course of steroids.

Drugs to modify the course of the disease

Over the last two decades, a large number of medications has been researched and approved for the management of MS.[19] Currently, at least ten medications are licensed for use around the world as DMDs—more in some countries. All have been shown in randomised controlled trials to have a significant short-term effect in reducing the rate of relapses for people with relapsing-remitting MS. Long-term benefit in slowing disease progression somewhat has been demonstrated for a number, although not all, as most of the clinical trials have been relatively short term, and few of the medications have been shown to have any significant effect on progressive forms of the disease.[19]

Research from the Swedish MS Registry through the Karolinska Institute in Stockholm has provided a longer term view, however, and given some indication that early treatment with these immunomodulatory drugs may delay progression to disability for people with relapsing-remitting MS.[20] These researchers looked at people newly diagnosed with MS from 2001–05 in the Registry, and found that those taking the medications took 77 per cent longer to reach the EDSS score of 4.

Many neurologists feel they are seeing a change in the MS disease process for many PwMS due to the widespread use of the disease-modifying drugs, with people progressing to disability more slowly than in the pre-drug treatment era. One neurologist told me that he was so excited when the first of the DMDs became available, as he finally was able to provide some hope to PwMS that something could be done about the disease. Of course, today we can provide considerably more hope with our growing knowledge of the lifestyle risk factors that can be modified to change the course of the disease.

The medications are reasonably well tolerated, but the likelihood of long-term adherence to these medications is limited by a number of side-effects, some of them serious. There is a need for more research on use of the DMDs for MS outside of clinical trials to get a better sense of their efficacy in real-world situations.

The first-generation DMDs were released in the 1990s. Comprising three self-injected interferon beta medications and glatiramer acetate, these drugs were shown in clinical trials to result in a modest reduction in relapse rate of around 30 per cent, with little effect on disability. Their safety profiles were considered acceptable, although the interferons had significantly more systemic side-effects than glatiramer, the side-effects of which were largely limited to localised skin reactions. The interferons were injected every second day (Betaferon or Betaseron), three times a week (Rebif) or weekly (Avonex), whereas glatiramer (Copaxone) was injected daily. More recently, glatiramer has been shown to be effective with and licensed for second daily injection at double the original dose.[21, 22]

Second-generation DMDs include the monoclonal antibody natali-zumab (Tysabri), delivered by monthly intravenous infusion, and associated medications, including the recently licensed alemtuzumab (Lemtrada), and others still under investigation, such as daclizumab (Zenapax). A number of oral drugs have also recently been approved, including fingolimod (Gilenya), dimethyl fumarate (Tecfidera) and teri-flunomide (Aubagio), while oral cladribine (Movectro) was withdrawn following difficulties in licensing. Fingolimod and teriflunomide are taken once daily, and dimethyl fumarate twice daily.

These second-generation DMDs generally have been shown to reduce relapse rate considerably more than the first-generation drugs, but some have potentially more serious side-effects. While acknowledging the difficulty of detecting reductions in disease progression in short-term trials, and difficulties in comparing differing ways of measuring this, one large review concluded that trials of the second-generation DMDs fingolimod, alemtuzumab, natalizumab and laquinimod in people with relapsing-remitting MS reported significant reductions in confirmed disease progression, ranging from 40 to 60 per cent reductions.[23]

> Currently approved disease-modifying drugs have been shown
> to lower relapse rates, with some effect in reducing progression
> of the disease.

Other general immunosuppressant medications have also been used
in MS, with varying degrees of efficacy. Of these, only mitoxantrone
(Novantrone) has been approved for use for rapidly progressive MS, and
is the only agent approved for use in secondary progressive MS (SPMS).
It has clearly been shown to have the most significant effect in reducing
disease progression of all the approved MS therapies.[24] While effective in
stabilising the disease, serious side-effects—including serious weakening
of the heart muscle and leukaemia—have limited its use.[25]

While the advent of these medications for the management of MS has
been described as one of the most rapidly advancing areas in neurological
research,[26] peak regulatory bodies have cast doubt on the cost-effectiveness
of the first-generation DMDs, with the National Institute for Health and
Care Excellence (NICE) in the United Kingdom rating them the least cost-
effective of all marketed pharmaceuticals between 1996 and 2005.[27] Others
have raised serious concerns about the soaring costs of these pharmaceutical agents, well above the costs of similar classes of drugs.[28]

A recent review by the Cochrane Collaboration, the peak medical
evidence review body, examined the available evidence on the effects of
the DMDs on relapses, disability and safety, concluding that while some
of the common drugs seem to be useful in preventing relapses, the sometimes very serious side-effects are not well documented, and the long-term
effects are not clear.[24] The study noted that there was no clear evidence of
benefit beyond two years, despite these drugs often being taken for many
years, reflecting the paucity of long-term trials in the area. The authors
were very concerned that most (around three-quarters) of the research
into these drugs was funded by the very pharmaceutical companies that
make major profits by selling them. Despite these caveats, the experience
of most neurologists is that the prognosis of MS has changed dramatically
since the advent of the DMDs, particularly the second-generation drugs,
with MS now being a much more manageable disease that is considerably
slower in progression than it was in the pre-drug treatment era.

First-generation DMDs
Interferons

Interferons have now been used to treat MS for over two decades. Interferons belong to a class of chemical messengers in the body called cytokines. Interferon, first described in 1957, is secreted by cells exposed to viruses and interferes with replication of the virus—hence the name. Subsequently, three main species of interferon have been described in humans: alpha and beta interferon, belonging to type I; and gamma interferon, belonging to type II. The type I interferons tend to suppress the immune system, and have been studied in the treatment of MS, and the type II interferons tend to promote inflammation. The interferons in general have anti-viral actions, affect the immune system and inhibit the growth of tumours. It is not certain which action is responsible for their therapeutic effect in MS. The interferons have also been used in treating hepatitis C, malignant melanoma and granulomatous disease. In these diseases, there is usually considerable discussion with the patient before embarking on treatment with interferons because of their serious side-effects.

The first large-scale study was by the IFNB (Interferon Beta) Multiple Sclerosis Study Group, published in *Neurology* in 1993.[29] This was a study of 372 patients in eleven centres. Patients were randomly assigned to receive inactive placebo injection, IFN-b1b 1.6 million units or IFN-b1b 8 million units, given by subcutaneous injection every second day for two to three years. The relapse rate for the placebo (untreated) group was quite high at 1.27 relapses per year. With the lower dose of interferon, the relapse rate was reduced by about 8 per cent to 1.17 relapses a year, and with the bigger dose was reduced by about 34 per cent to 0.84 relapses a year. The severity of relapses was also reduced.

Two years later, the same investigators presented five-year follow up of these patients.[30] Interferon continued to reduce the relapse rate by about a third in the higher-dose group. However, differences were not significant after the second year, and only five patients completed the five years of the study. Importantly, the five-year study failed to show any significant decrease in progression of disability. The original investigators of this study later reported the sixteen-year follow up of a good proportion of the 372 patients originally randomised in this study.[31] Nearly

90 per cent of these people were contacted and around 70 per cent had clinical records. The investigators could find no difference in disability and MRI outcomes between the three groups.

One of the difficulties in this original trial was the size of the placebo response. This is something that is not often mentioned in discussions about the interferon or other drug studies, but there is every reason to suspect that the placebo response will be quite large in MS. In addition, the natural history of MS is that the number of annual relapses falls over time. This makes it hard to assess whether a drug is making any difference to what would have normally happened. In this study, taking data directly from the reported results, from the end of the first year to the fifth year in the study the placebo group went from an annual relapse rate of 1.44 to 0.81, a 44 per cent reduction. The high-dose interferon group went from 0.96 after the first year to 0.57 in the fifth, a 41 per cent reduction. Placebo appeared to have a greater effect after the first year of study than the drug, and reviewers subsequently cast doubt on whether interferon beta has any beneficial effect after the first year of therapy.

These findings have largely been reproduced in subsequent interferon studies, with minor differences. One trial, the European interferon b1b trial (this trial being in secondary progressive MS rather than relapsing-remitting MS), showed an effect on progression to disability.[32] The delay in progression achieved with three years of interferon treatment was of the order of nine to twelve months, with a drop in the percentage of patients becoming wheelchair bound from 25 per cent for the placebo group to 17 per cent for the interferon group.

In all the interferon studies, many patients had side-effects and subsequently pulled out of treatment. This means regular blood testing to detect any abnormalities caused by the drug. Because the studies have gone for up to five years at a maximum, we don't know how long the benefits in relapse rate reduction are sustained. As a result, the interferons are widely being superseded by newer-generation DMDs—particularly the oral drugs, because of their ease of administration.

Side-effects of interferons
While most PwMS taking interferons do not get most of the side-effects, flu-like illness is very common, as are headaches.[33] Most people feel ill

on the day of injection, with an acute flu-like syndrome consisting of fever, chills, headache, muscle pains, joint pains, nausea, and perhaps vomiting and diarrhoea. These effects can to some extent be minimised with other drugs. Most people find that they gradually become tolerant of the flu-like side-effects. Rather more serious are other side-effects such as liver damage and depression,[34, 35] with the latter confirmed by the HOLISM study,[35] and the fact that interferon can impair fertility and should not be used during pregnancy. One side-effect that is not often discussed is loss of hair. Over a third of patients have hair loss.[36, 37]

One of the few studies to report side-effects over the long term was a large Canadian study of 844 patients taking interferons.[38] Over a third (37 per cent) of patients on the interferons developed liver disease as measured by elevations in liver enzymes. Thyroid disease is also very common in people taking the interferons. In one large, long-term follow-up study, 24 per cent of patients taking the interferons for MS developed thyroid dysfunction—mostly under-activity of the thyroid—and 23 per cent developed thyroid auto-immunity.[39] Most (two-thirds) developed this within the first year of treatment. So people taking interferons should have their thyroid function monitored closely while on therapy, particularly in the first year.[40] This is not commonly done. Other serious potential side-effects are pancreatitis,[41] skin problems[42] and peripheral neuropathy, which can produce neurological effects difficult to distinguish from MS.[43]

The interferons modestly reduce relapse rate, but with significant side-effects.

Side-effects are more frequent in younger people and those with smaller body size, and seem to be the most common reason for stopping the drug in the first year or two of therapy. In one study, 28 per cent of people stopped taking the drug within five years of starting therapy.[44] Those stopping due to side-effects did so relatively early, at around a year, whereas those stopping due to failure of the treatment to be effective stopped at three years.

It should also be noted that interferons should be stopped by women with MS who are taking them if they try to get pregnant. One large study showed very significant increases in the rate of stillbirths and low-birth weight babies to women taking interferons.[45] There were also significant foetal malformations.

Concerns about the interferon studies

One major concern with the interferon studies is that, because the side-effects of the interferons were so prominent, most patients receiving interferon as opposed to inactive placebo guessed correctly that they were taking the active drug. This is of concern in studies that are supposed to be blinded—that is, the participants are not meant to know whether they are getting the active drug or placebo, and nor are their doctors, so as to reduce bias. The placebo response may result in substantial improvements in the course of a disease, and when a study is effectively 'unblinded' because people know that they are getting the active drug it raises the distinct possibility that the beneficial effects seen in the study may be partly or even completely due to the placebo effect. That is, the drug itself may not be particularly effective in treating the disease, and the benefits are being exaggerated by patients expecting to get better. If patients know they are getting the active treatment, it is also very likely that this information will be transmitted to the treating doctors, introducing bias into their assessments.

In the IFNB five-year study, for example,[30] 80 per cent of patients in the high-dose interferon group correctly guessed their treatment. This weakens the conclusion that interferon was effective in that study, as the placebo effect may have played a major role in producing this apparent benefit, given that the relapse rate fell markedly for the patients in the placebo group in that study. Another major weakness of the study was the high rate of patient drop out, with 20 per cent of those in the high-dose group dropping out of the study or being unavailable for follow-up and subsequent analysis. A possibility when the drop-out rate was so high is that the patients who continued to deteriorate despite treatment gave up and left the study. This would have the effect of artificially making the treatment look better than it really was by leaving those who did well in the study available for final analysis. This was the only interferon study to report what happened to patients who dropped out, and they did have a higher relapse rate, more active disease and became more disabled than those who remained in the study.

 The interferon studies were not properly blinded, reducing confidence in the results.

One review of the interferon studies found that the evidence from the studies was not strong enough to draw any conclusions about the benefit of interferons beyond the first year of treatment, and that even in the first year the interferons could only be said to reduce the number of patients who had relapses slightly.[46] The review showed the interferons had no effect on the number of hospital admissions the treated patients had, or their need for steroids for relapses. The review noted that the most common problem with the studies was the high rate of patient drop-out, leaving only three-quarters of those patients enrolled in the studies available for final analysis. They also found that the evidence the interferons delayed or prevented disease progression was inconclusive, and that the interferons had a negative effect on quality of life.

More recent evidence looking at the use of Betaferon, Rebif and Avonex in Italy showed that at four years, despite falls in relapse rates, there was still on average a significant increase in disability.[47] Approximately one in five of the patients on Betaferon pulled out of therapy because of side-effects, this being approximately three times the number of patients pulling out who were on the other drugs. Another Italian study reported that, in a large group of people treated with interferons, there was a substantial (59 per cent) reduction in relapse rate over the four years of the study; however, 35 per cent had at least one relapse a year and nearly 30 per cent had sustained progression of disability, indicating that they were not responding to the drug.[48]

A large, well-conducted study from British Columbia in Canada reported some concerns about interferon use, in following 868 PwMS treated with interferons over time, and comparing them with 829 untreated people from the same time period and 959 untreated people from an earlier period, showing no difference in the time taken to require a cane to walk 100 m for people treated with interferon compared to those not

treated.[49] Expert neurologists commenting on the study in an accompanying editorial agreed with the authors that the study could find no evidence
that the interferons reduced the progression of the disease to disability.[50]

Further data questioning the benefits of the interferons come from
an analysis of the risk-sharing scheme introduced by the National Health
Service in the United Kingdom when the DMDs Betaferon, Rebif, Avonex
and Copaxone were supported for use by PwMS.[51] This scheme subsidised the drugs, but this was dependent on a follow-up analysis of
cost-effectiveness. The first two-year analysis of data was published in the
British Medical Journal. Although too early to make definitive statements
about cost-effectiveness, some surprising data emerged. With over 5500
people with MS registered in the data-monitoring scheme, 85 per cent
of them with relapsing-remitting MS, there were enough subjects in the
study to come up with strong outcomes. The study found that at the
two-year mark, there was no evidence that the drugs were cost-effective.
Worse, the data suggested that the DMDs as a group did not delay disease
progression as some had expected.

Overall, important issues about taking the interferons for MS are
that the studies showing benefit are drug company–sponsored, reducing
confidence in their conclusions, and have methodological problems
particularly related to blinding and drop-outs. Importantly, the beneficial
effect is small, and they may not prevent the progression of disability significantly. Most importantly, side-effects are common and can be severe.
Indeed, research suggests that the quality of life of patients taking interferon is not improved despite the slowing of disease progression, largely
due to side-effects[52] and to fatigue and depression.[53] For these reasons
and others, the interferons have largely been superseded in the modern
drug treatments offered to PwMS.

Glatiramer

Glatiramer acetate is another first-generation DMD in common use. It
was originally called copolymer 1 and marketed by the trade name of
Copaxone. It appears that glatiramer somehow re-educates the immune
system because the drug has a similar structure to the base protein
of myelin. This base protein is thought by many to be the part of the
nerve that is attacked by the immune system in MS. In effect, glatiramer

tricks the immune system into somehow activating certain immune cells normally associated with the damage in MS. These cells go into the brain, and upon reaction with myelin base protein reduce the inflammation at the MS lesions. In a sense, it works a bit like the desensitisation injections that people with allergies to bee stings can have. Glatiramer ultimately shifts the immune system balance from a Th1 to a Th2 response.[54] At least part of its effect in the animal model of MS is to reduce demyelination and promote remyelination.[55] In humans, it appears to induce an anti-inflammatory state in the cerebrospinal fluid surrounding the brain,[56] and to reduce free radical formation in blood.[57] Recently, there has been considerable interest in its neuro-protective effects.[58, 59]

Studies on PwMS commencing glatiramer therapy and comparing them over time with people not taking glatiramer have shown that the axons of people taking glatiramer are protected and recover from injury whereas those from people not taking glatiramer tend to die from the injury.[60] Unlike the interferons, glatiramer doesn't appear to have any general effect on the immune system, and it certainly doesn't suppress the immune system. It therefore doesn't make people more susceptible to infections or affect their blood count. So regular blood tests are unnecessary because it has no measurable effect on any other body system. Again, this is in contrast to the interferons.

The first major study of glatiramer reported astounding improvements in 25 people with MS treated with glatiramer compared with those treated with placebo injections for two years.[61] Remarkably, the glatiramer treated patients had a 76 per cent reduction in relapse rate, from 1.35 attacks per year to just 0.3. The percentage who remained relapse-free over the two years in the treated group was more than double (56 per cent) that of the placebo group (26 per cent). The pivotal study was a randomised controlled trial in which 251 people with MS were either treated with glatiramer or inactive placebo for two years.[62] Like the interferon studies, there were about a third (29 per cent) fewer relapses in the treated group (0.59 versus 0.84). Importantly, unlike most of the interferon studies, treatment with glatiramer suggested a slowing of the progression of disability. Although this was not shown with the usual measures of disability, the authors analysed the number of patients who got worse, were unchanged or improved, and found significant benefit here for glatiramer. After two years, those treated with glatiramer had improved EDSS scores by 0.05 points, whereas those taking placebo had worsened by 0.21 points. MRI data from the pivotal study showed there was a 35 per cent reduction in the number of brain lesions. Of equal importance, there were relatively few side-effects and no abnormalities detected on blood tests.

The major European–Canadian MRI study on glatiramer enrolled 239 people with relapsing-remitting MS.[63] These people had had MS for about eight years on average, with a mean EDSS of 2.4 and an average relapse rate in the previous two years of 2.7 per year. Participants had MRI scans every four weeks. After nine months in the study, those people taking glatiramer had 29 per cent fewer new MRI lesions and about 50 per cent lower total MRI disease burden. The clinical relapse rates—unlike those in the interferon studies—also correlated well with the MRI changes. People taking glatiramer had 33 per cent fewer relapses. One particularly interesting feature was that it took some three months before any beneficial effect was seen, and six months before this difference between glatiramer and placebo was significant. The effect seemed to increase the longer people were on the drug.

There has now been considerable experience with glatiramer. People from the original 251-patient pivotal study have been followed for many years, with interesting results.[64] A total of 205 of these people have been studied. The longer people remained on the drug, the greater the benefit they experienced. Those continually on the drug for six years had an annual relapse rate in the sixth year of 0.23, or roughly one relapse every four to five years. This is markedly less than their starting relapse rate. After ten years, 108 of these people were still on glatiramer and being followed up, and continued to have sustained falls in relapse rates and severity and accumulation of disability.[65] French researchers have reported similar findings.[66]

Of great interest, approximately 70 per cent of people continually on the drug for six years were either the same in terms of disability as when they started, or were somewhat better. This is a great result for PwMS and should provide considerable confidence to those people taking glatiramer over an extended period. The same research group looked at people from the original trial of 251 people with MS eight years later, and compared those who started on glatiramer and continued with those who started on placebo but at the end of the trial were started on glatiramer. This 30-month delay in starting glatiramer therapy was associated with a significantly smaller proportion of people remaining stable in terms of their EDSS scores.[67]

Similarly, the European–Canadian study has been followed up long term, now for a mean time of 5.8 years for nearly two-thirds of the original study group.[68] In this study, those in the control group who originally took placebo were treated with glatiramer after nine months along with those in the treatment group, so effectively this group had a delay of nine months in starting treatment with glatiramer. Researchers then compared at 5.8 years these people with delayed treatment to those who had been receiving glatiramer all along. This group was significantly more likely to be using a walking cane at this stage than those who had been on glatiramer all along. Again, this points to a beneficial effect of glatiramer on disease progression.

Researchers looking overall at glatiramer trials concluded that the chance of a relapse at one year for a person on glatiramer was about one-sixth of that for someone not on glatiramer.[69] Another study showed that for people in one of the major glatiramer trials, the reduction in lesions after treatment with glatiramer ranged from 20 per cent to 54 per cent.[70] All these results in combination suggest that glatiramer therapy is effective and ought to be more widely prescribed.

As an indication of how difficult the concept of proof is in medicine, despite these trials now over a long period and general acceptance of the benefit of glatiramer by neurologists, a major evidence-based review of the effectiveness of glatiramer by the highly respected Cochrane Collaboration concluded that, overall, there was no evidence that the drug had any effect on reducing relapses or on disability.[71] The methodology of this review was, however, very poor in that the reviewers put all studies of glatiramer together for analysis, including trials in primary progressive MS where glatiramer has been shown to be ineffective. Including these trials diluted the benefit of the other trials where it was shown to be effective, resulting in the nil benefit conclusion. Others have argued that its effectiveness is equivalent to the interferons, on the basis of reviews of the same studies.[72] If the experts have such trouble agreeing, it is no wonder people find it difficult and confusing to make a decision about the therapy on which they should embark. More recent work on the cost-effectiveness of glatiramer compared with the interferons suggests that glatiramer is the preferred agent.[73]

Other research about glatiramer is somewhat contradictory. The PreCISe study examined people with a first episode and typical MRI brain lesions suggesting MS—that is, a Clinically Isolated Syndrome (CIS), or what may have previously been called transverse myelitis—and compared glatiramer to placebo to see whether glatiramer would reduce the proportion of people going on to a definite diagnosis of MS. Of the 481 people with CIS randomly assigned to receive glatiramer or inactive placebo, the proportion of people who developed MS was 43 per cent in the placebo group versus 25 per cent in the glatiramer group. The trial was in fact stopped early because of the clear benefit from glatiramer.[74]

In contrast, another study examined 163 people with a new diagnosis of CIS attending 29 MS clinics in Austria.[75] They were looking at whether and when standard DMDs, the interferons and glatiramer, were started for these people, why they were started and how the people progressed over the next two years of follow up. Generally, most authorities recommend starting DMDs as soon as possible after a CIS to prevent progression to MS, although it is not known how often this is done in practice. The decision to treat was made by the treating neurologist in discussion with the person with MS.

Around a third of people were treated immediately, a third after three months and a third not at all. Of those treated immediately, 36 per cent went on to develop definite MS, of those treated later 56 per cent developed MS, and of those never treated only 19 per cent developed MS. The immediately treated group had an average of 0.5 relapses per year during the study, the later-treated group had 1.0 relapses per year, and the never-treated group only 0.2 relapses per year. These differences were highly statistically significant. The treated patients also had worse EDSS (disability) scores at two years than the never-treated group.

While, to some extent, these differences reflect the fact that the people with CIS who were thought by the neurologists to have more severe disease (with more lesions on MRI, for example) were more likely to be put on DMDs early, the findings are not strongly supportive of the need for early institution of DMDs for people with a CIS suggestive of MS. While physicians often argue that people are taking a grave risk by not taking DMDs early, these data suggest that many do extremely well without any medication.

Side-effects of glatiramer

Glatiramer has few serious side-effects, and mostly people taking the drug don't feel any different and don't know they are taking the drug. In comparison with the interferons, this not only is important for the quality of life of people taking the drug, but also gives us confidence about the reliability of the study findings, given that in the interferon studies, participants mostly knew they were taking the drug, introducing bias into the studies.

Most people taking glatiramer get skin reactions, but this is often due to poor education about optimal injection techniques. A small number get a transient flushing feeling, with palpitations and shortness of breath. In particular, the flu-like symptoms so commonly seen with the interferons are not seen with glatiramer. There is no need for regular blood testing, as the drug has not been shown to cause any other abnormalities, and the development of antibodies does not affect the drug's performance.

Glatiramer has modest benefit in reducing relapse rates similar to the interferons but without significant side-effects.

Although neither glatiramer nor the interferons are recommended for use during pregnancy, we know that the interferons can definitely cause problems. Research has shown no higher incidence of abnormalities than usual for women getting pregnant while on glatiramer. One review concluded that glatiramer posed the least risk during pregnancy of the available disease-modifying drugs.[76] It is also safe to breastfeed while taking glatiramer, in contrast to the interferons.

Now that we have longer term experience with glatiramer, we are starting to see a few problems related to the effect it has on the balance between Th1 and Th2 lymphocytes. A few uncommon skin conditions related to the change in this balance caused by glatiramer have now been reported, including erythema nodosum (a serious skin rash) and more recently a skin lymphoma.[77] So it is important to keep in mind that, even for drugs as apparently innocuous in terms of side-effects as glatiramer, it is wise to balance the likely benefit of its use against the potential for side-effects.

The dosing schedule for glatiramer—that is, a daily injection—puts some people off and leads them to opt for the interferons, which may be given every second day or even weekly. However, there is evidence that injecting every second day is just as effective as daily injection.[78] Indeed, given the way it works, it may well be that an initial immunising course of, say, nine months of injections, followed by periodic boosters, will be all that is necessary. A further issue about dosage that has been investigated is doubling the dose. A very large international randomised controlled trial of 1155 PwMS recruited from centres all around the world has shown no difference in outcome between double the usual dose of glatiramer (40 mg) injected daily and the standard 20 mg dose.[22]

Drug combinations with glatiramer may hold some promise. Researchers have suggested using mitoxantrone, a chemotherapy drug discussed later, to get control of particularly severe MS and then follow on with glatiramer.[79] This has now been studied in detail in a randomised controlled trial of 40 PwMS. The combination of mitoxantrone followed by glatiramer (M-G) in this study was far superior to glatiramer alone in all measures of disease activity. Specifically, M-G produced an 89 per cent greater reduction in MRI lesions at six and nine months than glatiramer alone, and a 70 per cent greater reduction at twelve months; relapse rates in the M-G group were half that in the glatiramer alone group.

Researchers at Harvard University have succeeded in producing other random copolymers, different from glatiramer, which appear more effective at suppressing EAE in animals.[80] If this finding translates to humans, it may be considerably more effective treatment for MS. With advances in immunology, we may see even 'smarter' molecules that are more stable and more effective than these copolymers.[81] This has recently been demonstrated in two multi-centre studies of a high-molecular weight copolymer of the same four amino acids as glatiramer, a drug called pro-tiramer.[82] The drug was highly effective at reducing the number of CNS lesions over 36 weeks. Recently, the patent for Copaxone expired, and a generic form of glatiramer was released. Research has shown this generic form to be similar in benefit to the original Copaxone, offering a much less expensive option for therapy for PwMS.[83]

Overall, there is now a two-decade track record of glatiramer use confirming its safety and efficacy. Given that the side-effect profile is clearly superior to that of interferon, and that the studies on glatiramer were properly blinded and hence more likely to be valid than the interferon studies, it should be considered before the interferons. Recent research from the MSBase Registry confirms that glatiramer is associated with lower relapse frequency than two of the three commonly used interferon formulations, with no difference in progression to disability.[84]

Second-generation DMDs
Natalizumab

Natalizumab (trade name Tysabri) is a more potent medication given by monthly injection that works by specifically targeting and inhibiting a protein, alpha 4 integrin, which is present on the surface of immune system cells and helps them attach to blood vessel walls and get into the brain. The initial trial, published in the *New England Journal of Medicine*,[85] provided strong evidence of benefit in relapse rate reduction for this drug. In this study, 213 PwMS were randomly assigned to receive a low dose or high dose of natalizumab, or placebo. The drug was given IV and administered once every four weeks for six months, and people were followed with MRI scanning and clinical assessment. Those people on placebo had on average nearly ten new brain lesions at the end of the six months, compared with 0.7 for the low-dose group and just over one new lesion for the high-dose group. Twice the number of people in the placebo group had relapses than in either of the treatment groups. Importantly, those taking the drug generally reported improvement in their sense of well-being, and those in the placebo group reported the reverse. This suggests that the drug is quite well tolerated in the short term, and that side-effects are not too unpleasant.

Two further papers reported on the benefits of natalizumab in MS, one with natalizumab alone, the other in combination with an interferon.

In the former study, 627 people receiving natalizumab alone had a 68 per cent reduction in annual relapse rate, as well as less progression to disability than those receiving placebo.[86] The latter showed that the combination of natalizumab and interferon was significantly better than interferon alone, with the annual relapse rate dropping to 0.34 per year on the combination, compared with 0.75 on the interferon alone, and less progression to disability.[87] More recent MRI studies confirm that natalizumab is highly effective at preventing new MRI lesions, with between 76 per cent and 92 per cent fewer lesions (depending on lesion type) in those on natalizumab versus placebo.[88]

Side-effects of natalizumab

Natalizumab can have serious side-effects. This first came to light when the FDA in America fast-tracked the drug to general use in 2004, but removed it three weeks later because of safety concerns. Unexpectedly, two people who had taken natalizumab in combination with an interferon in MS trials developed a condition called progressive multifocal leukoencephalopathy (PML), an illness similar to very aggressive MS and previously only ever reported in AIDS patients. Shortly afterwards, a third person taking natalizumab alone in a trial for inflammatory bowel disease also died of the illness. Following suspension, there was very careful investigation of all people who had taken the drug in clinical trials to see whether there were other cases of PML that had not been reported.[89] This detailed review revealed no new cases, and concluded that the risk of PML was about one in 1000 for people treated for about eighteen months. The longer term risk was unknown.

Natalizumab reduces disease activity, but people cannot remain on it for long periods because of increased risk of a potentially fatal viral infection of the brain.

Since then, as the drug has become more widely used, many more cases of PML have come to light, and we now have good information about the factors that affect the risk of this potentially fatal complication. It is now known that the disease is much more common for those who test positive for the John Cunningham Virus (JCV), the virus responsible for the development of PML. The exact risk of PML in PwMS taking this drug was thought to be around one in 1000, although more recent data indicate that the overall risk is around one in 500. This climbs to about one in 100 or higher for people who test JCV positive (actually 70–90 per cent of the community is JCV positive), have been on the drug for two years or more, and have had previous immunosuppressant therapy (such as methotrexate or azathioprine). For people who test negative, the risk is very much lower, at around one in 10,000.

One very important ongoing study has, however, raised significant hope that PML can be avoided. Following around 2000 PwMS taking Tysabri, US researchers have noted that in those people taking it less frequently than every four weeks (31–60 days between infusions), there have been no new cases of PML at all, compared with four new cases over the same period for those taking it four-weekly as prescribed, but with no apparent diminution in the effectiveness of the drug. These results were presented at the European Committee for Treatment Research in Multiple Sclerosis (ECTRIMS) conference in Barcelona in 2015, and provide important new possibilities for the safer use of the drug. There is no question that natalizumab is a very effective drug option for many PwMS with active disease, rapidly stabilising their condition for many, and this longer dosing schedule offers the real possibility that the serious concern about developing PML might no longer be an issue. For those on Tysabri, it is worth discussing this in detail with your neurologist, particularly for those who are JCV positive and therefore at higher risk of PML.

Further serious concerns about its toxicity were raised after two people receiving the drug who had long-standing benign moles that were being kept under surveillance by their doctors had sudden cancerous changes in the moles and developed widespread melanoma.[90] The company marketing the drug followed this by announcing that one earlier similar case had occurred during randomised controlled trials of the drug. So authorities now suggest that people with a family history of malignant melanoma should not receive natalizumab.

One issue not often discussed with Tysabri is that the drug passes into breastmilk, and therefore its safety during breastfeeding cannot be guaranteed.[91] The infant may receive as much as 5 per cent of the adult's

dose via the breast milk. So there may be a number of negative consequences for mother and baby, given that breastfeeding is protective
against relapses, and that mothers may be advised to stop breastfeeding
because of this passage of natalizumab into the milk.

The concern about serious side-effects has made this drug a more
risky proposition for PwMS, although clearly some people with very
active disease will require a drug of this potency to gain control of the
situation. Talk to your neurologist about the risks and potential benefits
before making a decision about taking this drug.

Stopping natalizumab

There are also risks in stopping the drug, in that a syndrome of disease
reactivation—the immune reconstitution inflammatory syndrome (IRIS)—
can occur, and disease activity increases again to the level it was at prior
to starting therapy; careful planning with medical staff is required to
manage this potentially serious risk of deterioration on stopping the
drug. Some have also shown a rebound effect on stopping Tysabri, where
disease activity is increased to a level above that present when starting
the drug. Italian researchers have now examined clinical and radiological
data from 54 people beginning two years before starting Tysabri, data
while on treatment, and data for a year after stopping Tysabri.[92] Their
results confirm the concerns about disease reactivation after stopping
the drug.

This group of PwMS had particularly active disease—that presumably being the reason they were started on this drug. Their relapse rate
as a group was around 1.7 relapses a year prior to starting Tysabri.
The drug appeared highly effective in controlling this disease activity,
with the relapse rate falling for the group to around 0.2 per year while
on the drug, staying at this level for the first three months after stopping
the drug. But then, the disease activity increased markedly for the group,
climbing to a relapse rate of around one per year. This was still below
the pre-treatment level of around 1.7 per year, but represented a very
marked reactivation of the disease process. Importantly, treatment with
any of the immune-modifying therapies after stopping Tysabri did not
prevent this increase in disease activity, except restarting Tysabri, which
was effective.

So, while people on Tysabri are often advised to stop the drug or have a break from it because of the increasing risk with time on the drug of developing PML, this is not feasible for most people because of disease reactivation. Spanish researchers aimed to prevent this by examining the effect of three doses of steroids at monthly intervals, followed by Copaxone therapy, after stopping Tysabri at the two-year mark.[93] Unfortunately, the study showed that people returned to their previous inflammatory activity quite quickly after stopping, despite this add-on therapy. While there were no new lesions or clinical activity at three months, at six months one in six people had had a relapse and over half had new lesions on MRI, and after six months, one in three people had a further relapse.

One large Italian study of 110 PwMS stopping Tysabri after at least one year on the drug showed that, despite the majority taking an alternative DMD when stopping, there was a dramatic (fourteen-fold) reactivation of disease activity overall, peaking at between two and eight months after stopping.[94] During this period, most people returned to the level of disease activity they had before starting Tysabri, but 10 per cent had a higher level of disease activity than before starting— the so-called rebound effect. The researchers concluded that no current treatments provided protection against this reactivation in disease activity and that this period was potentially risky for those stopping the drug.

Stopping natalizumab can result in significant rebound in disease activity.

Neurologists everywhere have been concerned about finding some other treatment to prescribe after stopping Tysabri to stop this reactivation, and many appear to be trying Gilenya (fingolimod). In one Italian study of 22 PwMS on Tysabri stopping the drug and taking Gilenya instead, reactivation occurred in eleven (50 per cent) and rebound in three (14 per cent).[95] Given that not all of these people had MRIs, this might have under-estimated the true incidence of reactivation and rebound. The conclusion of the researchers was that Gilenya doesn't become effective quickly enough for it to be used to prevent disease reactivation after stopping Tysabri.

Another study also looked at starting people ceasing Tysabri on Gilenya orally three months after stopping Tysabri, but after first giving them monthly doses of high-dose steroids to suppress disease activity.[96] Eight PwMS who stopped Tysabri and started Gilenya were compared with nine who stayed on Tysabri. Five of the eight stopping Tysabri and starting Gilenya had relapses, and six of the eight showed MRI evidence of disease activity. None of those staying on Tysabri had relapses or MRI evidence of disease activity.

Most recently, a large international study looked at 142 PwMS stopping Tysabri and switching to fingolimod after one of three periods off Tysabri before starting the new drug: eight, twelve and sixteen weeks.[97] Of the 142 participants, 112 people completed the study. There was a substantial number of relapses in all three groups, but the eight-and twelve-week groups did better than the sixteen-week group, with around 90 per cent of those in the eight- and twelve-week groups relapse-free, versus 84 per cent of those in the sixteen-week group. The lowest number of new MRI lesions was in the eight-week group. While there was a return of disease activity in all three groups, this provides evidence that a shorter gap is preferable before starting new therapy after stopping Tysabri. One review, by German neuroimmunologists, looked at the various options that have been tried in an attempt to reduce the risk of increasing disease activity on stopping Tysabri.[98] They noted that most were ineffective, but that the most promising appeared to be Gilenya; however, it needed to be started shortly (around eight weeks) after stopping Tysabri.

What does this mean for those considering stopping Tysabri? First, neurologists have concluded that none of the currently available therapies that have been tried to suppress disease activity and reactivation after stopping Tysabri seems to be effective, and that further studies of other avenues are needed to control this reactivation.[96] Second, it is very important for PwMS about to embark on drug treatment to be aware of this serious risk should they need to stop the drug in the future. This should be discussed with the treating neurologist and considered before starting therapy, bearing in mind the effectiveness and side-effect profiles of other available medications. Further, if people taking Tysabri do test positive for JCV, they need to seriously consider whether it is safer to stay on the drug, even with the risk of PML, or stop it, knowing that there is a strong chance that relapses and disease activation will occur after stopping the drug. Currently, there are no obvious solutions to what can be done about the risks of stopping Tysabri, although early initiation of treatment with Gilenya offers the best chance of reducing the rebound effect.

Fingolimod

Fingolimod (also called FTY720, trade name Gilenya), a newer drug taken by mouth, has a novel mechanism of action. It works on the immune system but, rather than suppressing it or modifying its function, it binds to a receptor on a proportion of circulating lymphocytes and temporarily traps them in lymph nodes. This means a lower number of activated T-cells are available to get into the central nervous system, so inflammation and myelin damage in the brain and spinal cord are reduced. Because the lymphocytes are reversibly trapped in lymph nodes, they are potentially available if needed by the immune system.

Fingolimod was approved worldwide as the first oral agent to treat relapsing-remitting MS. This followed two major randomised controlled trials of fingolimod against placebo and interferon beta 1a (Avonex). The FREEDOMS trial showed a relapse rate reduction of around 54–60 per cent with reduced progression of disability when compared with placebo.[99, 100] The TRANSFORMS trial was a twelve-month study of 1292 people with relapsing-remitting MS with a history of at least one relapse.[101] These people were randomly allocated to oral fingolimod (0.5 or 1.25 mg daily) or IFN-β1a (Avonex) once weekly. A total of 1153 people completed the study, so there was an 11 per cent drop-out rate. The relapse rate was 39 per cent lower in people treated with fingolimod in the 1.25 mg group and 52 per cent lower in the 5 mg group than the group treated with Avonex, but there was no significant effect on disability. Both studies found significantly reduced numbers of new MRI lesions and reductions in shrinkage of the brain in fingolimod-treated participants. These studies were followed by FREEDOMS II, another placebo-controlled trial confirming the safety and effectiveness of fingolimod found in the original study, but not showing any benefit for disability progression.[102]

Side-effects of fingolimod

Side-effects in the studies were not serious, consisting mostly of mild infections like colds and flu, and headaches. Certain viral infections—particularly herpes viruses, such as shingles—were more common and severe with fingolimod. Authorities hence recommend that people not immunised against varicella (the virus that causes chicken pox and shingles) should be vaccinated before treatment with fingolimod. Other important side-effects include the occurrence, following administration of the first dose, of very slow heart rates. A six-hour monitoring period is advised after administration of the first dose, so that such a heart rhythm disturbance can be detected and treated if needed. This effect appears to disappear with subsequent doses. One effect on the heart that remains with longer use, however, is a weakening of the contraction strength of the heart. In a group of 53 PwMS taking fingolimod, Italian researchers noted that the volume of blood pumped out of the heart with each contraction was significantly lower than a comparable group of 25 PwMS taking natalizumab.[103] While this can be tolerated by people with normal hearts, it suggests that anyone with MS who has heart failure who is considering taking fingolimod should take great care, and perhaps consider a different DMD in consultation with their neurologist.

More recently, some side-effects have been noted as people discontinue the drug for a variety of reasons. Neurologists have reported the case of a 45-year-old man—a participant in the original FREEDOMS trial—who developed malignant melanoma while on the study drug, and was forced to stop the medication.[104] There has already been concern raised about the possibility that fingolimod may be associated with a higher incidence of this cancer, given that in the TRANSFORMS trial, three PwMS in the fingolimod group developed malignant melanoma. The important part of this case report was that this man suffered a relapse two weeks after stopping fingolimod, followed by a further relapse at three months, with more than 20 new lesions on MRI and a dramatic worsening of disability (from 2.5 to 4.5 on the EDSS). This rebound of disease activity was far more severe than his disease activity before starting on the fingolimod.

While this appears unusual, it may therefore be important for people being offered fingolimod to consider an exit strategy for when they might wish to discontinue the drug, because of potential side-effects, or for other reasons. Like natalizumab, there may be the potential for worsening of the illness on stopping the drug. Decisions to stop these potent medications should be made in consultation with a neurologist who can closely monitor disease activity, and potentially vigorously manage any rebound in disease activity.

Neurologists have since reported the histories of a series of six PwMS who had to stop fingolimod.[105] All commenced an alternative disease-modifying drug when stopping; however, within three months of stopping, five returned to pre-treatment levels of disease activity and one experienced a rebound—that is, the disease flared up. This phenomenon may represent the immune system being essentially reconstituted after a period of suppression. The case series highlights the importance of making a very considered decision when starting one of the newer DMDs for MS, given the potential that many people will either be forced, or will eventually choose, to stop treatment.

Another important concern is the potential for foetal abnormalities when women taking fingolimod fall pregnant. There is strong evidence from animal studies that fingolimod is potentially damaging for the developing foetus if taken during the first trimester of pregnancy, when the foetus is rapidly developing and growing new organ systems. Human data has, however, been lacking until recently. A recently published paper underlines the importance of taking every precaution not to get pregnant while on the drug.[106] The paper describes the pregnancy outcomes of women who inadvertently fell pregnant during the pivotal controlled fingolimod trials that first showed the efficacy of the drug in MS.

The paper noted that women in these trials were advised to take precautions against falling pregnant. Despite this, 89 women did fall pregnant, the great majority (74) in the fingolimod group. This is surprising; there is no obvious reason for the discrepancy between the small number of women taking placebo who fell pregnant (11) and the large number taking fingolimod who fell pregnant (74). Of the 74 pregnancies in the fingolimod group, 66 were exposed to fingolimod during the pregnancy. Of these 66, one outcome was unknown; of the remaining 65, there were 28 live births (two with deformities, one very serious), nine spontaneous miscarriages, 24 planned abortions and, at the time of writing, four pregnancies still going. In the group who had planned abortions, there was one serious congenital abnormality, a death in utero and one failure to grow. This study raises safety concerns about fingolimod during pregnancy; women of childbearing age taking the drug for MS should take every possible precaution not to fall pregnant, or consider switching to one of the MS drugs that is safer during pregnancy.

Teriflunomide

Teriflunomide (trade name Aubagio) was first approved in 2012 for the treatment of relapsing forms of MS. It is taken as a once–daily tablet. While the exact mechanism of action is unknown, teriflunomide reduces the number of immune cells involved in the MS response (it is known to reduce proliferation of lymphocytes by blocking a certain enzyme). The most common side-effects are upper respiratory tract infections, urinary tract infections, nausea and vomiting, paraesthesiae (pins and needles), hair loss and abnormal liver enzymes, indicating liver damage.

Teriflunomide is the active metabolite of leflunomide, a drug used in the treatment of inflammatory arthritis. There are established concerns over leflunomide. It is thought to have the potential to promote blood cancers or solid malignancies. However, a large US observational study found only an increase in skin cancers (including melanomas). Post-marketing cases of lymphoma have been reported. Severe liver damage is thought to occur in 0.5 per cent and cases of serious lung disease have been reported.[107, 108] Because we have limited experience to date with the use of teriflunomide, it is important to consider the side-effects of the parent drug and the potential that these may also apply to teriflunomide. Those taking the drug are advised to avoid alcohol, other drugs that affect the immune system and live viral vaccines.

Teriflunomide itself has been the subject of a number of randomised controlled trials. The first of these, the TEMSO (Teriflunomide Multiple Sclerosis Oral Trial), was published in 2011.[109] It studied 1088 PwMS randomly assigned to either placebo, 7 mg or 14 mg of teriflunomide, and followed up for 108 weeks. Drop-out rates were similar for all three groups at around 30 per cent. There was around a 30 per cent reduction in annual relapse rate in both treatment groups, with a trend for a reduced disability progression in the treatment groups, although these differences weren't significant. There was no difference in fatigue levels between the three groups.

Another study investigated the safety and efficacy of teriflunomide as add-on therapy to interferon beta.[110] A total of 188 PwMS received either interferon plus teriflunomide or interferon plus placebo. The initial study was for 24 weeks with the PwMS having the option to continue for a further 24 weeks if they elected to do so. There were lower relapse rates in the teriflunomide groups, but these were not significant. There were, however, significantly fewer lesions on MRI scanning in the terifluno- mide treatment groups.

The results of all studies of teriflunomide in MS have been reviewed by an independent Cochrane review. The authors were 'unable to give any clear recommendations for the use of teriflunomide as a disease modifying therapy for MS because the studies had limited quality, were of short duration and were funded by a pharmaceutical company'.[111] The authors cited concerns over the high rates of drop-outs in both studies, although these were lower than in studies of many of the other MS drugs, and a lack of information about why PwMS dropped out as well as a lack of clarity over how PwMS were randomised to groups, what the criteria were for excluding PwMS for the trial extension and how this was blinded. This information was requested by the Cochrane reviewers, but not provided by either the researchers or Sanofi, the company sponsoring the trial. Overall, while teriflunomide appears reasonably safe in MS, it probably has relatively limited benefit.

BG-12 (dimethyl fumarate)

Dimethyl fumarate (also known as BG-12, trade name Tecfidera) is another oral treatment, this time first approved in 2013 for relapsing forms of MS. It is taken as a twice daily capsule and appears to have both anti-inflammatory and neuroprotective effects.[112] There is a long track record of safety for a very similar drug consisting of dimethyl fumarate in combination with three other fumaric acid esters; this treatment has been used for many years for the skin condition psoriasis, also thought to be an auto-immune inflammatory disease.

There have been two large studies that have investigated its role in MS. These were both short-term studies with a maximum follow up of

two years. The DEFINE study published in 2012 followed 1234 PwMS
for up to two years, looking at the proportion of participants who had
a relapse.[113] PwMS received either placebo or twice or three times daily
BG-12. The twice daily dosage seemed at least as effective as three times
daily—in fact, a little better. There was a 53 per cent relapse rate reduction compared with placebo, and BG-12 reduced the risk of confirmed
progression of disability of more than one point on the EDSS scale, which
was sustained for twelve weeks by 38 per cent compared with placebo.
There were also markedly fewer MRI lesions for those on BG-12.

The second study was the CONFIRM study, examining 1417 people
with relapsing-remitting MS; it was similar in design to DEFINE, but with
an additional group of people who took Copaxone for comparison.[114]
Both BG-12 and Copaxone groups were evaluated against a placebo.
At two years, BG-12 reduced annual relapse rate by 44 per cent for
the twice-daily dose, compared with placebo. In comparison, Copaxone
reduced relapse rates by 29 per cent. All treatments reduced the number
of new lesion formations: BG-12 reduced new lesions by 57 per cent
while Copaxone provided a 41 per cent reduction. Reductions in disability progression were seen, but these didn't reach significance.

 Dimethyl fumarate is taken as a pill and works reasonably well,
with limited side-effects.

Adverse events were common in both studies, and resulted in cessation of treatment in 16 per cent (DEFINE) and 10 per cent (CONFIRM)
of those taking BG-12. The most common side-effects were flushing,
gastrointestinal upsets, upper respiratory tract and urinary tract infections, protein in the urine (potentially indicating some kidney damage)
and generalised itching. There were falls in the white cell counts of
those taking the medication, considered toxic, in up to 10 per cent
of those treated with BG-12.

The number of PwMS withdrawing from the studies was very high:
around 25 per cent in DEFINE and 30 per cent in CONFIRM. During the
short study periods, neither study showed an increase in cancer risk or the
risk of infections commonly associated with suppressed immune system.

Previous data from use in psoriasis hasn't indicated any issues with this immunosupression.[115, 116, 117] However, the majority of these people were treated for short periods only, and BG-12 has yet to be studied in a long-term trial. The issue of immunosuppression is a concern and 2013 saw the first published case of PML reported in a person with psoriasis using the psoriasis formulation of BG-12 (with other fumaric acid esters).[118]

Overall, BG-12 has been shown to reduce relapse rates by around 50 per cent over short study periods of up to two years—although, due to high drop-out rates, the real figure may be somewhat lower. Side-effects such as flushing, gastrointestinal upsets and minor infections are common, and the longer-term effects of immunosuppression with BG-12 are not yet known. Recent analyses show that BG-12 begins working very quickly after starting the drug, with relapse frequency dropping within weeks and, in the large clinical trials, a drop in lesion numbers by the first MRI scan at 24 weeks.[119] It represents a relatively safe and effective drug option if the side-effects can be tolerated, and is well worth discussing with your neurologist.

Alemtuzumab and related drugs

Alemtuzumab, originally developed under the trade name Campath, more recently Lemtrada, was licensed for use in people with relapsing-remitting MS in 2014 in the United States and United Kingdom. Its initial development for use in MS began at Cambridge University over 35 years ago. First used to treat some leukaemias and lymphomas, it is a highly specific type of antibody that binds to lymphocytes, slowing down their passage into the brain and hence reducing myelin damage. Alemtuzumab is given as an intravenous infusion on five consecutive days, and then twelve months later as a second course on three consecutive days. Generally no further doses are said to be required for life, although recent data raise doubts about this. This is felt by many neurologists to represent a big advantage over other medications that need to be given regularly to maintain their effect—although obviously, once it has been given, it can't be removed from the body.

Randomised controlled trials have shown that alemtuzumab markedly reduces relapse rates, with some effect in slowing progression to disability, when compared with one of the interferons. The CARE-MS 1 trial compared alemtuzumab with Rebif in people with relapsing-remitting MS who had not been previously treated with a DMD.[120] Those in the alemtuzumab group had about 55 per cent fewer relapses over the two years of the study, but no effect on disability progression could be found. The CARE-MS 2 trial compared alemtuzumab with Rebif in people with relapsing-remitting MS who had active disease, as shown by relapsing while on therapy.[121] Those in the alemtuzumab group had about 50 per cent fewer relapses than the interferon-treated group, and were about 40 per cent less likely to progress in disability over the two years of the study.

In 2015, a seven-year follow-up study of PwMS taking alemtuzumab was published.[122] In this group of 87 PwMS in Cambridge receiving alemtuzumab for between three and twelve years, with an average of seven years, two-thirds were the same or better in terms of disability at the end of follow up. Because the length of the study was much longer than the earlier trials, it became obvious that many people needed more than the two intravenous infusions because they were having relapses. Nearly half the participants had more than two cycles of dosing, with one receiving five cycles of dosing.

This drug has several advantages over other DMDs, and appears to be quite effective. However, as with all MS medicines, the issue of side-effects needs to be considered. One constant feature of the side-effect profile of MS drugs is that the more potent they are at suppressing the immune system, the more immune-related side-effects they cause. In this case, the earlier shorter duration trials showed a worrying pattern. One-third of participants developed auto-immune thyroid disease, mostly requiring significant medical treatment in its own right. Some also developed an otherwise uncommon bleeding disorder, idiopathic thrombocytopaenic purpura, an auto-immune disorder resulting in a reduced number of platelets, and hence the potential for bleeding complications.

There are significant safety concerns about alemtuzumab related to thyroid and other auto-immune disease.

The seven-year study put this into further perspective, with a more realistic view of the potential for side-effects to show up. In this study, almost half the participants developed auto-immune disease of other bodily organs—usually the thyroid gland. Most people considering a new medication would be concerned about a one-in-two chance of getting a serious auto-immune condition in addition to MS as a result of treatment, and many neurologists are reluctant to prescribe the drug for that reason. This side-effect profile led to licensing alemtuzumab for more severe MS where the person has failed to respond to two previous disease-modifying drugs. PwMS considering this medication should ensure they discuss these side-effects with their neurologist before embarking on this therapy. Other common side-effects include feeling sick, headaches, rash, hives, fever, itching, insomnia and fatigue, and less common side-effects are frequent infections of the lungs, sinuses and urinary tract, in addition to herpes infections. It is also important to remember that a comprehensive monitoring program has to continue for at least four years after the last alemtuzumab dose to detect auto-immune adverse events.[123]

Another related drug, daclizumab (trade name Zenapax), appears to be a very promising option. A major randomised controlled trial, reported in 2010, comparing daclizumab as an add-on treatment for a group of people already on interferon beta, compared with people on interferon beta alone, showed 72 per cent fewer new MS lesions in the group taking additional high-dose daclizumab, and 25 per cent fewer lesions in those taking low-dose daclizumab.[124] In contrast to alemtuzumab, however, the safety profile was much better, without similar serious side-effects.

A further randomised controlled trial of over 1800 people with relapsing-remitting MS was reported in 2015.[125] In this study, researchers randomly allocated these PwMS to either daclizumab 150 mg given by subcutaneous injection every four weeks or interferon beta-1a (Avonex) given weekly. Those receiving daclizumab had 45 per cent fewer relapses and 54 per cent fewer MRI lesions than those in the interferon group, without serious safety concerns apart from a small increase in the number of serious infections. No difference was found between the two treatments in progression to disability. Daclizumab may represent an important treatment option once the drug is licensed, which one would expect to occur relatively soon. Monthly subcutaneous dosing certainly makes it more convenient than natalizumab, for instance, and without similar potentially lethal side-effects.

Ocrelizumab, another related drug, is a humanised immunoglobulin antibody currently being evaluated for treatment of relapsing MS that targets B cells rather than T cells. The drug is given as an intravenous infusion every six months, in a similar way to Tysabri. In initial studies, intravenous ocrelizumab reduced relapse rates and was well tolerated.[126] Further trials are underway. At the time of writing, the results of these had not been published; however, one major study had been presented at the ECTRIMS conference in Barcelona in October 2015. In the reported study, it was trialled in 2300 PwMS around the world. Importantly, the drug appeared to be somewhat effective in slowing disease progression for people with primary progressive MS, which to date has no effective drug therapies. It should be noted, however, that trials of the same drug in rheumatoid arthritis and lupus were stopped because of unacceptably high rates of infection that caused some deaths. Until the results of this study are published in a peer-reviewed journal, the place of ocrelizumab in the treatment of MS remains uncertain, but these data provide great hope that there will soon be at least partly effective drug treatment for people with primary progressive MS.

Laquinimod

Laquinimod (trade name Nerventra) is a derivative of linomide, a drug previously trialled in MS but never licensed. It is an immunomodulatory agent which, like fingolimod and teriflunomide, is taken as a once-daily oral drug. Laquinimod treatment results in an anti-inflammatory cytokine profile in immune cells and appears to have some protective effects on nerve cells. It has been studied in relapsing-remitting MS but is also under study in progressive forms of the disease. The randomised, double-blind, placebo-controlled ALLEGRO study enrolled 1106 patients with relapsing-remitting MS, receiving 0.6 mg laquinimod once daily or placebo.[127, 128] Laquinimod treatment resulted in a modest reduction in relapse rate versus placebo of around 23 per cent and about a one-third reduction in disability progression. Those treated with laquinimod had fewer MRI lesions and a one-third reduction in progression of brain atrophy compared with placebo.

The BRAVO study also evaluated laquinimod, but failed to show any significant reduction in relapse rate compared with placebo, whereas interferon beta 1a (Avonex), which was also being tested in the study, did show a 26 per cent reduction.[129] Laquinimod also failed to show any reduction in disability progression, although it did reduce the amount of brain shrinkage compared with placebo. A third trial, CONCERTO, is underway; however, these results are somewhat disappointing to date, and it seems unlikely that the drug will be licensed. Common side-effects include headaches, abdominal pain, back and neck pain, appendicitis and blood abnormalities, including liver enzyme elevations.

Immunosuppressant drugs
Mitoxantrone

This is a potent drug related to those used in chemotherapy. It is chemically similar to doxorubicin, which is used for acute leukaemias and lymphomas. Mitoxantrone has been used mainly for acute leukaemia, but, because it powerfully suppresses the immune system, it has also been trialled in MS. One randomised controlled study examined 51 people with MS randomly allocated to mitoxantrone once a month intravenously or placebo.[130] There was a major reduction (66 per cent) in the number of relapses in the treated group after two years, and a significant reduction in the proportion of patients with confirmed disease progression at two years.

Another study compared the results of people treated with mitoxantrone plus steroids with a control group of people treated with just steroids.[131] Forty-two people with clinically very active, progressive disease were randomly allocated to the two groups. After six months, there were very large differences between the groups. Ninety per cent of the mitoxantrone plus steroid group had no new MRI lesions versus only 31 per cent of the steroid-only group. There were also significant improvements in disability for people in the mitoxantrone group at months two to six, with a final mean improvement of more than one point. Additionally, there were significantly fewer relapses, and more people had not relapsed in the mitoxantrone group. Five people in the steroid-only group dropped out of the trial because they were deteriorating so badly.

In 2002, a large study of mitoxantrone in people with secondary progressive MS showed for the first time that this type of MS could be treated with disease-modifying medication.[132] This form of MS has been very difficult to treat to date. The study randomly allocated 194 people with secondary progressive MS to treatment with mitoxantrone or to placebo. The drug was given intravenously every three months for two years. People in the mitoxantrone group had very significant reductions in disease progression, with about one-quarter the worsening of the EDSS measure of disability, about a third fewer relapses and about a quarter of the worsening of their neurological status compared with the people taking placebo. Importantly, there were no serious side-effects or cardiac problems, which have been a concern with this drug. A French study followed up 304 PwMS who had been treated with mitoxantrone.[133] It found that the disease activity was markedly reduced for about two years before it became active again, and suggested that other therapies needed to be commenced during that time. These studies together are highly significant, showing that even progressive MS can to some extent be controlled.

Mitoxantrone is highly effective in reducing MS disease activity, even in secondary progressive MS, but can have significant side-effects.

One study showed that for people deteriorating despite treatment with interferon beta, mitoxantrone safely stabilised their condition.[134] Another study in 45 people with early but very active MS showed that mito-xantrone also stabilised their condition.[135] One of the people, however, developed leukaemia shortly after treatment. Further trials are needed, but at this stage it is certainly not a drug that should be considered for the average person with MS. If the disease becomes very active and progressive, at least there is something that can be done—albeit at some cost.

Unfortunately, side-effects can be a major problem. People taking this drug can get some of the effects regularly seen with chemotherapy, such as hair falling out, nausea, vomiting and loss of appetite. Bone marrow suppression is common, meaning that people are more susceptible to infections. Heart muscle toxicity has not yet been seen, although it is often seen in related drugs.

Influential Cochrane Reviews in 2005 and 2013 concluded that mitoxantrone is moderately effective in reducing relapse rate and disease progression in relapsing-remitting, primary progressive and secondary progressive MS in the short terms studied to date (two years), although longer trials are needed.[25, 136] No major side-effects related to cancer or cardiotoxicity were reported from the trials studied; however, the authors did note that, in other studies, heart muscle damage was relatively common, occurring in about one in eight people, while acute leukaemia due to the drug occurred in about one in 120 people.

Mitoxantrone therapy opens up an extremely promising avenue for treatment of patients with aggressive forms of MS and secondary progressive MS who would otherwise rapidly deteriorate or have few treatment options. There are obviously concerns about its safety, especially with long-term use. One review concluded that the benefits of mitoxantrone therapy outweighed the risks, especially for people not responding to the usual disease-modifying therapies.[137]

Many neurologists faced with the dilemma of a young person with MS with seriously active disease that has not responded to standard DMDs may have to consider the difficult decision of starting treatment with this very potent drug, in the full knowledge of the potential for serious side-effects. These are very difficult decisions for both patient and neurologist; detailed discussion of the risks and benefits is an important consideration before starting mitoxantrone, but many people in this situation will find that they can achieve some stability, having been in a dire position. They then have time to institute concerted lifestyle measures to enhance their control of the disease. The potential for heart muscle toxicity is an important consideration when deciding whether to prescribe this drug. Researchers are currently working on analogues of mitoxantrone that do not possess similar cardiotoxicity. One such drug is pixantrone, which appears very promising in animal studies, and may be trialled in humans.[138, 139]

One of the basic issues with drug therapy in MS is that the more potent a drug is at suppressing the immune system—which is a vital part of the balance in our body in preventing infection, cancer and other illnesses—the more severe its side-effects are likely to be. While we know that mitoxantrone is a potent immunosuppressant used as a chemotherapy agent, and that it causes the familiar toxicity associated with other chemotherapy agents, new research shows that it commonly causes cancers in its own right some years after treatment. Pascual and co-researchers followed up two groups of people receiving the drug, and found that after three to four years of follow up, the cumulative incidence of acute leukaemia was over 2 per cent.[140] This is a serious concern, as adult leukaemia is often fatal. The researchers recommended that people receiving mitoxantrone for MS be followed up for at least five years to ensure detection of this malignancy. People who are rapidly deteriorating with MS may well accept this risk, however, in an effort to do whatever it takes to get better.

Cladribine

This drug used in chemotherapy, effective in the treatment of certain leukaemias and lymphomas, was approved (as Movectro) in Russia and Australia in 2010 as the first oral pill for MS to be approved anywhere. It was, however, later withdrawn from the market by Merck Serono because European and US regulators insisted on further trials of the drug. Merck Serono felt that by the time these were undertaken, other oral drugs would have already found wide acceptance and the drug would hence not be profitable. The drug was designed to be given in short courses of only four to five days at the start of every month. It appeared to make a significant difference to the number of new MRI lesions, increased the time to relapse and increased the number of relapse-free patients, but was also relatively toxic.

In the clinical trials, shingles was quite common, and in some cases severe. Of more concern, in the pivotal CLARITY trial, there were ten cases of cancer developing in people in the cladribine groups, and none in the placebo groups.[141] It is not certain whether this was just chance, or cladribine caused the cancers, but given that the development of cancers is not unusual as a result of chemotherapy, it is important to be very cautious about this possible side-effect. Half of the cancers were benign, but the others were melanoma, pancreatic cancer, ovarian cancer, cervical cancer in situ and choriocarcinoma.

It is unlikely that cladribine will be reintroduced to the market, given that other oral drugs are now quite commonly prescribed and are less toxic.

Other potential drug therapies that affect the immune system
Cyclophosphamide
This is a rather toxic anti-cancer drug used for such diseases as lymphomas, multiple myeloma, breast, lung, cervix and ovary cancer, and several childhood cancers. Unlike most of the other anti-cancer agents, it has the advantage of being able to be given by mouth rather than injection only. In MS, cyclophosphamide has mostly been used for progressive forms. Several randomised controlled trials have not shown any benefit for either cyclophosphamide alone compared with placebo,[142] or different combinations of cyclophosphamide, steroids and other techniques.[143] One study, however, showed that people who had cyclophosphamide and steroids to induce immunosuppression, and then had booster doses of cyclophosphamide every other month for two years, had slower progression of disease than those without the boosters.[144] While the group of people who had the booster injections had slower progression of disability at 24 and 30 months, the effect was confined to those people under 40 years of age. For this group, the effect was very significant.

Another study looked at people not responding well to interferon therapy—that is, their disease was still quite active.[145] They randomised them to receive either monthly cyclophosphamide and steroids or monthly steroids alone in addition to their interferon therapy. The cyclophosphamide group did considerably better, presenting another treatment option for people not responding well to interferons alone. Another study monitored ten people with rapidly progressive MS who were given monthly doses of cyclophosphamide in combination with interferon beta, and then maintained on interferon beta alone.[146] They were quite stable both clinically and on MRI at 36 months. One report noted that a 48-year-old woman who had accidentally been given a very high single dose of cyclophosphamide three years after diagnosis had not had any disease activity of any sort seven years later.[147]

Unfortunately, cyclophosphamide has major side-effects—both short and long term. It causes hair to fall out, nausea and vomiting, ulceration of the mouth and other mucous membranes, dizziness and increased skin pigmentation. More serious effects are bladder irritation, with blood in the urine, and bone marrow suppression, with increased susceptibility to infections. In the longer term, it can cause a variety of cancers in its own right. These side-effects seriously limit its usefulness for PwMS.

Intravenous immunoglobulins (IVIgs)

Immunoglobulins (Igs) are the natural antibodies made in humans by certain immune system cells in response to infection or a foreign substance. Human Igs have been extracted from plasma and pooled, and used by intravenously (IV) injection to treat several conditions. High-dose IVIgs have been used to treat conditions including Guillain-Barré syndrome, chronic inflammatory demyelinating polyneuropathy, multifocal motor neuropathy and MS. Because they are a natural human product, they are virtually free of side-effects, and so offer advantages over some other therapies that affect the immune system. With human products, though, there is always the minor risk of transmission of infectious agents through the serum.

A large randomised controlled trial by the Austrian Immunoglobulin in Multiple Sclerosis Study Group looked at a monthly dose of IVIg for two years compared with inactive placebo.[148] A total of 148 people with relapsing-remitting MS were enrolled in the study. Results showed that the disability score decreased significantly in the treated group and got worse in the placebo group, and there was a 59 per cent reduction in the number of relapses in the treated group. Importantly, there were no adverse effects. Another study looked at MRI lesions during IVIg treatment.[149] There were fewer new MRI lesions with IVIg than on placebo (0.4 versus 1.3) and considerably fewer relapses.

Intravenous immunoglobulins are safe and effective, and should be prescribed more widely.

Another study of 91 people soon after a Clinically Isolated Syndrome reported the results of treating with IVIgs every six weeks.[150] The researchers showed that those treated were only one-third as likely as people not treated to progress to definite MS within a year. Further, they had fewer lesions on MRI. There were no significant side-effects with the treatment.

Another very interesting study combined IVIg and an immunosuppressant drug called azathioprine.[151] Although the study was not a randomised controlled trial, it followed 38 people with relapsing-remitting MS for three years of this combined therapy. Before starting therapy, these people had been having an average of 1.7 relapses a year. This fell to none by the end of the study, and the disability scale score improved overall.

There has been speculation that some of the benefits seen with IVIgs may be caused by not only immune system effects, but also improved remyelination of MS lesions. Certainly, at present, the mechanism by which IVIg works is unclear. Nevertheless, the studies show a significant reduction in relapse rates, and improvements in disability scores. Given the low toxicity of this therapy, it makes a very worthwhile addition to the expanding list of agents that can be used for MS when the disease is very active or severe.

However, IVIgs appear to be ineffective in secondary progressive MS.[152, 153] A summary of published work on IVIgs concluded that they are a second-line treatment in relapsing-remitting MS when other treatments are not available, that they have no role in progressive MS or acute attacks, but that they may be useful after childbirth to prevent relapses, and can delay the onset of definite MS after a first attack.[154] Relatively mild side-effects have been documented. These include fever, chills, fatigue, joint and muscle pain, abdominal pain and headache. Serious side-effects have included seizures, heart failure and kidney failure, but they have been rare. One report on the long-term side-effects of IVIg therapy reported 293 PwMS treated for up to ten years.[155] The drug was safe even when given over long periods.

More recently, a large placebo-controlled study in people with primary and secondary progressive MS showed a significant benefit for IVIgs in primary, but not secondary, progressive MS.[156] Given how few effective treatments there are for primary progressive MS, this should be investigated further, and offered to people who are deteriorating with this type of MS, although it is not currently available for use in many countries, including Australia.

Others

A number of other therapies that affect the immune system have been tried in MS, mostly with less impressive or doubtful results in comparison with those already discussed. Azathioprine on its own has not been shown conclusively to have benefit in several trials. There is also an associated risk of cancers developing. One did, however, show that azathioprine significantly reduced the number of new lesions.[157] Further work by the same research group showed that azathioprine was actually as effective as the beta interferons and, because it was a tablet as opposed to an injection, and much cheaper than the interferons, it ought to be considered as an alternative to the interferons.[158] Side-effects were, however, much more common than with the interferons.

An article in *Time* magazine in 2002 sparked worldwide interest in research conducted in Sydney, Australia. It reported that three patients had been treated with a combination of azathioprine and either glatiramer or one of the interferons, and that the patients had made dramatic recoveries from quite severe MS, to the point of being able to walk or jog after being confined to wheelchairs. Only one patient was, however, reported on in the medical literature by the same neurologist.[159] This was a 24-year-old woman with eye problems and great difficulty walking who was treated with glatiramer and azathioprine, and was able to jog again. Another group reported results from a study of azathioprine and Betaferon in ten people with secondary progressive MS.[160] Only eight stayed in the study, but these people had a 50 per cent reduction in relapse rate and significant improvement in EDSS. There does appear to be some promise here for the treatment of secondary progressive MS, although the combination of drugs is relatively toxic.

Other researchers have reported that the combination of azathioprine and Betaferon, used in patients who had continuing disease activity while on Betaferon, resulted in a 65 per cent reduction in the number of lesions on MRI.[161] There has not been much follow up of this possible therapy.

Methotrexate is another immunosuppressant drug used in inflammatory disorders with an immune system basis. Although one study of oral methotrexate in chronic progressive MS showed a reduced rate of progression of disability as assessed by observers, participants in the study noticed no difference.[162] The drug is fairly toxic, with bone marrow depression, liver cirrhosis and kidney damage its main side-effects, and regular blood testing is necessary. This reduces the utility of the therapy.

Other drugs under investigation
Oestrogens and testosterone

Recently, there has been a lot of interest in the female hormone oestrogen and its possible effect on the course of MS. Oestrogen is commonly found in oral contraceptive pills. It seems the oestrogens have a modulating effect on the immune system through a number of mechanisms, including a shift from a Th1 to Th2 cytokine balance, and their effects on other immune related hormones.[163] It has long been known that there is a decrease in MS activity in pregnancy when the levels of this hormone are quite high.[164]

Researchers have found that feeding oestrogen to mice with the animal model of MS dramatically reduces the severity of the illness.[165] These researchers suggested that oestrogen may be used as a treatment for MS—perhaps in low doses together with other disease-modifying therapy to minimise side-effects.[166] On the other hand, the US Nurses Health Study failed to show any difference in MS incidence between nurses taking oral contraceptives or the number of pregnancies they had experienced.[167] More recent work found a 40 per cent lower incidence of MS in women who had been on the oral contraceptive pill in the previous three years.[168] One recent study lent some support to a possible benefit, showing that women allocated to treatment with interferon plus one of the higher-dose oestrogen oral contraceptives had fewer new lesions on MRI scanning over the course of the study than those on interferon alone.[169] More human research on oestrogens is needed before it becomes clear whether they will be beneficial for PwMS.

Interestingly, the male sex hormone, testosterone, may also be of benefit to men with MS. Researchers have shown in a study of ten men that with daily application of testosterone gel over twelve months, cognitive ability was improved and there was a slowing of brain shrinkage.[170] Larger studies are needed before this can be recommended.

Minocycline

A novel drug approach to treating MS is minocycline, a widely used antibiotic taken by mouth for acne, which also has the effect of reducing the ability of immune cells to get into the brain by inhibiting enzymes called matrix metalloproteinases. These enzymes have been shown to be involved in the development of lesions in MS.[171]

The drug initially was shown to be effective in experimental animals,[172] and then followed up in a small study in ten PwMS. This showed that there was a significant effect on MRI, and that the drug was well tolerated in standard anti-acne doses.[173] There was an 84 per cent reduction in the number of MRI lesions while on minocycline. This is substantially higher than other therapies currently available. The same researchers followed these people for two years, and found that they remained essentially relapse- and lesion-free, with biochemical tests showing a positive effect of treatment on the immune system.[174] At the three-year follow up, a further report was published indicating a fall in relapse rate from 1.2 per year to 0.25.[175]

More recent research in the animal model of MS has shown that, in combination with interferons, the drug significantly improves immune responses and outcomes.[176] It has also been shown, in combination with one of the statins (cholesterol-lowering drugs), to improve the animal form of MS.[177] Canadian researchers have now shown a large improvement in PwMS taking minocycline in combination with glatiramer, compared with those taking glatiramer alone. The study outcomes for the minocycline-plus-glatiramer group were a 63–65 per cent reduction in MRI lesions compared to the glatiramer group, and a 54 per cent reduction in relapses. The problems with the study unfortunately mean that very few, if any, neurologists will prescribe minocycline for PwMS. Why is this?

First, minocycline should have been tested against placebo. There are still many people who opt not to take the injectable drugs, and so it would not have been unethical to have a placebo group. But it is very important that we know whether this drug actually works in MS (which appears almost certain), because it is very cheap, widely available, taken by mouth and has few significant side-effects. On all these counts, it is ahead of the new generation of drugs for MS that are taken by mouth. From preliminary studies, it is quite likely that minocycline would have been shown to be more effective against placebo than Copaxone—which would have been a disaster for Teva had this been reported.

Second, the study was set up with too few participants to find anything but a very large effect; this is one of the key issues about statistical analysis of clinical trials of which the drug company must have been aware. Typically, when setting up a study, the researchers hypothesise how big a difference they are likely to find, then enrol sufficient numbers of patients so that if they find this difference, it will be statistically significant. That is why the early glatiramer and interferon studies had so many participants. So the results the researchers found in this study in reductions in lesions and relapses were actually very large, but could not be 'proven' because there were only 44 PwMS in the study. If you have so few participants in a study, you will not find a statistically significant effect unless the size of the effect is huge. In fact, it is likely that the drug company got a surprise, as the size of the effect was so large that the results almost achieved statistical significance.

Most recently, the same Canadian researchers have trialled minocycline in people with Clinically Isolated Syndrome to see whether it will prevent progression to full MS. This study, reported at the ECTRIMS Conference in Barcelona in October 2015, showed a dramatic reduction in progression to diagnosed MS for those taking minocycline compared with those taking placebo. The researchers enrolled 142 people with a first demyelinating event likely to be a first attack of MS to receive either minocycline 100 mg twice daily or placebo. The proportion going on to develop MS within the next six months was 45 per cent lower in the minocycline group that the placebo group, and by one year 38 per cent lower, prompting lead researcher Dr Luanne Metz to say that this cheap, safe drug should be considered as a treatment for MS.

These very positive and potentially beneficial effects of minocycline in preventing the development of and treating MS, unfortunately, have been consigned to the 'further study is warranted' basket, rather than being immediately adopted by doctors, and widely taken up by PwMS. Because minocycline cannot be patented (it has been around for decades as an anti-acne drug, and is therefore prescribed as a generic brand and very cheaply), it is unlikely that any drug company will be rushing to continue these studies. It is highly likely that this safe medication is very effective in MS, with the potential to take over from many of the common medications currently used. What a great shame that the pharmaceutical industry has such control of the research agenda in MS (and indeed in many other areas of medicine) that little funding is available to study it further.

Promising generic drugs, including minocycline and low-dose naltrexone, have not been well studied—probably due to lack of financial incentive.

Low-dose naltrexone (LDN)

One of the more contentious but promising potential therapies for MS is low-dose naltrexone. Naltrexone is a drug that reverses the effects of opiates like morphine or heroin. It is used in clinical practice in people trying to rid themselves of addiction to opiates. How it works in MS and other immune-mediated diseases—if it does—is the subject of some conjecture. But there seems to be very considerable anecdotal evidence that it prevents relapses and also reduces disease progression.[178] It has been suggested that it acts by reducing cell death in oligodendrocytes. There is considerable evidence available for its apparent benefit in individual cases published in a number of sites on the internet, but to date there are limited data from randomised controlled trials, although several are in progress.

Basic research in the animal model of MS has shown that LDN halted progression of the disease, and reversed neurological deficits over an extended period, without any significant side-effects.[179] An Italian study enrolling 40 people with primary progressive MS showed that LDN is safe and well tolerated by PwMS.[180] It also showed a beneficial effect on spasticity. One very short duration study (seventeen weeks) found no difference in measures of quality of life comparing LDN with placebo, but that is not an unexpected finding for such a short period of time taking the medication.[181]

The first randomised controlled trial of LDN in MS randomised 80 PwMS to receive LDN or placebo in a cross-over study where people took the LDN or placebo for eight weeks, then swapped to the other study drug.[182] This appears to be the first major drug trial in MS that was not funded by the pharmaceutical industry, but by the participants themselves. The researchers found significant improvements for LDN over placebo in several mental health quality of life measures. This should be the beginning of formal research into LDN in MS, and further trials are awaited by the research community.

Despite the lack of research, the drug does seem promising. An important aspect of this treatment is that it is relatively free of side-effects, unlike many of the other heavily promoted immune-modulating therapies on the market. In addition, because it is a generic drug that cannot now be patented it is very cheap—far cheaper than other currently available drugs. Sadly, this also explains why it hasn't been studied much to date. The research and MS communities may well be frustrated for many years due to lack of adequate research into this promising therapy.

Statins

The statins (cholesterol-lowering drugs) also show some promise for the treatment of MS. There is a wealth of evidence from animal studies that they suppress inflammation and reduce the severity of EAE. One study showed that atorvastatin, one of this class of drugs, prevented or even reversed paralysis in laboratory animals with the animal model of MS.[183] There is experimental work to show that these drugs stabilise the blood–brain barrier, and so should be helpful in MS.[184]

One study showed that simvastatin, one of the statins, improved outcomes significantly for PwMS having an acute attack of optic neuritis.[185] The randomised controlled trial allocated people to receive 80 mg daily of simvastatin for six months or a placebo. None of the people in the study received steroids. A number of measures of the damage caused by the optic neuritis showed significant improvement, and people taking the simvastatin rated their vision as better than that of the placebo group. While there has long been interest in the possibility of using statins as a disease-modifying treatment to reduce the number of relapses in PwMS, this is the first study to use these drugs as an acute treatment for a particular relapse. It adds to the likelihood of the statins being useful for MS, and also underscores the likely role of fats in the disease.

Probably of greater significance was the research on 140 people with progressive MS treated over two years with one of the statins.[186] In a randomised controlled trial with people in the control group taking a placebo, the researchers found that MRI scanning showed 43 per cent less brain shrinkage in the group on the statins than those on placebo. Brain shrinkage in people with progressive MS has been shown in the past to correlate with worsening disability. In this study—presumably because of the short timeframe—they were only able to show a very slight improvement in disability in the treated group of a quarter of a point on the twelve-point EDSS. To date, no drug has been unequivocally shown to affect the worsening course in progressive MS, except mitoxantrone.

 Statins probably reduce brain shrinkage in progressive MS.

The researchers found no difference in any of the immune parameters they measured—that is, the balance between Th1 and Th2 cytokines— showing that the drug appeared to have no real effect on the tendency towards inflammation. They argued that perhaps the drug worked through protecting nerve cells, previously documented with this drug. Finally, they suggested that because it is known that PwMS have more cardiovascular disease, statins might be working through this effect, given that the drug is used to treat cardiovascular disease, and the fact that they did notice a drop in cholesterol in the group taking the statins. In fact, when you looked at it closely, it was a very large drop in cholesterol in the treated group, of around 25 per cent.

But what are the real implications of this study? Statins have their beneficial effect in heart disease through several mechanisms, the major one being an improvement in the lipid profile (balance of good and bad fats in the blood). Until recently, when statins seem to have become the first-line treatment for heart disease, doctors have always advised people with poor lipid profiles and high risk of heart disease to modify their diets to reduce saturated fat, among other lifestyle changes. This dietary change can improve lipid profiles and lower cholesterol more than the statins do if applied rigorously. What this study really reaffirms is that changing the lipid profile towards a healthier balance of good and bad fats results in significant slowing of disease progression, even for people with progressive MS.

This is exactly in accord with the findings of Swank and the OMS recommendations, except that I suggest using diet to achieve this improved lipid profile, because a very low-saturated fat diet is also associated with many other health benefits (reduced risk of many other chronic Western diseases) and has only beneficial side-effects, unlike the statins. It is somewhat surprising that these researchers did not discuss this in the paper. It is highly likely that many doctors treating people with progressive MS will now start offering statins to them, while continuing to ignore the more fundamental approach to good health and slowed MS progression: a rigorously applied ultra-healthy plant-based wholefood diet plus seafood.

Given the experience we have with this group of drugs and their documented safety profile, however, this is a promising avenue for treating MS—particularly as many people find it easier to take a medication than to make significant lifestyle changes.

Cannabis-related drugs

There has been interest in evaluating drugs that are extracted from cannabis (cannabinoids) in treating certain aspects of MS, particularly pain and spasticity. Indeed, results of clinical trials have been so promising that a drug consisting of various extracts of the cannabis plant (Sativex) was made available by prescription in Canada in 2005. The drug is delivered as a spray under the tongue. A review of the trials involving cannabinoids in MS notes that five randomised controlled trials have been performed comparing the spray against placebo.[187] Generally, pain, spasticity, muscle cramps and sleep disturbance were all improved. Side-effects included dizziness, fatigue and feeling intoxicated.

The Cannabinoids in MS (CAMS) Study, examined 630 PwMS from 33 UK centres.[188] It found some benefit for spasticity, and patients felt the drug was helpful. More detailed study has shown that cannabinoids shift the Th1/Th2 balance towards a Th2 profile, and thus may be of benefit in the immunomodulation of MS. Further, they may have a beneficial effect on the degenerative aspects of the disease.[189, 190]

Haematopoietic stem cell transplantation (HSCT)

Also known as bone marrow transplantation, centres offering this therapy have sprung up around the world in recent years. A number of researchers have suggested that, since MS is effectively an error in the programming of the immune system, a possible treatment would be to destroy all the bone marrow, either with chemotherapy like some blood cancer treatments or with radiation, and then start again with a 'new' rebooted immune system.

HSCT is a high-risk treatment that involves collecting stem cells from the bone marrow or blood, purifying them in the laboratory, giving chemotherapy to destroy the immune system and then putting the stem cells back into the person by intravenous infusion. A number of studies around the world have shown that the procedure can be effective for rebooting the immune system and markedly stabilising the progression of MS. In Australia, fewer than 40 PwMS with active, aggressive MS not responding to usual medications have been treated with HSCT. In the whole world, only a few hundred patients have been documented to have received this treatment.

This is a very high-risk treatment. The profound immune suppression caused by the chemotherapy can result in severe life-threatening infections and bleeding. While the death rate for people receiving this therapy was of the order of around 5 per cent initially, with better treatment in reputable centres, it is now closer to 2 per cent in the first 100 days after treatment. This treatment option is dangerous and should be considered experimental; currently, it is reserved for PwMS with a rapidly progressive, aggressive form of the disease.

Several reports have, however, documented promising results. One described 21 people with very severe MS unresponsive to other treatments who had received HSCT.[191] There was a dramatic improvement, with MRI evidence of brain inflammation virtually disappearing. The Australian media have reported the case of Ben Leahy, a twenty-year-old man from Canberra, who was diagnosed with MS in 2008, followed by a rapidly progressive course resulting in him being in a wheelchair and even in intensive care for a period with trouble breathing.[192] Because the disease was so rapidly progressive and his future was so bleak, his treating neurologist, Dr Colin Andrews, decided to try HSCT. The procedure was a great success, and Ben was rapidly up and about, walking, with only a bit of residual weakness in one leg and some visual disturbance from the old lesions. As techniques of bone marrow transplantation continue to improve, the fatality rate from the procedure continues to fall. Dr Andrews from Canberra quotes a figure of 1 per cent currently.

Another study followed PwMS after stem cell transplantation from one hospital in Greece. The hospital began stem cell transplantation for people with aggressive MS not responding to other standard therapies in 1995; this study reports a median follow-up time of eleven years.[193] The results suggest that while some people do die after the procedure, in general there is a sustained reduction in progression to disability for these people with very aggressive disease who might otherwise quickly get profoundly disabled. Thirty-five people were followed after the procedure. Two people died as a direct result of therapy, a somewhat higher death rate than the 2 per cent generally reported from other European centres. In general, the researchers concluded that stem cell transplantation is not a therapy for most PwMS, but should be reserved for aggressive cases, generally early in the disease, but where disease is progressing rapidly. In very severe forms, it can be life-saving. Transplantation had an impressive and sustained effect in suppressing disease activity. This may be something to consider for young people with rapidly progressing disease.

A 2015 US report of 24 PwMS with very active disease who were treated with high-dose immunosuppression followed by their own stem cells showed highly encouraging improvements in neurologic function, quality of life and lack of disease activity and progression.[194] Over three-quarters had no further lesions, relapses or further loss of neurologic function at the three-year follow up. While the authors reported that treatment was associated with 'few serious early complications or unexpected adverse events', there were many adverse events that were expected, given the serious toxicity of those immunosuppressant drugs. This clearly limits the application of this therapy to those with very rapidly progressive disease that is not responding to standard preventive medicine and drug therapy.

Stem cell therapy is highly promising, but currently quite toxic, with many unethical centres offering sub-standard versions of the therapy.

Some centres have cashed in on the reports of these successful procedures by offering 'stem cell' therapy, but without the pre-treatment to knock out the immune system. These centres have sprung up in places like Ukraine, Barbados, Mexico and China. Sometimes they offer stem cells collected from foetuses, claiming that these foetal stem cells have no side-effects. They often list an impressive array of diseases that this treatment can cure, charging in the order of US$20,000–25,000, usually paid in advance. None of these clinics has published any results of this therapy in any medical journals, and at best they may do no harm. But there is really no chance that they can help improve MS.

T-cell vaccination

Modern medicine is getting very close to manipulating the immune response to produce specific outcomes. Scientists chose a group of twenty PwMS who had not responded to standard disease-modifying drugs, and tried a completely new technique.[195] Here they removed T-cells from these people, activated them with synthetic myelin base protein and myelin oligodendrocyte glycoprotein, the proteins thought to be the targets of the immune response in MS. They then inactivated the cells and injected them back into the patients. The idea behind this is complex, but basically the body should then develop an immune response to the T-cells, reducing their number and activity, and thus reducing the activity of the illness. This is indeed what happened. The annual relapse rate fell from 2.6 to 1.1—a dramatic drop—and there was a reduction in the number of new lesions on MRI. While the long-term consequences of altering the immune response in this way are unknown, the treatment holds promise, certainly for those people who do not respond to drug therapies. A study of this group who had not responded to conventional therapies was very promising, with an 85 per cent reduction in relapse rate by the end of a year of treatment.[196]

Another study recruited 26 people with relapsing-progressive MS, whose T cells were shown to respond to these or other specific proteins known to be involved in the MS immune response.[197] They then grew these cells outside the body, and irradiated them to stop them functioning properly. At time points of one day, two months, three months and six months, they injected these patients' own irradiated cells under their skin as a vaccination. For the group who received only the control injections (salt water rather than the irradiated cells), there was a continuing steady deterioration of half a point on the EDSS scale, and a slight worsening in 10 m walking time. For the vaccinated group, disability improved by nearly half a point, and there was nearly a one-second improvement in 10 m walking time.

Further, as these were people with progressive disease but still having relapses, it was possible to compare relapse rates. There was only one relapse in the vaccinated group over the year of the study, whereas the seven people in the control group had six relapses. Importantly, no one suffered any significant side-effect of the treatment. This is really important news, particularly for people with progressive MS. Of course, there is still considerable work to be done to confirm these findings in a larger group before such therapy might become available clinically; however, this study opens up the potential of highly specific treatments for PwMS that are tailored to their own particular immune response.

Skin patches of myelin peptides

Other researchers have adopted a different immune-based approach to treating MS. They used a number of the proteins in myelin in a skin patch to induce immune system tolerance to the body's own myelin as a way of controlling the immune reaction to myelin in PwMS.[198] The patches were changed weekly initially, and then monthly. In comparison to a group applying placebo patches, the group with the myelin peptides showed a favourable anti-inflammatory immune response that would be expected to make a difference to the progress of MS. The results of the actual clinical progress haven't yet been published.

An editorial commenting on the article notes that only a few groups are adopting this approach to MS, but that it holds great promise.[199] Certainly, it is likely to have far fewer side-effects than the current disease-modifying medications, which the authors describe as 'heavy weapons' in contrast to the 'magic bullet' represented by the skin patches. Of course, DMDs would become a thing of the past if this approach works. Tailored immune therapy such as this may well become an important additional avenue for managing MS.

DNA vaccination

Another very exciting prospect for PwMS is that of DNA vaccination. This basically takes the part of the genetic sequence of a person with MS that codes for myelin base protein and uses it to vaccinate the person, so that they develop an immune response against that part of their own DNA. It is very experimental, but in one study researchers vaccinated a person with MS with this experimental vaccine and found a decrease in inflammatory cytokines as well as decreased antibodies to myelin in the spinal fluid.[200]

A number of exciting new possible therapies for MS are in advanced stages of testing.

This has now been explored further in a large randomised controlled trial. Using two different doses of the DNA vaccine BHT–3009 compared with placebo in 267 PwMS, the researchers found that after eight weeks there was a statistically significant 61 per cent reduction in the number of new lesions, but only with the lower dose.[201] The method of administration was by intramuscular injection at weeks 0, 2, 4 and every four weeks thereafter. This treatment appears to hold great promise. It is not clear whether it will cause any side-effects in the long term, although it appears very safe in the short-term clinical trial.

Synthetic peptide MBP8298

This is a human-made molecule designed to be very similar to myelin base protein (MBP), one of the likely targets of auto-immunity in MS. In theory, giving a big dose of this peptide periodically should cause the immune system to become tolerant of its own myelin and lessen its attack on it. A major study comparing intravenous injections of MBP8298 every six months with placebo showed that in certain sub-groups of PwMS there was a dramatic (over 75 per cent) reduction in the progression of disability in progressive MS.[202] These results are impressive, and offer great hope for people with progressive MS.

Intestinal parasites

It has recently been argued that the hygiene hypothesis may explain part of the pattern of MS incidence around the world. MS is a disease of affluent countries where sanitation has effectively eliminated many of the organisms that previously inhabited the human gastrointestinal tract. Previous data have suggested that MS is less active in individuals with some of these infestations, in particular worm infestations of the bowel. One small pilot study of five PwMS given an oral suspension of porcine whipworm, a non-toxic parasite that doesn't infect humans and is not contagious, but does provoke an immune reaction, showed that this administration provoked a strongly anti-inflammatory reaction, reducing the number of new MS lesions from 6.8 on average before administration to two after administration, with a return to previous disease activity once the administration was stopped.[203] This paves the way for large-scale trials of the whipworm administration.

Masitinib
People with progressive forms of MS (primary and secondary progressive MS) have long been concerned about the lack of medications that might help slow the progression of the disease. While there are many medications now that have some modest effect in relapsing-remitting MS, there has been little progress in developing any medication that might help progressive MS. One preliminary study, without adequate numbers to prove a benefit, was designed to see whether the drug masitinib did affect the course of progressive MS in a small sample of people with that disease.[204] Masitinib is a drug that is taken by mouth and inhibits an enzyme called tyrosine kinase, ultimately leading to the inhibition or death of mast cells, certain cells in the immune system intimately involved in the progression of MS.

The researchers randomly allocated 35 people with progressive forms of MS to the treatment group (27) or placebo (8). While there were side-effects in those treated, there was also a substantial improvement in their functional scores compared with when they started the trial, as opposed to a worsening of the functional scores in those receiving placebo. There were some serious adverse reactions to the drug, including marked reductions in the white cell count, predisposing these people to the potential for serious infections, but these disappeared rapidly on discontinuing the drug.

While there are clearly problems related to this toxicity, which still need to be worked through, this constitutes real hope of a drug treatment for progressive forms of MS, and is likely to be welcome news to many people with this form of the disease. This study paves the way for a larger randomised controlled trial of masitinib.

Anti-viral agents

Most virus infections are not treatable. While we have really good anti-biotics for a whole range of bacterial infections, such as those causing pneumonia, boils and ear infections, rendering many of these diseases a nuisance instead of the lethal diseases of the past, we are still search-ing for effective anti-viral agents. The common cold still affects millions of people each year, and we are powerless to prevent it. One virus for which this is not true is the herpes virus. A range of anti-viral agents typified by acyclovir have become available for the treatment of herpes virus infections. These agents are highly effective, and are relatively free from side-effects. They are thought to hold promise for the treatment of MS.

Acyclovir has been used to treat cold sores, shingles and genital herpes, as well as herpes encephalitis. However, it has a relatively short-lived effect in the body and must be taken five times a day for full benefit. A newer range of these drugs has more recently become available. The most commonly prescribed of these is famciclovir. This drug has been shown to suppress genital herpes when taken twice daily in a dose of 250 mg. Again, it is very safe and can be taken long term.

Given the likely role of herpes viruses in the development of MS, anti-viral treatment with acyclovir-like drugs against herpes viruses may hold some promise. The initial randomised controlled trial in the area suffered from having only a small number of patients.[205] The research-ers randomised 60 PwMS to receive either acyclovir 800 mg three times a day, or placebo three times a day for two years. Those treated with acyclovir had 34 per cent fewer relapses than the placebo group, but because of the small numbers of people in the study, this difference was not statistically significant, despite a treatment effect comparable in size to interferon and glatiramer. If patients were grouped accord-ing to relapse rates into low (0–2), medium (3–5) and high (6–8) rate groups, the difference between acyclovir and placebo treatment was significant. Looking at only those patients in the study who had had MS for over two years, so that a previous relapse rate could be determined, the acyclovir-treated group had a statistically significant reduction in relapse rate.

Another trial using valacyclovir in 58 PwMS found a trend towards better outcomes with treatment.[206] The data really suggest that the studies are too small to detect a significant treatment effect, and that bigger studies are needed. There is substantial evidence that the herpes virus is involved in the development of MS, and the few small studies suggest that treatment may reduce relapse rates; however, there is little inclination by industry to follow these studies up, given that the medication is generic and cheap in comparison with licensed DMDs. There seems little downside risk to these medications, unlike some of the more accepted therapies, and they can be taken orally.

HOLISM study findings on medications used in MS

Our research from the large group of PwMS we assembled for the HOLISM study from 57 countries worldwide provided a real-world picture of how these drugs are performing in practice. Data from clinical trials are important, but the trials—with their rigid inclusion and exclusion criteria—often recruit highly selected patients who are not really representative of PwMS in the community, and the drugs are often not able to be compared with each other in the trials, mostly just against a placebo. So it is hard to get a sense of which drugs perform better. Similarly, quality of life is often not measured in the trials—just relapse rate reduction, which many have argued is a poor measure, as it has little correlation with long-term disability, the real issue for most PwMS.[207]

In our sample of 2276 PwMS answering the relevant questions about medications, a third had never taken one of the 24 listed DMDs, 17 per cent had previously used a DMD but had discontinued use and were no longer taking a DMD, 18 per cent had previously taken a DMD but had discontinued it and were now taking another DMD, while another third were currently taking a DMD having not taken one previously. Glatiramer (Copaxone) was the most commonly used drug, taken by 21 per cent of those taking a drug, followed by one of the interferons (19 per cent). Of the newer drugs, natalizumab (Tysabri) was being taken by 6 per cent and fingolimod (Gilenya) by 4 per cent. Interestingly, 7 per cent of PwMS taking a medication in our study were taking low-dose naltrexone (LDN). So our snapshot of medication use by PwMS worldwide reflected a less current profile of prescribing than it would today, with the majority of drugs being first-generation DMDs; currently, the more effective oral medications are far more widely used.

The number of participants taking over the counter, prescription and herbal agents for various complaints was very high, with 19 per cent of participants taking one agent, 16 per cent taking two, 13 per cent taking three, 8 per cent taking four, 6 per cent taking five, 4.5 per cent taking six and 4.5 per cent taking seven or more, up to a maximum of fourteen agents for one participant. Generally, polypharmacy is defined as five or more concurrent drugs, and is considered a serious issue in modern medicine, given the potential for drug interactions. A total of 29 per cent of people in our study did not take any agent.

Quality of life was not consistently associated with the use of a DMD in our study. There were trends—some significant—to worse quality of life across the four domains (mental health composite, physical health composite, overall quality of life sub-score and health perception sub-score) for the interferons, fingolimod and natalizumab, when compared with the other DMDs, and more so when compared with no DMD use (see Figure 14). In contrast, glatiramer showed favourable trends for quality of life when compared with the other DMDs across these domains, and was the only medication for which quality of life was higher in any of the domains than for those taking no DMDs. The size of these differences overall, however, was small despite being statistically significant. LDN was frequently being used in addition to one of the first- or second-generation DMDs, but quality of life for LDN was significantly lower across many domains than for those taking 'other DMDs' and those not taking any DMDs.

We also compared each of the commonly used DMDs against each other across the full range of domains in quality of life. Glatiramer was associated with better quality of life than the other DMDs across most domains. Sophisticated regression analyses, after controlling for a range of relatively stable factors (age, marital status, employment status, education, number of close relationships, disability and number of comorbidities),

Figure 14: Quality of life, comparing individual DMDs with all other DMDs and no DMD use

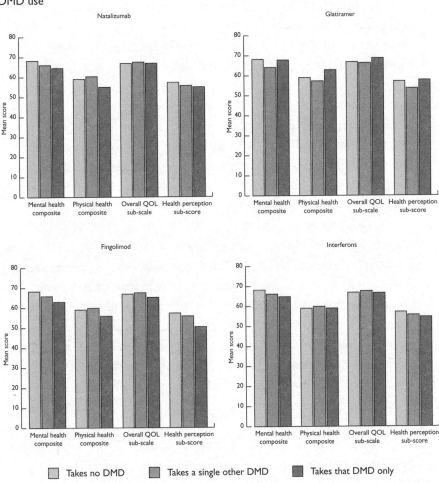

found a small (two points each on a 100-point scale) but significantly worse quality of life, both physically and mentally, for those taking a DMD.

Those PwMS taking five or more over-the-counter, prescription or herbal agents—that is, those with polypharmacy, irrespective of DMD use—scored significantly lower for every domain of quality of life than those not reporting polypharmacy use, up to a massive 31.5-point reduction.

A lower relapse rate was detected for those taking a DMD compared with those not taking one only for those taking the DMD for longer than twelve months. The reduction was about 24 per cent, comparable with the difference found in the interferon and glatiramer trials. There were no significant differences in relapse rates associated with each of the individual major DMDs (glatiramer, interferons, fingolimod and natalizumab) when compared with relapse rates for those taking any other single DMD, or with relapse rates for those not taking any DMD, and for those taking a single DMD for longer than twelve months. Relapse rate, however, was over 50 per cent higher for those taking five or more over-the-counter medicines, whether or not the person also took a DMD. DMD use didn't have any real association with disability that we could detect in our study. But again, those with polypharmacy—irrespective of DMD use—were more disabled.

Our HOLISM study provided a golden opportunity to see what these medications were doing in a real-world setting for PwMS. With about half the sample taking one of the DMDs, this gave us a chance to compare disease outcomes by whether or not PwMS were using medication, and by particular medications. With most medication studies funded by the pharmaceutical industry, few independent studies of a similar scale to our study have addressed the challenging issue of assessing real-world DMD associations with quality of life, disease activity and disability.

The pattern of medication use by PwMS in our sample provided some unique perspectives on their medication choices and the prescribing habits of their clinicians. The first-generation, self-injected DMDs were still the most commonly used medications in our sample, with a significant proportion of respondents having taken them for longer than a decade, although most had taken them for between one and ten years. Doctors treating PwMS are commonly still prescribing these medications, despite the arrival of a range of oral DMDs, as around a quarter of those taking these medicines had been taking them for less than a year. This may be contributed to by the fact that, in some countries, the newer oral agents are not subsidised by government and may be cost-prohibitive, but also that the study was conducted in 2012 and the oral medications have now been prescribed more widely.

Natalizumab was also frequently prescribed; however, many people had taken the drug for some years, raising concerns about the potential for the development of progressive multifocal leukoencephalopathy (PML), known to occur more frequently with prolonged use.[19] Fingolimod was used more frequently than the other approved oral medications, reflecting its earlier licensing approval in most countries. It was interesting to note how commonly LDN was used in this cohort, despite not being licensed for use in MS in any country. Despite limited evidence from randomised controlled trials of a possible benefit for quality of life with this medication,[182] we detected no positive associations of LDN with quality of life or relapse rate in our sample.

It is well known that many PwMS choose to discontinue their DMDs.[208] In our study, over 15 per cent had ceased a previous DMD and not taken an alternative medication, and a slightly larger proportion had replaced a previous DMD with another medication. Mostly this involved people ceasing one of the interferons (nearly a quarter of the sample). This is likely to reflect side-effects, known to be more common with the interferons than the other DMDs. Other data from our HOLISM study also suggest a negative effect on mood,[35] and this may have contributed to discontinuation of the drug. It probably also reflects preferences for oral agents over injectable drugs.

A large proportion of PwMS in our sample were taking over-the-counter, prescription and herbal agents for the common symptoms that accompany MS, particularly depression, pain and spasticity. Many were taking large numbers of such agents, raising the issue of drug interactions and side-effects. Similarly, a large proportion were taking medication for fatigue, despite a lack of evidence for any benefit from such medications.[209] This contrasts with the strong associations found between healthy lifestyle choices and reduced fatigue in our study.[210] Given previous data suggesting worse fatigue and cognitive deficit in those PwMS on multiple pharmacological agents,[211] the extent of polypharmacy in this cohort was of great concern, with over a third of the cohort taking three or more over-the-counter, prescription or herbal agents for symptom management, and around 15 per cent taking five or more, excluding their use of DMDs.

Our study represented a unique snapshot of medication use from a geographically diverse population, and allowed examination of the association between medication use and health outcomes important to PwMS and their clinicians. Quality of life outcomes have previously been highlighted as an unmet need in current MS management.[212, 213] Apart from glatiramer, none of the DMDs, or LDN, was associated with better quality of life in our study, and for glatiramer the size of this positive benefit for quality of life was very small. These marginally positive quality of life associations are in keeping with previous literature,[214] and fit with recent data on 672 PwMS from 148 centres worldwide, showing improvements in health outcomes, including quality of life, for those switching from other medications to glatiramer.[215] This fits with our recommendation that glatiramer ought to be used more as a first-choice drug therapy, particularly also given its long-established safety profile. We confirmed previous concerns about polypharmacy for the quality of life of PwMS,[211] and raised concerns about higher relapse rates and more disability.

We concluded that our real-world snapshot of self-reported medication use by a large sample of PwMS worldwide detected only a small signal of benefit in relapse rate reduction for those taking a single DMD for longer than twelve months, and inconsistent and generally minor associations with quality of life. Our follow-up data at 2.5 years will enable us to better determine any effect on progression of disability. So our data didn't show the medications commonly used for MS providing benefit for quality of life, except for Copaxone. With only a small reduction in relapse rate for those taking the DMDs for a year or more, and similar or worse quality of life than experienced by those not taking a DMD, our data on this group of over 2000 PwMS didn't really confirm clinical trial data. That may reflect the fact the sicker people were being prescribed the DMDs, and those who were doing better were not.

This part of the HOLISM study lent some support to the use of one of the major DMDs, in that relapse rate may be reduced with these drugs, in keeping with results of the clinical trials. In the spirit of doing 'whatever it takes' to get well after a diagnosis of MS, many PwMS will opt to take a DMD in addition to a preventive medicine approach; the HOLISM study data support the view that this is an individual decision. Similarly, for PwMS who opt to take one of the DMDs, the evidence about quality of life differences between the medications should be borne in mind when choosing which one to take.

HOW

Introduction

Important questions that a person with MS must answer after diagnosis are whether to take one of the DMDs and, if so, how to choose which one. While they are important questions, it is crucial to make a start on the preventive medicine lifestyle changes first, and as soon as possible after diagnosis, while taking some time to consider these medication questions and getting some sense of how the disease is likely to progress (or, hopefully, not progress). For some people, it will be evident that the disease is very active right from the outset, and prompt use of a DMD may be necessary. It is important to work closely with a neurologist to get a sense of how active the disease may be for the individual before embarking on these treatment decisions.

In a nutshell

- The first question to answer is, 'Should I take a disease-modifying drug?'
- This choice is very personal, and for most people does not need to be rushed.
- If the answer is yes, the next question is, 'Which one?'
- This choice should be based on careful balancing of benefits against risks.
- HOLISM showed that glatiramer (Copaxone) is the only commonly used medication associated with better quality of life, has very few serious side-effects, and is therefore a good choice for many people—although it does have to be injected.
- Many will prefer the convenience of one of the oral medications.

To take, or not to take, a DMD?

Many doctors, after looking at the evidence from clinical trials of the DMDs, will say to PwMS that they must start on a DMD as soon as possible after diagnosis, and must stay on that DMD for life, unless something better comes along. Medications certainly have an important role to play, and are a legitimate part of a comprehensive secondary preventive medicine approach to managing MS for many people, just as they are in many other chronic diseases like heart disease and diabetes. But starting a DMD as soon as possible after diagnosis is just one of many possible approaches, and it is not a sound approach if done in isolation with no attention to lifestyle risk factors for disease progression. This drug-only approach is based on a narrow view of the medical literature influenced by the many clinical trials that have shown that those PwMS starting on a particular DMD early do better over the long term than those starting later. This view, however, fails to take into account a great deal of other important information.

First, it fails to recognise the variability in the course of MS from person to person, and the changing natural history of MS in the twenty-first century. MS is a highly variable disease, manifesting differently from person to person. Some people have an attack, are diagnosed on the basis of that attack and MRI changes, but never have another one. Others have highly active, aggressive disease and progress to disability very rapidly. In my clinical practice, I have seen a woman in her forties who was wheelchair bound within six months of diagnosis. This sort of rapid progression is a real challenge for neurologists, who have to weigh up the risks of very potent medication with the likelihood of rapid development of permanent disability. Of course, very potent medication has to be considered. It makes no sense, though, to take the same therapeutic approach to people at both ends of this spectrum. Exposing the first person to all the side-effects of a DMD when they were not going to be significantly affected by MS is clearly not good medicine. Not offering the woman every available medical therapy is also not good medicine, after careful consideration of the side-effects of the various drugs.

The natural history of MS is changing rapidly. While the reasons are unclear, MS appears to be becoming a disease with a better outlook. A smaller proportion of PwMS now progress to a cane or wheelchair than occurred in the last century. That may be due to earlier diagnosis since the advent of MRI scanning, diagnosis of some people in whom the diagnosis was never made in earlier times because their illness was so mild, or other factors—probably including the more widespread use of DMDs. Whatever the reason, the outlook for PwMS today is not nearly so poor as it was last century, quite apart from the major advances in preventive medicine that this book describes that can modify the course of the disease. If progression to disability is becoming less common and varies considerably from person to person, does a 'one size fits all' approach of putting everyone on a DMD make sense?

 Whether to take a DMD after MS diagnosis is an individual decision requiring careful consideration; it should not be rushed.

It is probably worth thinking about the spectrum of PwMS as being like a bell curve in a graph of number of people progressing to disability versus time (see Figure 15). The left group will progress rapidly, the middle (largest) group will progress more slowly over a number of years, and the right group will progress very slowly and possibly never be disabled, even without any intervention. Those on the left may well need the help of the more potent MS medications like natalizumab,

Figure 15: The roller-coaster to stability

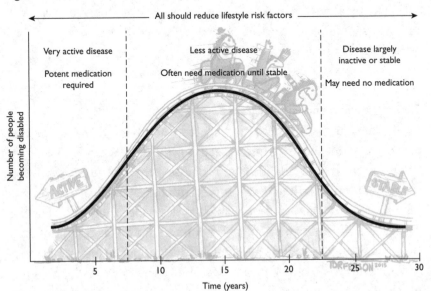

alemtuzumab or even mitoxantrone if they are really deteriorating quickly—certainly soon after diagnosis before a lifestyle approach has really had time to contribute to stability of the disease. Those on the right may well never need medication, especially if they adopt a secondary preventive approach and gain control over the disease. The situation is somewhat more flexible for those in the middle. Consultation with an experienced neurologist is especially important for people in this group. Some may require one of the DMDs to get some stability while a secondary preventive approach is instituted—perhaps one of the less-toxic ones, like glatiramer, or fingolimod if the disease is more active. Others may prefer a wait-and-see approach while they take stock of how quickly things are progressing.

Importantly, one of the difficulties in making this decision relates to the fact that it is currently not possible to provide an accurate prognosis at the time of diagnosis. We currently do not have any tests or other tools to tell how quickly or slowly a person with a new diagnosis of MS might progress to disability. That is the reason licensing authorities worldwide suggest reserving the more potent immune-modulating medications for those who have aggressive, rapidly progressing disease, as the side-effects of the more potent medications are more severe, in line with their more potent action in modifying the way the immune system functions. But how does one know how aggressive the disease is and how quickly it will progress without observing the natural history of the illness over at least some period of time?

Timing of commencing a DMD

PwMS are often advised to start disease-modifying drugs *as soon as possible* after diagnosis. Quite apart from the decision about whether drugs are needed at all in individual cases, the question of whether starting early is important has not been discussed widely. Publishing in *Multiple Sclerosis International*, Canadian neurologists suggest that this is indeed a difficult question.[216] The authors note that timing of such treatment should be highly individualised, and the person with MS very well informed before making any decision. They note that their reading of the literature only partly supports early treatment after clinical onset of multiple sclerosis. Of course, a neurologist might consider that many active lesions on MRI scanning, and two relapses in rapid succession prior to diagnosis constitutes active disease, and would recommend starting a medication with some urgency—and that is clearly appropriate. I would argue that it is also important to be active early in modifying those risk factors that are known to affect disease progression, as discussed in the other steps of the OMS Recovery Program. Many people stabilise the illness in this way, and find that they do not require medication.

So a personalised approach is needed, one that takes the unique circumstances of the individual into account, putting the person with the illness at the centre of the treatment, and considering the preferences and choices of the individual. Many neurologists and other doctors—particularly those in primary care and family practice—are very good at this sort of doctor–patient interaction. Today there are also many online resources that can help, both in finding a doctor who uses such a patient-centred individualised approach, and in making the choice about whether and when to start on a DMD. Research shows that while doctors offer the most trusted source of information for PwMS, most actually get their information from the internet.[217]

One useful site is Healthline, <www.healthline.com>, a reputable online resource with a sound medical advisory board that provides helpful information on which to base such a decision. Under Multiple Sclerosis, for example, the site discusses what a primary care doctor can offer, what finding an MS specialist doctor can add, and issues around whether to start a DMD.

The site poses questions like:

- What is your own position or attitude on treatments? Do you want a doctor who goes for aggressive treatments, or one who takes a 'wait and see' approach?
- Would you like an integrative approach? You may or may not like the idea of having access to in-house mental health practitioners, rehabilitation specialists, nutritionists, and other experts.

A wait-and-see approach has been advocated by a number of authorities, despite the dire warnings of some doctors who focus on the narrow industry-sponsored clinical trial data showing a divergence of outcomes for those who wait versus those who commence pharmaceutical treatment immediately. For many years, the Mayo Clinic, <www.mayoclinic.org>, recommended a 'wait and see approach', although in recent years it has stopped using this terminology, and simply spells out the issues.[218] The site notes that MS is so unpredictable that devising a treatment approach is challenging, and that currently there is no way to reliably predict whether a particular medication will work or not for any individual. So it recommends basing the decision on several factors, particularly how aggressive the disease is—including recent attack frequency, severity and recovery—personal preferences, side-effects of the DMD and whether these side-effects or the requirements for taking the DMD or monitoring its side-effects cause undue hardship for the person. It notes that sharing decision-making between the person and the doctor is critical, as each person's situation is unique, and the best approach is a tailored one, specifically designed for the individual. Choosing the right doctor is an important part of this equation.

A key issue here is the current lack of translation into clinical practice of the evidence around the potential for a preventive medicine approach to make a major difference to disease progression, and hence to be taken into account when making a decision about whether or not to take a DMD. As outlined in this book, there is now a comprehensive, congruent evidence base supporting the value of a secondary preventive medicine approach to MS management. While some of it is relatively new—much of it derived from the HOLISM study—a lot of it has been around for decades, and so should be considered as part of any treatment plan for someone diagnosed with MS.

To not consider this approach and its ramifications when making the decision about whether or not to take a DMD is simply not using all the tools we have at our disposal to manage this illness. Unfortunately, this approach is sometimes seen as being in conflict with responsible advice about using proven medications to manage MS. There does not need to be any conflict or polarisation of views if the person with the illness is kept central to the decision-making process, taking into account the person's individual situation, and their personal characteristics and preferences.

An important consideration is that very few of the clinical trials of the various licensed DMDs for MS have included any consideration of the preventive lifestyle characteristics of the people participating in the trials, or included significant lifestyle risk-factor modification. Where these have been studied, they have been shown to make treatment more effective—for instance, adding vitamin D supplementation to therapy with interferon.[219] The HOLISM study has controlled for lifestyle behaviours and risk factors in its holistic investigation of all the factors that might influence disease outcome. The data assembled in this book clearly suggest that the magnitude of benefit from such a preventive medicine approach is large—potentially as large or larger than that of the more recent DMDs, and probably with a significant benefit in delaying disease progression. So a decision about taking a DMD based solely on the clinical trial data showing a worse outcome for those not taking a DMD, in the absence of any knowledge or data about the potential difference that diet, exercise, sun exposure, vitamin D, omega-3 intake, meditation and so on could have made to participants in either treatment or control groups is not sound.

A person with MS could be convinced that the untreated group may have done better than the treated group had they adopted a preventive medicine approach. Equally, another person could be convinced that the treatment group would have done better again had they too adopted a preventive medicine approach, and that the best strategy would be to do both. There is evidence to support such a conviction.

As with the management of any chronic disease, however, some PwMS will find the option of making significant lifestyle changes too daunting or difficult, and will prefer to take a medication. Others will be immensely grateful to find that there are choices, and will grasp the opportunity to make a difference to their own health with both hands. Whether or not to add a DMD in that situation will come down, for some people, to their own background and trust in pharmaceutical agents, and for others to the degree to which they wish to do 'whatever it takes' to stay or get well, and this may reflect their own experience and knowledge of MS and how disabling it can be, or considerations such as the cost and availability of the medicines. Most PwMS, in my experience, consider the issue of side-effects for any particular drug to be crucial to making the decision—particularly in deciding which of the DMDs to take once a decision has been made to go ahead with a medication. Side-effects vary from annoying (skin reactions) to potentially fatal (PML), and this needs to be carefully factored into any decision about whether to take a DMD, and which one.

Which DMD to take?

So, if after all the consideration and weighing up of evidence and balancing personal choices, one decides to take a DMD, which one? This can be a difficult decision, and again there are a lot of factors to consider. An initial consideration is deciding whether there is a drug that can help for the particular type of MS that one has. So for people with PPMS, for example, there are very few choices; indeed, many neurologists would say there are no medications that help for this type of MS. I disagree, in that while there are none licensed for use in PPMS, there is considerable anecdotal evidence that LDN may be of value. As previously noted, for a variety of reasons, LDN has not been well studied. But many people with all types of MS have reported significant benefit from LDN. Importantly, there is no real downside to taking it, as it has negligible side-effects. This is one of the key considerations in choosing a drug: balancing the potential benefits against the like-lihood and severity of side-effects. In very general terms, the more potent a medication is, the more likely it is to have serious side-effects. Recent news about the potential benefits of ocrelizumab for people with primary progressive MS also provides a good deal of hope for people in that situation.

> Which drug to take is also a serious decision that should be given ample time.

Similarly, there are very few options for people with SPMS. In some countries, interferons have been licensed for use in SPMS, and that may be an option. Mitoxantrone, a potent chemotherapy agent, appears to offer some possibility of halting progression and recovering some function, although that needs to be balanced against the serious side-effects of treatment-induced leukaemia that occurs in around one in 50 people given the drug. It should really be reserved for those who are progressing rapidly.

If one has relapsing-remitting MS, the number of potential medications is now very large, depending on the country in which one is living, and the extent to which the drug is subsidised by government, making it affordable. Most of the MS drugs are prohibitively expensive if they are not subsidised. For people with relapsing-remitting MS in most Western countries, many or all of the medications for relapsing-remitting MS are subsidised. In Australia, for example, the cost of even the most expensive of the MS medications is around A$30 per month, or around A$6 if one has a Health Care Card. That means medicines that might cost A$20,000 a year or more if one was paying full price are readily affordable for nearly everyone. Choosing the right medication is a key decision, and a very personal one that should be made in conjunction with the treating neurologist, taking into account the person's medical history, preferences, personality and views.

The decision should not be made lightly, and should be given ample time. There may be pressure to choose a medication quickly, with a suggestion that the longer one waits, the more damage one incurs. But whether starting early with treatment includes a medication or not, and how soon that is started, is a decision that does not have to be made immediately unless one has very active disease. Secondary prevention strategies are legitimate treatment options for MS, even if not yet widely recommended. It is certainly a legitimate choice to start with a preventive medicine strategy and make a decision about medication use after some period has elapsed during which to assess the effectiveness of prevention.

So which medication? Some of the issues to consider are effectiveness, track record of safety, cost, convenience, route of administration, need for monitoring or hospital attendances and, critically, the potential for and severity of side-effects. One expert review concluded that multiple disease, drug and patient-related factors should be considered when selecting the appropriate drug and treatment strategy for the appropriate patient, suggesting that this would accord with a personalised medicine approach to managing MS.[220]

Safety and side-effects are critical issues in deciding which DMD to take.

Unfortunately, there are few if any head-to-head trials of the various licensed medications, for obvious reasons to do with marketing of company products. If a drug company shows its drug is inferior to that of a competitor, it will be very hard to sell. A drug like glatiramer or one of the interferons, with a demonstrated 30 per cent relapse rate reduction in clinical trials, may only result, for someone having, say, ten relapses over ten years, in a reduction to seven relapses over ten years, with little influence on progression to disability. These older DMDs are not highly effective medications, which is the first point to consider. More recent drugs like fingolimod or natalizumab appear to result in more potent reductions in relapse rates, and this may be a consideration in choosing which drug to take; they may well also have an effect on progression to disability.

Track record of safety is important. We know from 20 years of experience with glatiramer that it is a safe drug. Serious side-effects have not become apparent over those two decades; if there was a major safety issue, we would have seen it by now. A more recently released drug like daclizumab, although heavily promoted, has very little track record on which to base an assessment of long-term safety, but even over the short term there are worrying safety issues.

For a great majority of PwMS, the issue of convenience—particularly related to route of administration—is a key consideration. The newer oral agents like fingolimod, teriflunomide and dimethyl fumarate have the great advantage of being in pill form, so injections are avoided. This is important not only practically, in terms of injection site reactions and needle phobia, but also psychologically. Most people feel much less like a 'patient' taking a tablet than taking an injection; put simply, they don't see themselves so much as a sick person. So fingolimod, which is taken only once a day, is simply more convenient for many people than dimethyl fumarate, which is taken twice a day. Most people find having to medicate once a day easier. Similarly, a person may opt for the safety and track record of a long established drug like glatiramer, but be put

STEP 5: TAKE MEDICATION IF NEEDED

off by the daily injection, preferring one of the interferons that involve second daily, thrice weekly or weekly injection. But the issue of greater likelihood of side-effects with the interferons, and the need for regular blood testing to detect these side-effects, may sway the decision back to glatiramer, despite the inconvenience of more frequent administration.

This is the sort of weighing up process that is required in order to make a decision with which one is happy, and likely to stick to in the long term. It really is important to have invested this sort of consideration and personal weighing up if one is to have the best chance of the medication working, and of tolerating any side-effects that may appear. Just like the OMS Recovery Program, the decision to take a medication should be embraced, looking forward to the potential benefits of getting the disease under control, rather than feeling that the decision has been foisted upon you—that you are passively and perhaps reluctantly accepting a decision made by someone else, with greater authority. The personal investment of spending time looking into all the issues around each of the considered drugs, making an active choice and embracing the medication is likely to make the drug work better. While some may call this a placebo response, it is really using mind–body medicine to its best effect to get the best out of all the avenues employed to recover from MS.

The issue of side-effects is a critical one to consider for PwMS when choosing a medication. This applies to not only what side-effects a particular drug has, and how severe they might be, but also the likelihood of developing them. So, for instance, while one may say that the flu-like illness that one gets every time one of the interferons is injected is only a nuisance, and not a really severe side-effect, the fact that around half the people who take the drug get the side-effect is a serious consideration, and enough to convince a great proportion of people who start on this drug to stop taking it. At the other extreme, PML only happens on average to around one in 500 people who take the drug natalizumab; however, when it does happen, it is frequently fatal! For a disease that in many cases doesn't cause serious problems for decades after diagnosis, the possibility of dying from the treatment has to be seriously considered; really, it has to restricted to PwMS who have very active disease and have tried other less toxic drugs without success. So PwMS need to be extremely critical about the choice of drug once they make a decision to take one.

OMS drug recommendations

I am often asked for my opinion of the various drugs. I have no conflict of interest in this, and have not undertaken any research funded by companies marketing these drugs. I do have personal experience of having taken glatiramer for some years, and so am perhaps biased towards that drug as I did not experience any side-effects when using it. When looking at the same information, though, ten different people or scientists are likely to reach ten slightly different conclusions. This is particularly so when the information varies markedly, depending on the source of the information.

So one's doctor may have formed a certain view about a drug that is different from those of other doctors—or indeed the average person with MS—depending on their background, understanding of the clinical trials, exposure to drug company marketing and motivation. A person with MS receiving that information needs to be aware that it represents only one opinion, and is almost certainly somewhat different from many other doctors' opinions. Making an informed choice means arming oneself with the necessary background information to balance a medical recommendation with what is in the literature and with a person's own beliefs, values and preferences. In the end, the choice is yours.

My own personal assessment of the various medications is relatively simple, and is of course not able to be influenced by your particular situation and preferences. These need to be borne in mind when looking at the advice I offer. However, I do not feel that the interferons have any role to play in managing MS in the modern era. There are safer drugs with good safety records and fewer side-effects. Far too many people develop depression while taking these drugs, as confirmed by our HOLISM study, and that is a serious concern—quite apart from the serious physical side-effects. Of course, if you are taking one of the interferons and feel happy with the medication, and are not deteriorating or depressed, then there is no reason to stop it just because of my take on these drugs.

In my view, if an injectable drug is chosen, for whatever reason, then glatiramer is preferable. It has a long safety record, has no serious side-effects, doesn't make people feel sick and is modestly helpful in reducing relapses. It may also have some benefit in slowing progression. It is also now available as a relatively cheap generic drug. Head-to-head research showed that, in a large cohort of 845 PwMS taking glatiramer or interferon, using 'intention to treat' analysis (that is, ignoring the drop-outs and analysing everyone who started on the drugs), the two-year risk of relapse with glatiramer was nearly half that for the interferon (6 per cent vs 11 per cent).[221] In those who used the drug continuously for the period, the difference was even greater in favour of glatiramer (2 per cent vs 9 per cent). Glatiramer is also more than twice as likely as the interferons to reduce fatigue from MS.[36] A more recent study showed that glatiramer and the interferons were roughly comparable in benefit,[222] but, of course, glatiramer far outweighs the interferons in terms of safety.

 Of the injectable DMDs, glatiramer's safety is a great advantage.

The other injectables, natalizumab and daclizumab, are too toxic to recommend for the average person with MS, but may be needed for those whose illness is particularly active and progressing. Natalizumab results in the often fatal PML for around one in 500 people who take it—up to one in 100 if one is JCV positive and has previously taken immunosuppressants, as many PwMS have done. Alemtuzumab causes serious illness in around a third to a half of all people taking it, principally auto-immune thyroid disease. Of course, some people with aggressive disease may require something more potent, and may be willing to accept the risk of these serious side-effects for the potentially better control of the illness.

From the available oral drugs, the pick is probably dimethyl fumarate, although it is somewhat less convenient than fingolimod and teriflunomide in that it is taken twice, rather than once, a day. It does have a very long safety record, though, in that a very similar drug has been used for the treatment of psoriasis over some decades now without serious safety concerns. Some people may opt for fingolimod, although that has potentially more serious side-effects, and doesn't have such a long safety record. There is not much in it, however, and the ease of once a day medication may be enough to swing the decision to fingolimod for many people. Teriflunomide just doesn't appear to work very well.

One issue that hasn't really been addressed in the medical literature is the consideration of problems that might occur if one needs to stop one of the drugs. This is a key issue for the drug natalizumab, given that the incidence of PML continues to grow with time, to the point where most authorities recommend it should not be taken for longer than two years. For every single person starting the drug, there will come a time when consideration needs to be given to stopping it. And this raises the issue of the disease rebounding in terms of activity—that is, becoming suddenly more active on stopping the drug. This can also be a problem, but occurs much less commonly with fingolimod.

Having chosen a drug, a further consideration for PwMS is what to do if the drug doesn't appear to be working. This may require switching to another medication. One study showed that 30 per cent of people taking either interferons or glatiramer stopped them for one reason or another within five years, but around half shifted to another agent.[223] A US study showed that for patients switching from interferon therapy to glatiramer due to lack of effectiveness of the interferon, the relapse rate dropped dramatically on glatiramer.[224] Another study showed that people who not only switched from interferons to glatiramer but also vice versa actually did really well, with annual relapse rates falling by about half to three-quarters in the three years after switching.[225] This has been confirmed by more recent work.[226] It is important for PwMS and their doctors to be aware that if the chosen drug is not working, there are always other options, and they usually work.[227]

OVERVIEW

There has been an explosion of drug therapies for MS over the past two decades; some have proven more effective than others, with varying side-effects. Detailed information about the drugs needs to be carefully considered before starting a medication for MS. Some people with very active disease, in close consultation with their neurologist, will decide to start on a medication with some urgency immediately after diagnosis. Many others, after careful consideration over a period of time, will opt for one of the DMDs in addition to the lifestyle changes recommended here, but that decision often does not have to be made urgently or hastily after diagnosis. As many people stay on these medicines for years, the initial decision has to be carefully weighed. Others may opt not to take a medication. These are individual choices. But taking a DMD should not in any way reduce the importance of adopting a preventive medicine strategy that reduces the impact of important lifestyle risk factors. While a drug-only approach is not good medicine, the medications have a significant role as part of an integrated preventive medicine strategy to assist recovery for many people with MS.

STEP 6

PREVENT FAMILY MEMBERS FROM GETTING MS

Prevention of MS by modifying an important environmental factor (sunlight exposure and vitamin D level) offers a practical and cost-effective way to reduce the burden of the disease in the future generations.

Dr Abhijit Chaudhuri

INTRODUCTION

One may wonder why preventing others from getting MS should form part of the OMS Recovery Program. The risk of close family members developing MS is extremely high, and this provides us as PwMS, and our doctors, with an important, not-to-be-missed primary prevention opportunity that can markedly reduce the incidence of MS in the world, and importantly in our close relatives. This has benefits not only for those whom we help in preventing the disease through active intervention in their lifestyles but also for those of us with MS. One person in a family developing MS can be difficult enough for everyone in the family, in addition to the person with MS; one or more of the other family members also developing MS adds greatly to the potential burden for everybody. The complex psychological responses we may have to such developments can trigger serious mental illness and worsen MS. There are many families where several people have developed the disease; today, we have enough sound evidence to make recommendations that can minimise the risk of this happening again.

WHY

In a nutshell
- A diagnosis of MS identifies a group of people at high risk of getting the disease: our relatives.
- Not only is preventing MS in family members good for them, but it is also good for everyone.
- Key factors increasing the risk of MS in these relatives are sun avoidance, low vitamin D levels, smoking—both active and passive—and a high-saturated fat diet.

The risk

Once a person is diagnosed with MS, this immediately identifies a high-risk group of people around them. All those people related to the person with MS have a higher risk of getting the disease—some more so than others. As such, they form group that is perfectly suited to primary prevention. This possibility of reducing the burden of disease due to MS in our close community has been sorely neglected in the past, despite clear evidence that such an approach will be effective. For those of us diagnosed with MS, this is a golden opportunity to use the best available medical evidence to reduce their risk, particularly through modifying their lifestyles.

Primary prevention of MS in relatives of those diagnosed should be a priority.

The size of that increased risk depends on how close a relative they are to the person who has MS: the closer the relative, the higher the risk. So, as previously outlined, children of a parent diagnosed with MS are at 20–40 times higher risk, higher again if they are female. If there are other risk factors, and the population is one where the background incidence of MS is already high such as in Canada or Scotland or southern Tasmania (where the risk for the general population can be as high as one in 300), the risk to the relative of someone with MS can be very substantial—as high as one in four or five for a first-degree relative such as a sister who smokes. So it is critically important for those of us who have been diagnosed with MS to consider the issue of prevention in our close relatives.

Fortunately, as I have outlined in this book, the risk factors for development of MS are really quite well understood. While not much can be done about certain environmental risks like the risk of developing certain viral infections, a lot can be done about others, such as diet, sun exposure, vitamin D supplementation, stress reduction and smoking. The Third Nordic MS Symposium in 2015 concluded that evidence supported modifying a number of lifestyle risk factors, including not allowing children to become overweight, abstaining from smoking, vitamin D supplementation to aim for blood levels of up to 125–250 nmol/L and adequate sun exposure.[1] Of these, we have the most concrete data on smoking, so let's start there. It's also an opportunity to discuss the risks of smoking for the person with MS.

Smoking

Smoking is a major lifestyle issue for those who seek optimal health, whether or not they have MS, but we now have evidence of a very specific detrimental effect for PwMS and their relatives. While we are focusing here on the issue of preventing MS in our close relatives, it is useful to look at its harmful effects for PwMS as well. An important point to emerge from a large study on nurses' health was this very clear association between cigarette smoking and the risk of developing MS.[2] The Nurses Health Study found that, compared with women who had never smoked, the risk of getting MS was 1.6 times greater for current smokers and 1.2 times greater for past smokers. There was also a clear relationship between the duration of smoking and risk of MS. The risk was highest (1.7 times) for those who had smoked for over 25 years. This was strongly supported by a Norwegian study that showed an almost identical risk, with smokers 1.8 times more likely to develop MS than non-smokers.[3] Another study showed that for people who had Clinically Isolated Syndrome, smokers were nearly twice as likely to go on to develop definite MS, and to develop it earlier than non-smokers.[4]

A meta-analysis of all studies on smoking showed a significantly elevated risk of MS with smoking.[5] The author felt that the most likely reason for the association was unhealthy lifestyle behaviours of the smoking group, but most opinion leaders would suggest that the more likely cause is the toxic effect on health of the deliberate inhalation of the very potent cocktail of poisons involved in cigarette smoke. This study didn't look at whether smoking worsens existing MS, just at whether it is associated with its initial development, but more recent studies have now examined the issue of how smoking influences MS progression.

Researchers at Harvard School of Public Health conducted a well-designed case-control study on smokers with MS.[6] PwMS who had ever smoked were three to four times more likely to develop secondary

Figure 16: Smoking—both active and passive—is an important risk factor in MS

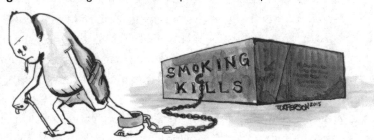

progressive MS than those who had never smoked. Another study confirmed, in a group of 122 PwMS for a mean duration of six years, that smokers were significantly more likely to have progressive disease and to progress at an earlier age.[7] Another important reason not to smoke if one has MS is that researchers have shown that people who smoke after MS diagnosis have a 23 per cent higher chance than those who don't of developing another additional auto-immune disease.[8]

> Smoking precipitates and worsens MS, and increases the risk of developing another auto-immune disease.

Perhaps the strongest evidence supporting the harmful effects of smoking were published from the Karolinska Institute in Sweden in 2015.[9] Examining 728 PwMS who smoked at diagnosis of MS, and following them over time, the researchers noted that those who continued smoking developed secondary progressive MS eight years earlier than those who quit smoking. Each additional year of smoking after diagnosis accelerated the time to conversion from relapsing-remitting MS to secondary progressive MS by about 5 per cent. As Professor George Ebers has previously said, time to development of secondary progressive MS is a far more important measure of disease activity for PwMS than relapse rate.[10] The researchers' clear recommendation was to advise PwMS who smoked at the time of diagnosis to quit, not only to prevent getting other smoking-related diseases but also to slow the progression of MS.

What about the effect of smoking on other family members? A case-control study showed that children were more than twice as likely to get MS if their parents smoked, and the longer they were exposed the more likely MS was to develop.[11] So passive smoking is harmful in MS as well. This has important implications for relatives of PwMS, and the issue of passive smoking. One study has confirmed that passive smoking—for example, by children in families where a parent smokes—raises the risk of developing MS by about 30 per cent.[12]

For those of us diagnosed with MS, these are very good reasons not to smoke so as to minimise the risk of progression of the illness. Now there are even more compelling reasons. We know that our children and other near relatives are already at considerably higher risk than the rest of the population of developing MS; it is extremely important that adults in the house do not smoke so as not to raise the risk even further. And this goes much deeper. Smoking by parents models this as an acceptable behaviour for children. So not only does the passive smoking harm our children and raise their risk of developing MS, but it also makes it more likely that the children themselves will start smoking, raising their risk further.

HOLISM study findings on smoking

We examined this issue in some detail in the HOLISM study, asking participants whether they were current smokers, former smokers or had never smoked any tobacco products; how frequently they smoked, whether former or current smokers; and time since quitting for former smokers. In keeping with our other data showing how healthy and educated a group of PwMS we had surveyed, only 12 per cent of our respondents were current smokers, while just over 40 per cent had smoked previously, indicating that a great many had quit. This figure of 12 per cent of the population smoking is substantially lower than the smoking rate of the countries involved in the HOLISM study. A higher proportion of HOLISM participants in the United States smoked compared with those in Australia.

Smoking status, amount smoked and time since quitting were significantly associated with level of disability. Never-smokers were more likely to have minimal disability, while current smokers were more likely to be more disabled, and the likelihood of this increased with amount smoked per day. Those who had quit ten or more years earlier were still more likely to require major mobility support. In sophisticated regression analyses, being a current smoker increased the odds of major disability almost twofold compared with those who had never smoked, while being a former smoker increased the odds by a quarter compared with those who had never smoked. So quitting does appear to significantly reduce the likelihood of becoming disabled.

Many people who smoke say that smoking makes them feel better, and quitting would deprive them of one of their 'pleasures' and worsen their quality of life. We found exactly the opposite. Those who had never smoked had significantly better quality of life across the board compared with former smokers and current smokers, and former smokers had significantly better quality of life when compared with current smokers (see Figure 17). Actually, quitting one of life's 'pleasures' makes life more pleasurable!

Compared with those PwMS who currently smoked one to fifteen, or sixteen or more, cigarettes a day, non-smokers (both former smokers and those who had never smoked) had significantly better quality of life across all areas examined. A longer time since quitting was significantly associated with better mental and emotional health and quality of life. Overall, the data clearly indicate a detrimental effect of smoking, not only on disability, but also on quality of life.

Figure 17: Quality of life by smoking status

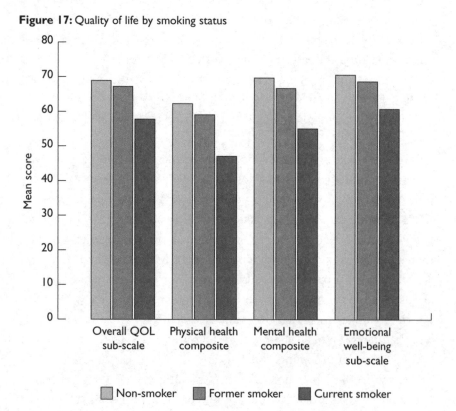

Vitamin D and sun exposure

There are now good research data on sunlight and vitamin D preventing MS, and this is now an important avenue for disease prevention for relatives of PwMS. All doctors managing PwMS now have a responsibility to advise parents with MS that the evidence is clear that they can greatly reduce the risk of their children getting MS with sun exposure or vitamin D supplements, or both. There is now research underway worldwide examining the magnitude of the benefit of supplementing with vitamin D to prevent MS in those at risk. In Australia, the PrevANZ Trial, funded by MS Research Australia, is looking at a closely related issue— that is, preventing the development of MS in those people diagnosed with a CIS who have not yet developed MS. This trial will report in 2017, and its findings should add weight to the primary prevention potential of vitamin D for those with CIS. But we already have enough data to be confident that vitamin D supplementation at adequate dosage will reduce the risk of MS developing in relatives of PwMS.

A Tasmanian study showed a major reduction in risk of MS for those who got adequate sun exposure, particularly in childhood in winter.[13] For those who live in areas where getting adequate sunlight is a problem, or for those who wish to avoid the sun for other health reasons, the US Nurses Health Study has clearly shown that MS risk can be nearly halved by taking a small supplement (anything over 400 IU) of vitamin D.[14] From our knowledge of vitamin D effects on the body and immune system, it is likely that a higher dose would have even more significant protective effects. A review of the literature concludes that vitamin D supplementation may prevent the development of MS.[15] Another study demonstrated a direct genetic mechanism that may explain why vitamin D prevents MS, by showing its functional interaction with the genes that most influence the onset of MS.[16]

Both adequate sun exposure and vitamin D supplementation reduce the risk of developing MS.

Swedish researchers have provided more proof of the protective effect of adequate vitamin D levels.[17] They studied a very large sample of people who had provided blood specimens in Sweden since 1975, but only 192 in fact had MS. They used a case-control study design, matching these 192 people with twice the number of people without MS who had also provided samples, and compared vitamin D blood levels prior to the diagnosis of MS. There were some disturbing findings, most particularly that the average level in blood in winter for the population was around 30 nmol/L, a staggeringly low level that predisposes this population not only to MS, but also to a range of other diseases, including type 1 diabetes and rheumatoid arthritis. Further, they found that the average blood level of vitamin D had been dropping steadily since 1975, and hypothesised that this might be the reason for the explosion in MS incidence in that part of the world.

In terms of MS risk, they found that a blood level of 75 nmol/L or above was highly protective against the development of MS, reducing the risk by 61 per cent. At OMS, we recommend 100 nmol/L based on the US army recruit study previously discussed, and this paper adds further evidence to support the maintenance of a higher than usual vitamin D level in blood. The Swedish researchers, unfortunately, simply did not have enough people with high enough levels of vitamin D to reach any conclusion about whether a higher level would be even more protective. Another disappointing finding was that they couldn't find any protective effect of adequate vitamin D levels in pregnancy on the risk of the baby later developing MS; however, that was almost certainly due to inadequate numbers.

Researchers from an Eye Research Centre in Iran have looked at this important issue in a slightly different way. Optic neuritis is well known to be a common first event in MS, being the first Clinically Isolated Syndrome with which PwMS present in 20 per cent of cases. Of people who develop optic neuritis, 50 per cent go on to be diagnosed with MS. These researchers enrolled 30 people with an attack of optic neuritis into a randomised controlled trial, where half received vitamin D3 at a dose of 50,000 IU a week, or around 7000 IU daily, and the other half received an inactive placebo.[18] They were seeking to determine whether a reasonable dose of vitamin D3 prevented conversion to MS and, if so, to what extent. Those receiving D3 had nearly a 70 per cent reduction in the risk of developing MS, and also had significantly fewer new brain lesions.

This was one of the first studies to use adequate doses of vitamin D3, which may explain why such a strong result was found.

Even though this study was small, it adds significantly to the compelling evidence of the benefits of vitamin D3 in preventing MS. The available evidence is strong enough to recommend that doctors making a diagnosis of optic neuritis start supplementation with vitamin D3. Many doctors would consider that any first demyelinating event now warrants commencement of supplementation with D3, given its lack of side-effects, and its potential health benefits over and above reduced risk of developing MS.

A 2015 review article from Swedish researchers concluded that, given the evidence and the lack of side-effects, there is every reason to supplement the relatives of PwMS with daily doses of vitamin D while awaiting more evidence.[19] The authors noted that the same applies to PwMS themselves. They stressed the importance of not using excessive doses when using vitamin D as a primary prevention strategy, and the doses suggested here are certainly not excessive.

Diet

Professor Swank points out in his book that he placed all family members on the same diet. This was likely for two reasons. First, it made it much easier when preparing meals. Separate meals for the affected family member would then not be an issue. But it also probably reduced their chances of getting MS. Swank points out that, in his experience of over 3500 PwMS and their families, not one of their relatives developed the disease, to his knowledge. This is quite extraordinary, given the high risk in relatives.

There is very little other interventional research work on modifying the diet of those at high risk of developing MS, despite all the solid population-based evidence of increased risk for those consuming diets high in saturated fat. Despite that, many PwMS adopting the OMS Recovery Program opt to modify the diets of their children, given the other health benefits of a plant-based wholefood diet plus seafood. Certainly it is easier to modify the diets of children than adolescents or adults, and often sets up healthy eating habits for life.

HOW

Introduction

Reducing the risk of our relatives developing MS after our own diagnosis is a matter of changing habits—our own and those of our relatives. The easiest way to substantially reduce the risk is simply to take a vitamin D supplement, but getting more sun, quitting smoking and changing our family's diet can also help.

In a nutshell
- Quit smoking.
- Remember that quitting is not a medical illness, and doesn't need medication or a doctor; the best way is just stopping, cold turkey.
- Encourage family members to quit smoking, get more sun, take vitamin D and change their diets.

Smoking

At the very least, when someone is diagnosed with MS, doctors and other health workers should provide some guidance about reducing the risks to other family members. This should include advice about the family members stopping smoking, in addition to the person with MS stopping smoking, given the increased risk associated with passive smoking. There is a lot of information about quitting smoking out there—perhaps too much. Most areas have services that can help with quitting, variously called Quitlines or Quit Smoking services, such as Quit Victoria at <www.quit.org.au>.

But it is important for smokers to realise that, although quitting smoking has become something of an industry, with doctors and drug companies involved, at its core smoking is just a habit. To some extent, industry has turned smoking into an illness in itself, one that needs medication as treatment. While sometimes it can be wise to get help to give up the habit, it is useful to remember that around three-quarters of all smokers stop without any help.[20] There is no question that it is possible.

It is certainly worth trying to just stop cold turkey, as this method simply works for more people than getting involved with a program or taking nicotine-replacement medication. Like the majority of industry-funded trials, those investigating nicotine-replacement therapy conclude that it is far more effective than it actually is.[21] Having a few attempts and failing is entirely normal; often people don't make a serious attempt until they have had a few failures. Actually, when asked, most ex-smokers in hindsight don't find stopping smoking as traumatic as they thought it would be before they tried.[22] While a lot is made of planning and setting a date in the many available quit campaigns and resources, people who have successfully stopped smoking often do so spontaneously, without a plan.[23] Just stopping actually works!

> The most commonly effective way of stopping smoking is simply to stop, cold turkey.

I have great difficulty in understanding why anyone who is committed to getting better after a diagnosis of MS would smoke, given its known harmful effects; however, obviously some people still do. Looking at the available evidence about what works, our advice is to simply stop. And this is not just for your own health, from both an MS and a general health point of view, but also to reduce the risk of relatives who are at higher risk of developing the disease. And, of course, these relatives should also quit if they currently smoke. It is a relatively simple way of reducing one's risk, so why not do it?

Sun exposure and vitamin D

Sensible advice should also be given about increased sun exposure and the maintenance of an adequate and protective vitamin D level in blood year round. Depending on geographical location, that usually involves some supplementation with vitamin D for at least part of the year.

Children should use sunscreen, hats and protective clothing at the beach only after the first fifteen minutes of full exposure in bathers, and in general they should be encouraged to spend time outdoors, if possible with a lot of skin exposed. Prolonged periods in the sun without protection are to be avoided, though, stopping sun exposure well short of what might cause skin redness. Low-dose, frequent sun exposure is ideal. A vitamin D supplement of 5000 IU a day is necessary in winter in most parts of the world where the UV index drops to 4 or less during winter, reduced proportionately for children. So, using 50 kg as the adult dose equivalent, a 25 kg child requires half this dosage. This can be omitted on days when there is adequate sun exposure. This should guarantee that the child's vitamin D level in blood remains above 100 nmol/L year round without the need for blood testing.

The right age to start vitamin D supplementation is minus nine months—that is, from conception. This is achieved by the mother having high vitamin D levels throughout pregnancy. It has been suggested that on a population basis, in areas of high MS prevalence, supplementing with vitamin D during pregnancy and early childhood could prevent a great proportion of the MS in the world.[23] The author suggests that, like folic acid, vitamin D supplementation should routinely be recommended in pregnancy. This is supported by many large epidemiological studies, including one showing that babies born at the end of winter were more likely to get MS later in life than those born at the end of summer.[24]

Dietary modification

The question of whether or not to modify children's and other close relatives' diets is harder. We all know what fussy eaters children can be. We also know how much kids these days like fast food. Rather than eliminating saturated fats from the diets of their children, some people opt to make their diets healthier in general, with more unsaturated essential fats and less saturated fat, but not eliminate fat altogether. If children are older and understand why their diets are being modified, or very small so that they don't really have a say in it, it can be a little easier, although still potentially a difficult issue. For teenage kids, it is generally harder. One day, of course, they will have the prerogative of making their own choice about this. Perhaps this book will help. It may be a good idea to discuss the risk figures presented here with your partner, and perhaps children if they are old enough, and then make a decision. Alternatively, a service offering genetic counselling may be able to offer advice.

OVERVIEW

A variety of interventions can reduce the risk of relatives of PwMS developing the disease. Mostly they simply involve changing habits. Taking sensible precautions to prevent others developing the disease helps everybody.

STEP 7

CHANGE YOUR LIFE, FOR LIFE

Be sceptical, ask questions, demand proof. Demand evidence. Don't take anything for granted. But here's the thing: When you get proof, you need to accept the proof. And we're not that good at doing that.

Michael Specter

INTRODUCTION

So you've been diagnosed with MS. Perhaps it has happened very recently, and you have stumbled upon the OMS Recovery Program. Or your neurologist may have recommended it, or perhaps you have heard about it through the media in relation to some of the research findings. You may have had the disease for some time—possibly many years, and have heard from others that it might be possible to turn your situation around with the OMS Program. Whatever the motivation for looking into this, it helps to be clear about why it is important to change your life, and why it is important to stick with the changes for life, not just try them out temporarily to see whether things improve. The reason for trying the OMS Program is simple: it works!

In a nutshell
- While there are no guarantees, the OMS Recovery Program offers people with MS a realistic chance of a normal, healthy life.
- The HOLISM and STOP-MS studies show that healthier lifestyles are strongly associated with better health for people with MS, including better quality of life, less depression and less fatigue.
- Taking disease-modifying medication is an important part of the OMS Program for many people.
- It is worth asking the question: why not change your lifestyle? The alternative is not very appealing.

WHY

With the ease of access we all have to social and other media, it is easy to be exposed to many sources of information claiming to be able to reverse or cure MS. Because the disease is so variable from person to person, and in a single person over time, it is quite possible for a person with MS to try some alternative therapy and then notice some improvement, as the disease would have improved anyway. It is natural for that person to then credit that therapy with that improvement. So single-person testimonials about a variety of therapies are easy to find. While that always provides an interested scientist with another potential lead to study in further research, on its own it doesn't constitute evidence or proof.

The OMS Recovery Program is a mainstream, evidence-based prevention program.

In distinct contrast, the OMS Recovery Program was developed from a detailed scientific analysis of the medical literature, prompted by my own MS diagnosis, made more compelling by my experience of my mother's death from the disease. I was in a somewhat unusual position in that I was a medical professor at the time of diagnosis, and editor of a major medical journal. I knew science. I knew how to critically appraise the medical literature. That, after all, was what I had been doing for a decade at that time, as medical researchers sent their papers to me to be considered for publication in the journal I edited. I had also been publishing my own medical research since 1987, so was well and truly familiar with both medical science and medical publishing, as well as with bias in medical literature and the conflicts of interest that might distort medical research findings. In short, I was in the ideal position to make sense of the medical literature on MS and how one might potentially stay well after an MS diagnosis.

So my synthesis of the literature, published first as the book and later the website *Taking Control of Multiple Sclerosis*, then as the book and website *Overcoming Multiple Sclerosis*, formulated a detailed lifestyle-modification program that was based on a rigorous assessment of the existing medical science about what factors might slow or stop the progression of MS to disability. For many PwMS, and certainly for the majority of those who came and continue to come to our OMS retreats, this was enough to convince them to adopt these changes and stick with them for life. Interestingly, the doctors in those groups were generally the most rapidly convinced by the evidence, perhaps because of their background knowledge about research, and they were the most staunchly adherent to the Recovery Program over the years. They have also had the best outcomes, with many recovering completely. The stories of three of them, Keryn Taylor, Sam Gartland and Ginny Billson, are told in the book *Recovering from Multiple Sclerosis*, although there have been many others with similar stories.

Other PwMS, who did not have direct exposure to the retreats, but instead read the book or used the website, did not have the same degree of engagement with the science, but many were also convinced and made the changes needed. Unfortunately, in those early years, many healthcare workers were not so convinced about the OMS Program and didn't offer support to patients on the Program. It was clear that many regarded this as an interesting hypothesis, but not a proven program. So it became clear to me over the years that I needed to conduct research evaluating the outcomes of PwMS who attended the retreats, and that I had to test the research-derived OMS hypothesis about these lifestyle factors, diet, exercise, sun exposure and vitamin D, smoking, omega-3 supplements and meditation in my own research before many PwMS would be convinced enough to make these changes, and many doctors would support their patients making these changes.

Stage of disease

What about the stage of disease people have reached when they consider starting this approach? Certainly Swank's original work on diet showed that those starting early had the best outcomes, but he also showed that those who were quite disabled when starting the diet had markedly less deterioration than those who didn't stick to the diet. Our research had comparable findings. Quality of life improvements, reductions in fatigue and depression, and other measures of health were as pronounced for those who were more disabled and for those with different types of MS as they were for the recently diagnosed; we controlled for these factors in our statistical analysis.

 It is never too late to start the OMS Program.

Our experience of those attending our retreats, with whom we keep in touch, is that many significantly disabled PwMS who come to a retreat and start on the Program find that they can stabilise the illness—that is, prevent further progression. It is more than that, though: many find that they actually start to recover, and a number find that the process of recovery just continues the longer they stay on the Program, to the point where, many years later, they have recovered much of what they lost before starting the Program—often almost imperceptibly. It is really important to emphasise that this Program is extremely helpful for those recently diagnosed who don't yet have significant disability or many symptoms (secondary prevention) as well as those with more advanced disease who come to the Program late with significant disability and many symptoms (tertiary prevention). In effect, it is never too late to start the OMS Recovery Program, but the earlier you start, the better chance you have of living a long and healthy life.

Will it work for me?

But will it work for me? It is important to note that, like any other mainstream medical treatment, nobody can guarantee that this preventive medicine approach will work for every individual who adopts the treatment. The Program is based around risk reduction. So adopting the Program, according to the best available evidence, should reduce a person's risk of deteriorating over time due to MS. For some, that means achieving stability; for others, it leads to recovery. For others, it means slowing the progression of the disease rather than any improvement. Our HOLISM data and our retreat follow-up study present the results as they apply to a whole group—effectively a summary of the average response across the group. As with all averages, some people do better than average, while some do worse. We can say, though, that our data strongly support the hypothesis that the more engagement a person with MS has with the Program, the better their outcome is likely to be.[1] This is similar to Dean Ornish's work showing that the more people adhered to his lifestyle plan, the better their outcomes from heart disease and prostate cancer were.[2, 3]

Across many of the lifestyle factors we studied, we found what is called a dose–response effect, otherwise known as a 'biologic gradient'. This refers to the observation in science of increased benefit in response to increased dose of or exposure to a particular factor—for instance, as one moves through a series of graded improvements in diet, the likelihood of depression and fatigue falls in a linear relationship, and quality of life improves in a step-wise fashion. This dose–response effect provides strong scientific evidence that improved diet causes these changes.

There are no guarantees, but the OMS Recovery Program is beneficial for most people with MS; the earlier you start, the better.

It also reinforces the point that one can always do better than average by being especially rigorous about the Program. More attention to a really healthy diet pays dividends. Many people who have been to the retreats report to us that they have adopted most of the Program, but often have an Achilles Heel; for many, that is meditation. Some people, despite the wonderful experiences they had on retreat meditating each day and feeling themselves changing in their view of the world and their perception of stress, get home and find they just can't squeeze meditation into their busy lives. As mentioned previously, a Buddhist monk once said, 'If you can't find time to meditate for half an hour a day, you need to meditate for an hour a day'; that sums it up beautifully. The Program is designed on the basis of a careful evaluation of the scientific literature, modifying all the risk factors that can affect staying well after a diagnosis of MS. The HOLISM research strongly validates the fact that all of these modalities work well in their own right, and our STOP-MS research shows that they work even better together. Why omit any part of the Program when they all work to keep you well?

Interestingly, we often see PwMS returning to a retreat for a refresher. It is not at all an uncommon story to find that seven or eight years have passed since the retreat and, while things were going extremely well for the first few years, some deterioration has now taken place and the participant has come back to be 're-energised'. When looking into this in detail, the story is remarkably consistent: the person invariably reports that they got complacent, sometimes thinking that they had 'beaten' the disease, and started to slip back into old habits. This fits perfectly with the work of Swank, who reported exactly the same phenomenon in his paper in The Lancet.[4]

The OMS Recovery Program is a total change of life, for life. It doesn't matter how well one feels, or how much one has recovered, just like with heart disease or type 2 diabetes, if one slips back into old dietary habits, becomes sedentary again, perhaps even starts smoking again or stops meditating, there is every chance that the disease will recur or worsen. It is possible to be completely well after a diagnosis of MS by following the OMS Recovery Program, but for it to work, you actually have to do it! And preferably, all of it. Our research confirms this very clearly.

The STOP–MS study findings

In our STOP-MS follow up of PwMS coming to our OMS retreats, by March 2008 we had 76 people who had completed baseline and one-year follow-up questionnaires, and 44 who had completed baseline and 2.5 year follow-ups, and felt that this was a sufficient number to get a sense of whether the program was working. With appropriate approvals from ethics committees, members of my research team analysed these data and published them in the journal *Quality in Primary Care*.[5] The cohort showed a significant improvement in health-related quality of life (quality of life) at one and 2.5 years' follow up compared with their health just before attending the retreat. After one year, overall quality of life increased 11 per cent from 73.4 to 81.7, physical health composite 15 per cent from 66.2 to 76.4 and mental health composite 13 per cent from 73.7 to 83.6. After 2.5 years, quality of life increased 5 per cent from 68.4 to 71.7, physical health 17 per cent from 59.7 to 70.0 and mental health 14 per cent from 66.9 to 76.6. These changes were all statistically significant.

We were delighted to see how big this improvement was in those who had agreed to participate in the study. Given the reduced quality of life seen in large populations of PwMS[6] and the decline in quality of life seen in a substantial proportion of PwMS over time,[7] these results were potentially ground-breaking. Not only did a single attendance at an intensive preventive medicine program for MS stop PwMS deteriorating as we had hoped, but also their health improved significantly, and the improvements continued to get bigger with time. We eagerly awaited enough PwMS to reach the five-year time point to allow us to see whether these effects on quality of life would plateau or even fall away with increasing time since the retreat. We were not disappointed!

By this time, we had decided to stop surveying people at the 2.5 year time point, so as to relieve the burden of surveys and hopefully increase the response rate from participants. And we had many more people at the one-year time point, so we knew we would get a much more accurate picture of just how much these PwMS had improved by that time, and much stronger data. By that time point, a total of 274 retreat participants had completed baseline questionnaires. The cohort demonstrated major statistically significant improvements in quality of life.[8] At one year after attending the retreat, improvements of 11 per cent were observed in the overall quality of life, 19 per cent in the physical health composite and 12 per cent in the mental health composite. In the 165 who had reached the five-year time point, there were even greater improvements, with a 19 per cent median improvement in overall quality of life; 18 per cent in the physical health composite and 23 per cent in the mental health composite, compared with baseline.

Where else in all the MS literature could one find an intervention that resulted in improvements in mental and physical health and overall quality of life that continued to grow over at least five years? Surely this would be a new wonder drug that would be heading every TV station's evening news? Or some new surgical procedure, like stem cell transplantation, where the great outcomes outweighed the serious risk of the procedure? Isn't it remarkable that our new research, published in the international journal, *Neurological Sciences*, showed that such an outcome could come from only a one-week live-in retreat where PwMS learn how to live well? No new technological or medical marvel, no surgery, no risk. Just mainstream good health from an optimal diet, free of saturated fat, optimal vitamin D levels, exercise and meditation. And with only positive side-effects. Figure 18 from the published paper shows this improvement very well.

Figure 18: Quality of life at one and five years after an OMS retreat

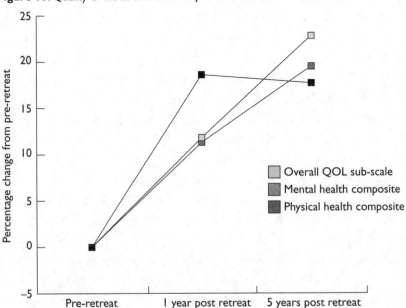

This result was really quite staggering. No other study of any other intervention in MS has shown such improvements; nor has any other study using the MSQOL-54 in a comparable cohort shown improvement at all, let alone such a large benefit. If someone said to you at diagnosis that you would be roughly 20 per cent better overall in five years' time, you would be overjoyed. Of course, these are average figures, and some people did not do as well, while others did correspondingly better. But, on average, they had very significant improvement.

 STOP-MS demonstrates that OMS retreats dramatically improve quality of life.

We closed the study off in May 2013, coinciding with me reducing my role from leading the retreats to a much smaller role presenting on just one day. That was the time when Dr Keryn Taylor took over facilitating the retreats. We felt at this time that we had enough participants overall for the data to be sufficiently robust to report in major journals, and also that, to be consistent, we should report on only those retreats that I personally had facilitated, so that not too many variables were changing during the course of the study.

At the time of writing, we have nearly enough numbers at the ten-year time point to analyse and report. That will certainly make interesting reading when published. Our five-year paper concluded that the study added to the evidence base supporting such a preventive medicine approach in the management of MS. Most importantly, it shows that the OMS Recovery Program isn't just an interesting theory, but that it can be done, and it works! Lifestyle risk-modification should form part of any comprehensive MS-management plan, just as it should for other chronic Western diseases and, given that there are likely to be other health benefits, this approach really must be offered to PwMS.

In addition to the benefits PwMS experience, there are also likely to be reduced healthcare costs and improved satisfaction with the health service. It is important to once again note that a secondary prevention approach to MS management is not in any sense in competition with the use of pharmacological therapies; both should be considered for their potential benefits and risks, with decisions tailored to the needs of the individual. We know, however, that clinical trials assessing the impact of lifestyle modification in the long term are actually really difficult to undertake; there are fewer financial incentives to invest in such research than for drug therapy, and there is little financial support to promote the results of such research. So many clinicians are not aware of this important treatment option.

To maximise the potential benefits of the study, we chose to amend it in 2010, adding very detailed questions about the lifestyle behaviours and medication use of PwMS in the sample. This would enable us to assess a key factor on which we had no data: how many people were adhering to the OMS Recovery Program, and whether adherence to the Program affected how well or badly people were doing after leaving the retreat. Those data will soon be published.

HOLISM study findings on the OMS Program and OMS retreats

The HOLISM study provided another opportunity to study the overarching hypothesis about prevention in managing MS developed back in 1999, not only through examining in detail the risk factors identified and subsequently refined, but also in looking at outcomes of those who had been to OMS retreats and comparing them with the outcomes of the other participants. HOLISM dramatically confirmed the original hypothesis. Really, apart from a very few minor nuances in supplementation with omega-3s (flaxseed oil proving to have much stronger associations with improved health than fish oil) and relatively weak evidence about sun exposure (probably reflecting the lack of a validated tool for measuring it in our study), the hypothesis was shown to hold up strongly in a very large international cohort of around two and a half thousand PwMS from 57 countries around the world. We can feel confident now in saying that the OMS Recovery Program works.

Interestingly, as part of this HOLISM research, we examined the importance of engagement with the various aspects of the Program. In other words, we investigated the question of whether the health of PwMS who came to the retreats, read the book and visited the website was better than those who didn't. The answer was crystal clear, and emphatically yes! Those who engaged with all three OMS resources had dramatically better quality of life—not just mentally, which one might expect, but physically.[1] High-level statistical techniques including regression analysis showed that, controlling for age and gender, compared with the highest level of engagement with all three resources of retreat, book and website, no engagement with the resources was associated with mental quality of life scores 15.6 points lower on a 100 point scale, and physical quality of life 19.5 points lower, and nearly three-fold higher odds of clinically significant fatigue and incredible ten-fold higher odds of depression risk. People not on the Program in this very large international sample were doing really badly compared with those on the Program in the facets of life that most PwMS rate as important: their quality of life, and whether they are fatigued or depressed.

Engaging with the OMS Recovery Program is associated with dramatically better health.

Other HOLISM papers looked more closely at these latter two debilitating features of the disease that so many PwMS seem to have: fatigue and depression. In the fatigue paper, published in the world's biggest medical journal, *PLOS ONE*, we found that about two-thirds of the PwMS in our sample (1402 out of 2138, or 66 per cent) screened positive for clinically significant fatigue.[9] Again, we did high-level statistical analysis of these results and, after controlling for a range of stable socio-demographic and disease-related variables, we found increased fatigue to be associated with obesity, use of the common DMDs, poor diet and little social support, and reduced fatigue with exercise, fish consumption, moderate alcohol use and supplementation with vitamin D and omega-3 fatty acids. In short, this confirmed the previous study on engagement with the Program, in that these were exactly the factors identified in 1999 and published in the first book and website; those PwMS in the HOLISM study who were doing what the Program suggested had dramatically lower levels of fatigue. It also highlighted the commonly reported situation of many PwMS: that their fatigue is worse while taking the usually prescribed MS drugs.

The depression paper, led by Dr Keryn Taylor, examined the risk of depression associated with these lifestyle factors. Published in one of the major psychiatry journals in the world, *BMC Psychiatry*, the research showed with sophisticated regression analyses that poor diet, low levels of exercise, obesity, smoking, marked social isolation and taking interferon were associated with greater depression risk, whereas supplementation with omega-3s—particularly flaxseed oil—frequent fish consumption, supplementation with vitamin D, meditation, and moderate alcohol consumption had significant and strong associations with reduced depression risk.[10] Again, this strongly confirmed the findings of the engagement paper: that higher levels of engagement with and adherence to the OMS Recovery Program were associated with much lower risk of depression.

The results of the HOLISM research were staggering. Not only did they provide strong validation and confirmation of the original elements of the OMS Program, but there was also really no unexpected finding about any particular component of the Program. The Program worked in practice in a large international group of PwMS, and really needed little modification. There could be no argument with the findings, as our data were simply a snapshot of the real world, reporting exactly what is happening to PwMS who do or don't adhere to or engage with the OMS lifestyle guidelines. Those who do adhere to the Program have much better health than those who don't. That is not a matter of opinion, but demonstrated by evidence. As a mainstream preventive medicine program to slow or stop the progression of the once-feared incurable disease MS, this was stunning evidence. And it was not only in quality of life, fatigue and depression that the HOLISM results validated the original Program. Many of the individual studies on diet, exercise, omega-3 supplementation, meditation, smoking and alcohol also showed significant associations with less disability and fewer relapses.

HOLISM validated all the key preventive medicine aspects of the OMS Recovery Program.

Overall, the HOLISM study strongly validated and confirmed the original OMS Recovery Program recommendations. So why is it important to get onto the OMS Program and stay on it for life? Because it works! There is no other approach associated with such marked health improvement for PwMS, and it has been studied in detail and stands up to rigorous scientific scrutiny, with the evidence published in the major neurology, psychiatry and general medical journals in the world. This is a critical point. In the internet age, it is easy to mistake blogs and forums for science; our results are published in some of the most important medical and neurology journals in the world. Going with less proven approaches simply poses too much of a risk when the OMS Program has been so thoroughly evaluated with such strong research findings.

Is the OMS Recovery Program proven?

This is an interesting question, and discussing it is very worthwhile. What is proof in medicine? Well, the answer is not as straightforward as one might think or hope. In fact, unlike mathematical theorems or hypotheses in physics, we can't design an experiment in medicine that will answer the question of whether something definitely works. We can only draw inferences; the more evidence we have in favour of a particular intervention, the stronger the inference we can draw that the intervention works. But we can't actually prove it. John Ioannidis, Professor of Preventive Medicine at Stanford University School of Medicine, in his wonderful paper in 2005 that has been downloaded over a million times, summarises the literature showing that the majority of published research claims are actually false.[11]

The problem is that, in medicine, if we design a trial where we test, say, treatment against an inactive placebo, and those people treated with treatment A are shown to have, say, 30 per cent better outcome than placebo, we use inferential statistics to tell us whether that result is statistically significant. By inferential, of course, we mean we make an inference based on the statistical test that the result did not happen by chance. We use p values in medicine to quantify this. So in the above study, the p value might have been p<.05. This means that a result showing that treatment A patients were 30 per cent better than placebo patients would happen by chance less than one in twenty times. So clearly this only shows that the probability that this occurred by chance is small. But it could still be a chance finding. In medicine, we tend to view this p<.05 value as important and inferring proof. But it is not proof. Even if the study is done another ten times, and they all show the same size treatment effect, it is still not proof. The probability that it has now happened by chance is smaller each time this result is obtained, but it could still be chance.

Things that make us more confident that the result is real include the size of the sample of people tested being very large, the result being replicated in subsequent studies, the study population being shown to be really representative of ordinary people in the real world rather than hand-picked research subjects, and no obvious bias existing. Bias is different from the chance variations that occur in the ways people respond to treatments. Where, for example, authors have a strong financial interest in the result being positive—such as in drug company trials, where the drug may well be licensed on the basis of positive research findings, and companies stand to make a lot of money from the drug—there is a strong bias in favour of a positive result. Ioannides lists several corollaries to his assertion that most research findings are false, including the smaller the size of the population being studied, the smaller the size of the effect found; and the greater the financial interest, the less likely the research result is likely to be true.

So what are we to make of the level of proof of the OMS Recovery Program? In 1999, I devised the Program, based on my research of the medical literature. Over subsequent years, with further evidence accumulating, I updated the Program, reporting the growing evidence base in *Taking Control of Multiple Sclerosis* and then *Overcoming Multiple Sclerosis*. There was no doubt that it was an evidence-based program, with many hundreds of studies from the medical literature cited in these books to support the Program, ranging from basic science studies showing the anti-inflammatory and immune modulating effects of diet and omega-3 supplementation to population and case-control studies of the various risk factors outlined, through to intervention trials, including trials on diet, vitamin D, exercise, meditation and the other elements of the Program. But as a whole program, it had not been tested.

Our two-pronged approach was first to teach the elements of the Program to groups of PwMS and follow them up at intervals to see what had happened to their quality of life—the STOP-MS Study—and to assemble a very large group of PwMS worldwide to examine the associations between the risk factors for progression that we had identified and a range of important health outcomes for PwMS, including quality of life, relapse rate and disability—the HOLISM Study. As an experienced researcher and academic, I was stunned at the results of these studies. Both arms of the research validated my initial findings on review of the literature. The inferential statistics that we employed showed that these results were highly unlikely to have occurred by chance.

There were many factors supporting a proven effect: the two studies, using different methodologies, had consistent and congruent findings; the size of the effect was large; the sample we used was very large and representative of ordinary PwMS at different illness stages with different types of MS; for a number of the risk factors, there was a dose–response effect—that is, for example, the better the diet, the better the quality of life; the findings were highly biologically plausible—that is, there were good physiological reasons the intervention might work; and the authors had no significant financial interest in the result, reducing the likeli-hood of bias—although, in my own case, I clearly had a very significant personal interest.

So, is the Program proven? Given that nothing in medicine is actually ever proven, it is a question of how much evidence an individual with MS needs before considering the Program proven and opting to make major lifestyle changes. While it will be important for my own research team at the University of Melbourne to continue these studies—particularly to look at the follow up of PwMS in the HOLISM study over the years, to observe what happens to their health as they change their lifestyle habits, and for other groups to research and replicate these findings—the strengths of the research mentioned, and the fact that these results so strongly confirm our initial hypotheses, mean that most people consider this proof when presented with the evidence.

The OMS Recovery Program is an evidence-based seven-step program for recovering from MS, with the supporting evidence pub-lished in some of the best medical journals in the world. And probably equally importantly, there is no down-side. The only risk PwMS take when adopting the OMS Recovery Program is that they might surprise themselves with how healthy they get, how many medications for a variety of common Western diseases they can throw away, and how good they feel!

HOW

Introduction

So how do you change your life so dramatically? What are the best ways, and how do you make it sustainable, so that when things go wrong—as they often do in life—you don't fall back into old habits and get sick again? Living with MS can be very difficult. From the moment of diagnosis, the whole world changes. It is never the same again. But that provides an incredible opportunity. Because so much is changing anyway, it is a good time to make major changes to the way we live at the same time. Most people notice that they get better and better at change the more of it they do. Approaching these major lifestyle changes in that light makes them much easier.

In a nutshell
- Attitude and motivation are critical; embrace the Program as a great, new way to live well.
- Bring your partner and family along on the journey if they are willing; it is easier to succeed with support.
- Get better at changing habits; the more you change, the easier it gets.
- Make looking after yourself a priority; that can be hard for many people.
- Face the reality of the diagnosis, express the grief and don't get trapped in denial.
- Consider coming to an OMS retreat to kick-start recovery.
- Become part of the OMS community; a retreat, the website, the forum, social media can all can be a great support on the road to recovery.

Making the change

First and foremost, motivation is really important. It is vital to see this whole change as something that comes from within—that is, as a choice that we make voluntarily and even eagerly, which has not been forced upon us by some external authority, like me or any other doctor. Really, it is something to get excited about. In the face of all the negativity around the diagnosis of MS, and the dire predictions of many around us, there is the real possibility that we can be well. What a wonderful opportunity! The change is much more sustainable if it comes from within rather than from externally. The language we use around the change reinforces this, and it is important to use language that supports the self-directed nature of the change. 'I eat fish but I don't eat meat' is far preferable to 'I can eat fish but I can't eat meat', or 'I know I shouldn't eat meat'. The word 'can't' should be dropped from the vocabulary when referring to the choices we make around our lifestyles.

It is useful to start examining objectively the basis for our likes and dislikes. I have a friend who says things like, 'But I love meat, why wouldn't I eat it?' Well, actually, after reading the evidence presented in this book, there are very persuasive reasons it is better not to eat meat— not only for PwMS, but also for anyone who wants to be optimally healthy. Often, the notion of liking something is actually more about a habit that we have rather than a particular enjoyment or preference. Most of us were brought up eating meat, believing that it was good for us. Our 'liking' of meat often stems from this. It is interesting that if one changes the habit of eating meat to a habit of not eating meat, that 'like' of meat soon gives way to a real dislike of meat.

Personally, I can't stand the smell of meat anymore; it is really obvious to me, after nearly twenty years without eating meat, that meat is the flesh of another animal, often burnt. It smells like burnt flesh, and I can only imagine it tastes like burnt flesh. After nearly two decades without it, I really can't remember what it tastes like anymore! I realise now that my previous 'like' for meat was simply a habit, and now that I have a new habit—a much healthier habit—of not eating meat, my 'like' has changed to 'dislike'. The same applies for many of the foods that people who adopt the OMS Program say they really miss, like cheese. After all these years of not eating cheese, I see it for what it really is: the congealed breast milk of another animal, full of animal fat, with an oddly solidly fatty consistency and an off-putting smell. After the self-discipline of simply not eating it for some years, my change in habit drove my change in taste, so that I now dislike even the thought of cheese, let alone eating it. There may well be good physiological reasons for this change, in that the OMS dietary change also changes the type and nature of the bacteria living within our digestive tracts, and that may well drive a change in taste and cravings.[12]

Habits

Habits are interesting. When something becomes a routine or a habit, we often no longer notice much about it; we just do it as a matter of course, because that is what we always do. There is often no logical reason the habit should persist; it just does. If there is a compelling reason to change the habit, such as a serious health crisis, often that is enough motivation to change. But for some people, even that is not enough, and they feel so strongly attached to the habit and other habits that it just feels like it is impossible to change. One thing that helps with changing habits is the development of flexibility and curiosity. Trying new things, sitting in a different chair at the table, walking a different way to work—really, almost anything can be done a little differently than we usually do it. After a while, developing this flexibility becomes fun. And it can have its rewards. We often notice new things when we do things differently. Logically, why would the way we have always done things be the best way? Often, after trying something different, we realise that it is a far better way of doing something.

 Changing habits gets easier the more one changes.

One example: I was in the habit of taking a shower after a swim at the local pool in one particular shower cubicle, because I felt it had a nice shower head that spread the water stream out in a way that covered me when I showered. I hadn't actually tried any of the other three cubicles. One day, as I was about to step in to my favourite cubicle, someone beat me to it. I waited outside the door a little while, but he was clearly in it for the long haul! The other cubicles were free, but quite irrationally I stood there, gradually getting colder. I soon realised how absurd this was and stepped into the next cubicle. I am sure you can guess what happened. The showerhead in the next cubicle was way better than the one I had always used; the water literally gushed out, and the original one was very measly in comparison. I quickly reflected on my lack of flexibility, and tried another cubicle the next time I was there. Eventually I found that a third cubicle had the very best shower head, and that became a favourite (see Figure 19). But I would never have known had I not been forced to break the habit.

Of course, an interesting phenomenon then follows: once you break a habit and develop a new one, the new one becomes just as hard to change as the old one. After all, it's just a habit! The important thing is that if you are going to make the effort to change a habit that is not serving you well, then make sure the new habit really is one that you want to keep, because it may also be just as hard to change the new habit. This is one way in which meditation can be such a helpful practice. Meditation involves just noticing how things are, with a sense of curiosity, without attachment to them. At its heart, it really encourages flexibility, curiosity and lack of attachment. Meditation actually makes it easier to change habits and to become more flexible.

On the OMS retreats, we encourage people to sit in a different seat every day, just to get used to being more flexible, to literally see things from another viewpoint. We also don't serve caffeinated beverages, again to promote flexibility and help people to become aware of their habits,

Figure 19: The old shower habit

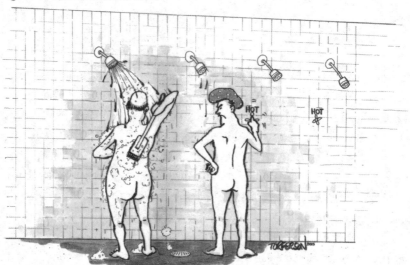

and make it easier to change them. Changing habits is an active task that requires some commitment and positive action. But it is also something that gets easier the more you do it.

An important part of changing habits is to make it easy to adopt the new habits. So some people might see the great benefit of eating wholefoods, but not find it easy to source a good supply of fresh fruit and vegetables. Finding an online organic grocer who delivers to your door can make such a change not only easier, but also fun and engaging. Ordering the mixed box of whatever is in season, delivered to your door on a weekly basis, can prompt the preparation of a whole new array of dishes, as you work out what to do with all the swedes or turnips that have turned up in today's box!

Priorities

Similarly, many people adopting the OMS Recovery Program rethink a lot of the traditional priorities in life. For some, for example, reducing their hours at work and spending more time with family and in recreational activities allows much more time for enjoyable tasks like exercise and meditation, or time spent with family or other parts of their social network. Many people doing this start to wonder how they ever managed to fit full-time work into their lives. This sort of active decision about changing life to suit one's new requirements and interests is vastly different from the feeling people get when their hours are reduced or they are retrenched at work. Many people following this lifestyle approach feel quite able to continue working full-time, but make a decision to reduce their hours simply to make life more enjoyable. We are living in a society where busy-ness is regarded as an admirable trait, and it is hard to disengage from that at times. But many people find that a simpler, less pressured life, with fewer hours devoted to work, is much more fulfilling.

Some people undertake a complete reappraisal of where work fits into life, resulting potentially in changing careers, reducing hours or giving up work altogether. It is important to put ourselves first when faced with such a difficult illness, and that is often something foreign to many of us. Apart from this active lifestyle choice to reduce working hours so as to enjoy life more, it is quite common for PwMS to find that they can no longer work full-time. It was often said in the past that 80 per cent of PwMS no longer work full-time within five years of diagnosis, although that is changing in the modern era. I feel it is important to be open and honest with employers about such difficulties. There is legislation to protect the working rights of those with disabling illness, and most employers—even if they are not particularly compassionate—will be aware of this. Colleagues, too, are often grateful to be told about the illness and about any difficulties it causes, as it gives them the opportunity to help.

 Resolve to do whatever it takes to stay well.

From the day of diagnosis, or the day of reading this book, it is important to decide to do whatever it takes to stop the disease from progressing. Resolving this moves one from being a passive to an active participant in life after the diagnosis. Adopting the position of waiting for deterioration, as is sometimes recommended, or worse still, denial of the illness, is a very negative, passive place to be and is not conducive to recovery. A major review on brain-immune function in MS has summarised the literature on this, noting that, 'In MS, a problem-focused coping style (e.g. an active effort to change a situation) has often been associated with better adjustment, less disability and less depressive symptoms. A more passive . . . strategy seems to be less adaptive and often goes along with increased psychological distress, increased levels of overall stress and negative mood and depression.'[13] In contrast to an approach of denial, it helps to become something of an expert on MS, to develop a really sound understanding of the disease process, the factors that contribute to its progression and the research behind these. Researchers have shown that PwMS as a group have high levels of such health literacy, but those who don't go on to develop unhealthy lifestyle habits and end up needing more medical care.[14]

Preventing cognitive decline
One problem many PwMS face when trying to engage with the evidence and become more literate about their health and their options is the

difficulty imposed by the cognitive decline that may accompany the illness. It may simply be very hard to follow the sometimes complex arguments and evidence about the causes of MS and the benefits of life-style change. So what can be done to contain or prevent gradual erosion of cognitive function so that this engagement is made easier? Apart from the adoption of the OMS Recovery Program to stabilise the illness and prevent the damage that occurs in the brain, there are more specific things that can be done to prevent cognitive decline.

It has long been held that, as far as the brain goes, one should 'use it or lose it'. Using functional MRI, where it is possible to view parts of the brain that are being used for certain activities, researchers have demonstrated that PwMS can protect against loss of cognitive function using the concept of intellectual enrichment.[15] These researchers showed that those with higher educational level and vocabulary (as a marker of how much use they used their brains) were much less likely to show signs of cognitive decline. Intellectual enrichment involves the development of the brain's default network—that is, the parts of the brain not commonly used from day to day, but used a lot in intellectual pursuits. So it may be possible to use 'brain training' (cognitive strategy training) to minimise the impact of the cognitive decline that is usually seen with MS as the disease progresses. In effect, the very process of engaging with the OMS Program, reading the evidence and getting involved in understanding the science can be highly beneficial in improving cognitive function—what a nice feedback loop!

Other researchers have examined the leisure activities that PwMS do in their spare time. In a group of 62 PwMS (41 relapsing-remitting and 21 secondary progressive), most of them on MS medications, researchers investigated whether these people had cognitive leisure activities—that is, intellectually enriching leisure activities, such as playing a musical instrument, keeping a diary or blog, having hobbies, maintaining a website and so on—and the effect of these on cognitive decline.[16] While they found that brain shrinkage did predict a decline in higher mental function, they showed that those with the highest levels of intellectually enriching leisure activities were most protected against this.

This research emphasises the importance of keeping involved in fulfilling activities that are stimulating and require intellectual effort.

This is doubly important in MS, because depression is so common with this illness, and once people are depressed, they are much less likely to continue with these intellectually enriching daily activities. Being pro-active about avoiding depression, with diet, omega-3 supplements, sun exposure, exercise and meditation, helps to maintain a positive attitude to continuing intellectually enriching activities and hobbies. Similarly, doing these activities helps avoid depression. So this is a highly bene-ficial positive feedback loop that feeds on itself to keep PwMS optimistic, positive and cognitively sharp. For those not keeping a diary, which I strongly recommend, this might be a good time to consider starting one. Other activities, like art, music and reading, also seem to have the same beneficial effects.

The authors concluded that, 'Lifestyle choices protect against cogni-tive impairment independently of genetic factors outside of one's control.' This is another important lifestyle choice that can contribute to recovery for PwMS.

Depression and grief

Another major impediment to successful lifestyle change is the negative or depressed mood that can come with a passive approach. Of course, depressed mood can also be the result of the natural grief that follows a diagnosis of MS. Trying to make lifestyle changes when one is depressed is very difficult indeed; even getting up in the morning can be extremely difficult. One of the keys to avoiding depression after MS diagnosis is to express the grief that follows the diagnosis. First, it is important to recognise that grief is a completely natural response to the potential loss that comes with a MS diagnosis. While most of us generally take our mobility and health for granted, the sudden potential loss of it can cause us to spiral downwards into profound grief. While that is normal, holding onto the grief and not expressing it can often turn this transient depressed mood into a more permanent state of depression. Express-ing the grief, the profound sense of loss that comes with the diagnosis of a disabling condition like MS, is critical to moving on with a healthy emotional state that allows us to embark on the exciting road to lifestyle change and recovery.

It is important to accept the diagnosis and express the grief after a diagnosis of MS; denial doesn't work.

Expressing the grief, however, first relies on an acceptance of the reality of the diagnosis, and of the reality of the potential losses we face from the illness. Denial—that is, simply ignoring the problem and getting on with things as if there isn't a problem—stands squarely in the way of acceptance of the diagnosis for many people; sadly, it is often encouraged as a strategy by our healthcare advisers. At the time of diagnosis, I asked my own neurologist, 'What do I do now?' Innately, I sensed that I needed to do something, that action was required. The response was 'Nothing . . . Wait until you get sick and come back and see me and we will see what can be done.' This is essentially a strategy of denial. Overcoming MS requires engagement with the illness, engagement with the emotions that well up in response to the diagnosis, engagement with all the ramifications of the diagnosis, the potential loss of our independence and mobility, our jobs—possibly even our enjoyment of life, or our life itself. Accepting these harsh realities is necessary so that the grief associated with that acceptance can be expressed, allowing us to move on and begin a process of recovery. One study showed well that avoidance or denial is strongly associated with depression;[17] denial is not a solution.

But many of us find it difficult to express grief. We may have been brought up in families where keeping a 'stiff upper lip' was considered a priority. Or we may find comfort in denial, in not having to face the truth. It is, however, very difficult to really start making the changes needed to recover from MS until the diagnosis and the associated potential loss have been faced and accepted, and the grief expressed. This may be through writing or music, keeping a diary, talking to loved ones and friends, seeing a counsellor or attending an MS group. Allowing the emotion to flow without resistance, and allowing it to drain away, is really important. Many people find that once they start this process of getting more in touch with their emotions, and letting them go, they find it easier to also confront other emotional problems that are more long-standing. It is useful to commit to a continuous process of exploring and resolving emotional and spiritual 'dis-ease' and unfinished business. Often these past, poorly resolved issues make and keep people sick. MS can provide the perfect excuse to do this inner work that is so necessary for recovery, mentally and physically, for a healthy life.

Some people find it comparatively easy to jump on board, accept the diagnosis and express their grief over a period of time, and make a dramatic whole-of-lifestyle change, altering their eating and living habits, and perhaps their work and their friendships and relationships. My experience is that this applies to a minority of people. Often people need a lot of help to make such changes in their lives. A key ingredient for most people is the level of support they have—from loved ones, friends and the wider community. Our HOLISM data show that for PwMS, a crucial factor in their health is the number of people they can count on to support them when the chips are down. It is so much easier to express the grief to people who are close to us; it is very much easier to change habits when our partners or close family are also making the same changes. One very helpful way of tapping into that support network is to attend an OMS retreat.

OMS retreats

As mentioned earlier, in April 2002 Ian Gawler and I began a series of live-in retreats for PwMS at the Gawler Foundation, about an hour south-east of Melbourne. Ian had been running residential retreats for people with cancer for many years. After he wrote the Foreword for my first book, *Taking Control of Multiple Sclerosis*, he and I got together and decided to set up retreats for PwMS along the same lines. The retreats last one week, and combine all the elements discussed in this book. These include daily meditations in the meditation sanctuary, communication exercises, education sessions about the techniques presented in this book, inspiring sessions with a range of counsellors and facilitators, and of course wonderful food prepared by the experienced cooks at the Foundation.

A few years later, I and my wife, Dr Sandra Neate, began running similar annual OMS retreats in the Coromandel in the North Island of New Zealand, in conjunction with the MS Society of Auckland and The North Shore. Professor Craig Hassed facilitated with us on a number of occasions, as did Paul and Maia Bedson from the Gawler Foundation. In 2013, Sandra, Craig and I ran the first OMS retreat in the United Kingdom, in Leicester, and since then several more have been run by Dr Keryn Taylor and Craig. More recently, smaller two- and three-day retreats have been run in the United Kingdom by Keryn and Phil Startin, who attended the Leicester retreat. Sandra and I, with Paul and Maia, ran the first European OMS retreat in Austria in 2015, attended by 37 participants from all over the world. Although not retreats, one-day OMS events have also been run through the United Kingdom, facilitated by Miranda Olding, an experienced specialist MS nurse, and Phil Startin.

Almost universally, people attending the retreats say that they are a life-changing experience, and that they provide a kick-start to help tackle the disease. Some of the written feedback from the Austrian retreat illustrates this well: 'This has been one of the most profoundly moving, spiritual, life-changing experiences of my life; easily on a par with giving birth, even! Thank you!'; 'Amazing in every way. If you have MS this is a must, so you can have hope for your future!'; and 'If you have the chance to take part in a retreat grab it with both hands. Finding OMS gave me hope. This retreat has been transformational, life changing. Thank you.'

Quite apart from all the practical information and food-preparation techniques they provide, the retreats work on a range of other levels. First, they normalise the disease. PwMS, particularly when first diagnosed, often feel very isolated and alone. Many have never met anyone with the illness before, and know very little about it. While it is no doubt confronting sitting in a group of around 25–30 other PwMS on the first morning of a retreat, this rapidly gives way to a recognition that these are all very ordinary people who just happened to develop a serious illness and, even more, that these people often have great depths to them— strengths that many people in the ordinary community do not have, as they have had the courage to face these difficulties, and to attend such a program.

 Come to an OMS retreat; people say it changes their lives.

Another enormously gratifying consequence of these retreats is to watch the close friendships that develop over the course of the week. Some of the exercises we facilitate encourage very close, personal communication and the sharing of sometimes painful emotions; people doing that together often develop very close friendships that last well beyond the retreat. Indeed, the group always stays in touch after the retreats by email or social media group, and often arranges periodic reunions or get-togethers. The support network that this creates is very strong. And these people genuinely understand the difficulties that can arise for PwMS, and usually provide great support for the inevitable ups and downs of life that follow. In our experience, many of these groups have now continued to interact via email or in person for over a decade. Now that is a support network!

The OMS organisation

Overcoming Multiple Sclerosis has now become a global organisation, so support is available to PwMS in many other countries. OMS has its headquarters in the United Kingdom. At the time of writing this book, OMS has a Chair (Linda Bloom, who participated in one of the earliest retreats at the Gawler Foundation), Chief Executive Officer (Gary McMahon, formerly General Manager of MS Auckland and the North Shore), with a personal assistant, and several volunteer workers, but also a full-time fundraiser and full-time social media officer. OMS also currently has registered UK and Australian charities to enable tax-deductible donations to further OMS's ability to provide support to PwMS. A US charity is in the process of being established.

The support network has now grown through our new improved website, <www.overcomingms.org>, which has over 100,000 visitors a month, over two-thirds of them new, and nearly half from the United States, with a very active forum of over 14,000 members, and various social media pages including the Facebook pages Overcoming Multiple Sclerosis (15,000 likes), a variety of country-specific Facebook OMS pages, two Twitter accounts, @georgejelinek (2,500 followers) and @OMS Stories where we post recovery stories, a number of Instagram accounts run by keen volunteers, and our regular newsletter, *Whatever*

It Takes (WIT). The website also has a regular blog from one of the OMS members or a guest blogger, as well as a series of podcasts where I go into particular issues that members raise.

Another feature of the website about which people have given really positive feedback is a series of Drawshop videos that outline the key tenets of the OMS Recovery Program, as well as a string of video interviews with people on the Program who provide insights into their journeys to health. The website also allows the opportunity to volunteer to help OMS, and to be an OMS Ambassador, where people on the Program can lead by example and help spread the message to other PwMS worldwide that overcoming MS is possible. Through our OMS Member Support section, one can get advice about setting up local OMS support groups and about free book offers. We also have a dedicated YouTube channel, OMSispossible, which is easily found by typing that into the search box.

One of the benefits of getting involved in the OMS movement is that it keeps one in touch with like-minded PwMS. Anyone with MS who spends any time on some of the conventional MS sites will attest to the fact that there can be a lot of negativity out there on the net. Contact with this negativity can eat away at the hope and positivity that is needed for recovery. Even doing a PubMed search on multiple sclerosis can lead to feelings of negativity and even depression, as so much of the medical literature is based on the paradigm of MS being a disease that progresses relentlessly to disability. While our research and that of others is starting to turn this paradigm around, and PwMS are starting to see that a preventive medicine approach to MS management can lead to a very different prognosis, most clinicians and PwMS still haven't been exposed to this new way of looking at the disease, and mostly the prognosis of inevitable disability is reinforced.

Recovering from MS

One way to counteract that is to surround oneself with good stories. This is not the same thing as denial. Facing the illness head on, accepting the reality of the potential losses that can flow from the illness and then engaging in a significant lifestyle change that provides realistic hope of a long, healthy life is anything but denial. But the hope and positivity do need reinforcement, and can suffer from being eaten away by negativity on social media, or even from well-meaning friends and relatives. Avoiding contact with these sites, and sometimes spending time with people who are supportive rather than negative, is a prudent thing to do. Sometimes this results in a reordering of friendships, which—like many of the other changes that come with a whole-of-life change—can be somewhat daunting for many people. On the plus side, people often discover unexpected friendships in their lives as a result of this reordering.

> Recovering from MS is definitely possible; don't be put off by those trapped in the old paradigm of relentless progression to disability.

There are other ways of surrounding yourself with good stories, too. Inspiring stories of recovery from diseases other than MS can help to cement the feeling that these things are possible. The inspiration that can act as motivation for this whole-of-life change can be drawn from many sources. There are many other books out there that chronicle individual recoveries from a range of common diseases. A great feature film by Shannon Harvey called *The Connection* pulls together the stories of five people, myself included, who have recovered against the odds from a variety of conditions. Go to <www.theconnection.tv> to download a copy.

The book that Karen Law and I wrote, *Recovering from Multiple Sclerosis: Real Life Stories of Hope and Inspiration* (published by Allen & Unwin) has the recovery stories of twelve people, three of them doctors, including Dr Keryn Taylor who now facilitates OMS retreats. It is always good to read about what is possible, and what has actually happened for other people who have adopted the OMS Recovery Program, and actually recovered. It is a very good antidote to the negativity that can surround this illness.

For some people, this sort of discussion raises the whole question of recovery. They can be convinced by many mainstream sources of MS information that it is not possible to recover from MS. The abstract of a review in the *Journal of Neurology*, for example, starts with the sentence, 'Multiple sclerosis is a lifelong, immune-mediated progressive disorder.'[18]

That is the current medical paradigm; most clinicians in the field believe it is not possible to recover from MS. Once you have MS, you always have MS. Similarly, the conventional answer to whether people can do anything themselves to slow or stop the progression of MS has also been no. It has even been said by reputable authorities that 'MS has a mind of its own', as if MS is some kind of external invader in the body, like a virus or bacterium, and not part of us. But even with a virus or bacterium, we know there are all sorts of 'host' factors that interact with the organism and change the way it behaves in a particular person.

So, if the conventional response is that recovery from MS is not possible, what do we make of people who make the whole raft of changes I have outlined here and stay well? Let's say, like me, they stay well for nearly twenty years. Or more. Or, like some of Swank's patients, for 50 years! What about people who have contacted us, or been to our retreats, who have had genuine diagnoses of MS, made all these changes and found that the lesions on their MRI scans clear, like Dr Sam Gartland or Linda Bloom? Or senior medical specialists who are very discerning in their view of medical evidence—even sceptical, like Dr Ginny Billson, who has been perfectly well since starting the Program after years of progressive difficulty. This tends to provoke a certain response from a clinician who doesn't believe this is possible: that the person must never have had MS.

We know if someone has cancer, for example, they would be considered cured if they had not had a recurrence and were still alive after five years. So why is MS different? The consequence of it being considered different is that PwMS can never really feel they are over it and get on with a new life free of illness. Surely there must come a point when someone who commits to all these changes and stays well, and commits to keeping on with the lifestyle program permanently, is considered to have recovered. But what is that point?

It is probably an individual thing, but for the sake of starting a discussion about this, why don't we take the ten-year mark, relapse-free, progression-free, as signifying recovery? This would be an enormously liberating thing for PwMS to aim for and achieve. And as long as they didn't then abandon all the things that have kept them well at that point, there is nothing to lose and everything to gain from considering themselves recovered.

If you ask Ian Gawler whether he has recovered from cancer, 40 years after being given three weeks to live,[19] he will say, tongue in cheek, 'I don't know; I'll know when I die of something else!' But of course he knows, as we do, that he has recovered. And he lives life as if he has recovered. But for PwMS, there is often the feeling that no matter how long they remain well they still live under the cloud of MS, that it could return at any time, that it is a lifelong disease. But recovery from MS is in fact just as possible as recovery from cancer. As we have seen, Dr Dean Ornish has shown that people who adopt an intensive lifestyle approach to prostate cancer similar to the Recovery Program actually change the way their genes are expressed.[20] Like Ian Gawler's recovery from 'terminal' bone cancer, where presumably his DNA actually changed so that the cancer was no longer expressed, it must be possible for PwMS who adopt a similar approach to Ornish and Gawler to change the way their genetic structure is expressed so they literally no longer have MS.

My own experience, and that of many of the people who are following the Recovery Program and staying well, is that it is certainly possible to remain well after a diagnosis of MS, and that after a period of time this constitutes recovery from the illness. For me, it took a long time to accept that this was a reasonable position to take. But the benefits of looking at it in that way are that a great weight is lifted off my shoulders. I don't jump at every little symptom, thinking I am going to have a relapse. Mind you, I am never tempted to go back to my old way of life, and I pay great attention to getting the detail of the lifestyle right, such as keeping my vitamin D levels in the right range.

Setting goals is a really good idea when adopting these lifestyle changes. A good goal to have to begin with is to get to six months as a first milestone, then two years and then ten years relapse-free. At that point, I feel it is quite appropriate to consider yourself recovered. And quite appropriate to celebrate that wonderful event, and look forward to a long, healthy and happy life! It's also good to set mini-goals along the way, like the frequency and duration of exercise or meditation, and so on. Mobile phone apps are getting better and better at assisting with monitoring these goals, so that weekly walking targets, or meditation targets, can be monitored and improved on. Our own OMS app can be really helpful; it can be found in the Apple App store or on Google Play for Android.

Support

Finding a good, supportive doctor is an important part of this recovery process. The ultimate aim, of course, should be to get so well that medical assistance is no longer required—just as it is the aim with all illnesses. But, at least initially, it is important to have the support of a trusted doctor who becomes a key part of your team in helping you to recover. It is important to remember, however, that you are the captain of your own health ship. The ultimate decisions about your treatments, lifestyle choices and health outcomes are yours. If a medical adviser is engaged with your Program, and actively supports it with helpful advice, performing appropriate tests periodically, such as vitamin D levels or vitamin B12 levels, and supporting treatment choices in regard to whether or not and which medication to take, the team will work optimally. If that is not the case, then it may be necessary to find another medical support person.

Doctors treating PwMS will be familiar with the fact that not all MS is the same. Some people seem to have more aggressive illness than others. A good doctor will tailor the pharmaceutical approach to each patient individually, so that those with more aggressive disease are treated with the more potent drugs, but it is always critical to simultaneously correct as many of the adverse lifestyle risk factors that exist for each person as well. So, it makes no sense to treat someone with aggressive MS with natalizumab but not help them give up smoking, manage stress better, exercise, optimise vitamin D status and so on. This would not be good medicine, and the same applies to most other chronic Western diseases.

Good doctors and our support network can also be really helpful during the inevitable difficult times that occur cyclically throughout life. MS relapses tend to occur between four and eight weeks after a triggering event—often a major, stressful event in our lives. So it is wise to take special care and get good help in the aftermath of trigger events, like sudden loss of a loved one, marriage breakdown, major emotional difficulties or even virus infections. Special care means being meticulous about diet, sunlight and meditation in particular. It is probably good advice in general to meditate more when things are difficult, but for PwMS this is particularly so. It may also be worth thinking about getting some help—perhaps from doctors, friends or counsellors—when things in life go badly wrong. And taking some leave from work may also be a good idea, and a supportive doctor can help with that.

Choices

PwMS have a wide range of choices about how to tackle the disease. The scientific evidence is now very clear. Starting with diet and getting adequate sunshine or vitamin D, there are many simple life-style changes that can significantly slow or halt the progression of the disease. Exercise, meditation, managing stress and difficult emotions, and avoiding depression are also important. In combination, this exceptionally healthy lifestyle is very likely to result in sustainable well-being for PwMS, and indeed for people without MS. For many people, this will lead to recovery.

One bonus of getting the disease under control with these interventions is the sense of positivity and achievement it brings. If that doesn't help, for whatever reason, or in people who from the beginning have very active disease, there is now a range of medical therapies, some more toxic than others, that have been shown to be effective in MS, even in very active disease. There is no conflict here; it is not a case of one or the other, lifestyle change or drugs. They are likely to be optimally effective in combination.[21] Although despair is an understandable initial response to diagnosis, the outlook is far from bleak. Armed with the information now available, people should be able to make an informed choice from the lifestyle changes and therapies offered, and live long, healthy and happy lives. MS is now a treatable disease, regardless of type or severity. And recovery from MS is now a realistic possibility; overcoming multiple sclerosis is possible.

The whole package: what can one expect?

So this detailed analysis of the medical literature, including our own STOP-MS and HOLISM studies, makes the case, quite unequivocally and emphatically, that it is possible to overcome MS, that it is possible to recover. What does that mean for individual PwMS?

We know that MS is often markedly different from person to person in terms of how it is expressed, how much disability a person has, how active the disease is and how quickly it progresses. There is simply no doubt, on the basis of the medical literature presented here, that for a group of PwMS who make major lifestyle changes in keeping with the seven steps of the OMS Recovery Program, the group will have a better outcome. On average, there will be fewer relapses, progression to disability will be slower and life will be better—that is, quality of life will improve. That is the conclusion from this analysis of the literature. But every group contains many individuals, and not all—or even most—respond in the average way. As with all medical treatments, some people do better than the group average, and some do worse.

 The majority of people following the OMS Recovery Program improve.

With the OMS approach, our data and experience suggest that the majority of PwMS following this approach improve, some more than the group average and some less than the group average. But will some people who faithfully follow the approach get worse? Our data aren't yet strong enough or long-term enough in follow up to determine this with any certainty. However, our feedback from PwMS who follow this approach is that some do gradually deteriorate; their general feedback is that they deteriorate considerably more slowly than they were deteriorating before they started the approach, but they still very gradually get worse. For many people, this is a major breakthrough, and they are extremely gratified to slow their decline. But for most, their goal is to actually stabilise—that is, to stop their decline—and for others still, recovery of function—partial or complete—is the goal.

It is important to set goals, and it is important to aim high. It is quite realistic to expect at least some recovery, and life being what it is, the higher we aim, the more we tend to succeed. But equally, it is important to acknowledge that slowing the rate of decline may be the best that some people experience—especially those who may have adopted the OMS Program late in the disease course, or who have started with rapidly progressive disease, or reached that phase after years with relapsing-remitting disease. It is, however, important to leave no stone unturned in the quest to recover, to do 'whatever it takes'. For some people, that involves adding a drug—sometimes one of the very powerful drugs, accepting the inevitable side-effects that accompany more potent medication. The OMS Program should at least make those side-effects less of an issue. For others, the road to improved health may involve seeking out more aggressive medical therapies like mitoxantrone or stem cell transplantation—but only in reputable centres—or less well proven avenues to facilitate healing. Where possible, this would best involve treatment modalities that don't have serious side-effects, that add to positivity and greater enjoyment of life.

Some, for instance, may embark on much deeper spiritual journeys in an attempt to overcome the inner obstacles they may feel they have to true healing. In my experience, of the many thousands of PwMS who have contacted me over the years, I have seen significant personal transformations as people engage with Buddhism, or very intensely with yoga or Qigong, or some other spiritual tradition. For some, this has led to great improvements in their physical as well as psychological well-being. Others have explored dietary issues in more depth, with major lifestyle changes such as excluding gluten from their diets, or adopting raw vegan diets, and such changes have led to them turning the corner in disease activity. Others still seek out not yet proven therapies such as hyperbaric oxygen therapy, helminth therapy or low-dose naltrexone.

The OMS Recovery Program is an evidence-based approach, and our seven-step approach does not include such alternatives, for which we feel there is insufficient evidence. But on a case-by-case basis—particularly when health does not improve substantially—there is no reason such alternatives cannot be tried, and a longer journey to health undertaken. PwMS trying some of these treatments need to be vigilant and cautious, however; industries have sprung up around venous angioplasty or stem cell treatment for PwMS, many in less than reputable centres, and often at great cost. Looking into these in detail and getting some objective advice are important before embarking on such potentially harmful and costly therapies, for which the evidence is currently not strong or in some cases completely lacking.

For most people, however, the standard OMS approach is effective. Of course, as with any medical treatment—even things such as surgical procedures and drug treatments for heart failure—not all people who are treated get better. Indeed, for some of these treatments, some people not only don't get better, but also have a serious complication—sometimes even death. One thing of which we can be very confident with the OMS Program is that the lifestyle risk factor modification approach, including the vitamin D and omega-3 supplementation, is not only safe and without substantial risk in itself, but for the majority of people should also result in improvements in overall health in addition to the potential benefits for MS.

Particularly in the early days of OMS, when the approach was perhaps not so well understood or supported by the doctors of PwMS, we had many anecdotes about consultations that went something like this: 'But Doc, how can you say that the OMS Program isn't helping me when you yourself have taken me off my statins, blood pressure–lowering medications and anti-depressants?' While there was initially some reservation or reluctance to concede the potential for this preventive medicine approach by some healthcare workers, over time, as they saw their patients' health improve and their quality of life get better, many became convinced.

OMS is mainstream

It is important to emphasise that this seven-step approach to overcoming MS is mainstream preventive medicine. The Program is so mainstream that in 2015, after a number of generous philanthropic donations, we established the world's first research unit at the University of Melbourne, Australia, devoted to investigating this preventive medicine approach to managing MS. At the end of my career in academic medicine, I decided to devote myself completely to this preventive medicine approach to MS management by establishing the Neuroepidemiology Unit within the Centre for Epidemiology and Biostatistics, in the Melbourne School of Population and Global Health, a landmark development incorporating preventive MS research into one of the more influential public health schools in the world. Through high-quality innovative research, our unit aims to expand the evidence base around the potential health benefits of a preventive medicine approach to the management of MS, and to communicate this to PwMS everywhere, and to their treating clinicians.

The latter part of our mission is critical. We know that translation of research findings into clinical practice is notoriously slow; one review reported that new research findings can take up to seventeen years to make their way into clinical practice, and that only 60 per cent of people with chronic conditions receive recommended care.[22] We are not only passionate about confirming which factors in our lifestyles pose the biggest risk for disease progression to PwMS, and showing that if people modify those factors, that they can recover; we are equally passionate about ensuring that this message gets out to PwMS everywhere. To do that, we utilise every medium open to us, from publishing in the medical literature so that this evidence gets to the key clinicians in the area, to presenting our findings at international conferences of involved clinicians, to speaking to groups of PwMS all over the world face to face or on radio or TV, to running OMS retreats of one, two, three or five days' duration providing concerted information to small groups of PwMS, to using social media such as Facebook, Twitter and Instagram to spread the message.

This is the critical message: that it is indeed possible to recover from MS if one modifies the key lifestyle risk factors responsible for the disease progressing. While much of the medical literature underpinning that message has actually been around for a long time, it has only now been put together in a simple format as a Program for PwMS to follow. And our own research continues to validate, refine and further develop that evidence base to inform modifications to the Program over time.

 Getting the OMS message out is now a crucial part of our mission; we'd love your help.

My mother had no such support. She died a painful death, her body ravaged by the effects of uncontrolled MS. She smoked, ate meat and spread lard on her bread until her death, did not go outdoors, get any sun or take vitamin D. She had every risk factor working against her. And there were no available medications in her day. And so her disability progressed very rapidly. But she did not know any of this evidence, and really, at that time, neither did anybody else.

That is all changing. A preventive medicine approach to recovering from MS will, I predict, be part of medical school teaching of students within my lifetime. The whole paradigm of MS being a chronic, relentlessly progressive disease leading almost inevitably to disability will shift; and it will not be because of some miraculous cure. It will be through the application of good, mainstream preventive medicine principles that we use as a profession throughout medicine, in heart disease, diabetes, hypertension, stroke, cancer and other chronic Western diseases. It isn't necessarily an easy approach. Taking some miracle cure sounds enormously attractive to many people. But the rewards of the OMS Recovery Program are amazing, not just in preventing MS from progressing, but also in getting control over the disease, in truly recovering. And also in really engaging with life—living a fuller, healthier life that is truly authentic and aligned with our emotions and our spirits.

OVERVIEW

Sometimes, it takes an enormous challenge like MS to knock you onto the path that you were meant to follow. I know it did for me. Anything less and I am sure I would still be living the stressful, unhealthy lifestyle I was before diagnosis—that is, if I was still alive! I feel pretty sure that heart disease or some other serious illness might well have claimed my life had I continued on the same path.

Many PwMS express gratitude that they had the shock of an MS diagnosis to wake them up, to make them realise how important they were, how important the small things in life that they took for granted were. Many have now recovered from MS. Recovery is actually a realistic possibility after a diagnosis of MS. Many are living more fulfilling, more authentic lives now that they have truly engaged with life. This opportunity is open to everyone. In seven relatively simple steps, it is possible to recover from MS and live a long, healthy and happy life. Why wait?

NOTES

Chapter 1

1. Buchter B, Dunkel M, Li J. Multiple sclerosis: a disease of affluence? *Neuro-epidemiology.* 2012;39(1):51–56.

2. Shapira Y, Agmon-Levin N, Shoenfeld Y. Defining and analyzing geoepidemiology and human auto-immunity. *J Auto-immun.* 2010;34(3):J168–177.

3. Erasmus, U. *Fats that Heal, Fats that Kill: The Complete Guide to Fats, Oils, Cholesterol and Human Health.* 3rd ed. Summertown, TN: Alive Books; 2010.

4. Chopra D. *Journey into Healing.* Sydney: Random House; 1994.

5. Patani R, Balaratnam M, Vora A, Reynolds R. Remyelination can be extensive in multiple sclerosis despite a long disease course. *Neuropathol Appl Neurobiol.* 2007.

6. Kerschensteiner M, Bareyre FM, Buddeberg BS, et al. Remodeling of axonal connections contributes to recovery in an animal model of multiple sclerosis. *J Exp Med.* 2004;200(8):1027–1038.

7. Doidge N. *The Brain that Changes Itself: Stories of Personal Triumph from the Frontiers of Brain Science.* New York: Penguin Books; 2007.

8. Atkins EJ, Biousse V, Newman NJ. Optic neuritis. *Semin Neurol.* 2007;27(3):211–220.

9. Milonas I, Georgiadis N. Role of optic neuritis diagnosis in the early identification and treatment of MS. *Int MS J.* 2008;15(2):69–79.

10. Optic Neuritis Study Group. Multiple sclerosis risk after optic neuritis: final optic neuritis treatment trial follow-up. *Arch Neurol.* 2008;65(6):727–732.

11. Swanton JK, Fernando KT, Dalton CM, et al. Early MRI in optic neuritis: the risk for disability. *Neurology.* 2009;72(6):542–550.

12. Gilbert ME, Sergott RC. New directions in optic neuritis and multiple sclerosis. *Curr Neurol Neurosci Rep.* 2007;7(3):259–264.

13. Optic Neuritis Study Group. Visual function 15 years after optic neuritis: a final follow-up report from the Optic Neuritis Treatment Trial. *Ophthalmology.* 2008; 115(6):1079–1082.

14. Costello F. Optic neuritis: The role of disease-modifying therapy in this Clinically Isolated Syndrome. *Curr Treat Options Neurol.* 2007;9(1):48–54.

15. Pelidou SH, Giannopoulos S, Tzavidi S, Lagos G, Kyritsis AP. Multiple sclerosis presented as Clinically Isolated Syndrome: the need for early diagnosis and treatment. *Ther Clin Risk Manag.* 2008;4(3):627–630.

16. Vedula SS, Brodney-Folse S, Gal RL, Beck R. Corticosteroids for treating optic neuritis. *Cochrane Database Syst Rev.* 2007(1):CD001430.

17. Marrie RA, Chelune GJ, Miller DM, Cohen JA. Subjective cognitive complaints relate to mild impairment of cognition in multiple sclerosis. *Mult Scler.* 2005;11(1):69–75.

18. Savettieri G, Messina D, Andreoli V, et al. Gender-related effect of clinical and genetic variables on the cognitive impairment in multiple sclerosis. *J Neurol.* 2004; 251(10):1208–1214.

19. Simioni S, Ruffieux C, Bruggimann L, Annoni JM, Schluep M. Cognition, mood and fatigue in patients in the early stage of multiple sclerosis. *Swiss Med Wkly.* 2007; 137(35–36):496–501.

20. Wallin MT, Wilken JA, Kane R. Cognitive dysfunction in multiple sclerosis: assessment, imaging, and risk factors. *J Rehabil Res Dev.* 2006;43(1):63–72.

21. Schulz D, Kopp B, Kunkel A, Faiss JH. Cognition in the early stage of multiple sclerosis. *J Neurol.* 2006;253(8):1002–1010.

22. Nilsson P, Rorsman I, Larsson EM, Norrving B, Sandberg-Wollheim M. Cognitive dysfunction 24–31 years after isolated optic neuritis. *Mult Scler.* 2008;14(7):913–918.

23. Haase CG, Tinnefeld M, Faustmann PM. The influence of immunomodulation on psycho-neuroimmunological functions in benign multiple sclerosis. *Neuroimmunomodulation.* 2004;11(6):365–372.

24. Kleeberg J, Bruggimann L, Annoni JM, van Melle G, Bogousslavsky J, Schluep M. Altered decision-making in multiple sclerosis: a sign of impaired emotional reactivity? *Ann Neurol.* 2004;56(6):787–795.

25. Campbell JD, Ghushchyan V, Brett McQueen R, et al. Burden of multiple sclerosis on direct, indirect costs and quality of life: National US estimates. *Multiple Sclerosis and Related Disorders.* 2014;3(2):227–236.

26. Wesler IS. Statistics of multiple sclerosis. *Am Med Assoc Arch Neurol Psych.* 1922; 8:59–63.

27. Swank RL, Dugan BB. *The Multiple Sclerosis Diet Book: A Low Fat Diet for the Treatment of MS.* New York: Doubleday; 1987.

28. Pugliatti M, Riise T, Sotgiu MA, et al. Increasing incidence of multiple sclerosis in the province of Sassari, Northern Sardinia. *Neuroepidemiology.* 2005;25(3):129–134.

29. Gray OM, McDonnell GV, Hawkins SA. Factors in the rising prevalence of multiple sclerosis in the north-east of Ireland. *Mult Scler.* 2008;14(7):880–886.

30. Houzen H, Niino M, Hata D, et al. Increasing prevalence and incidence of multiple sclerosis in northern Japan. *Mult Scler.* 2008;14(7):887–892.

31. Warren SA, Svenson LW, Warren KG. Contribution of incidence to increasing prevalence of multiple sclerosis in Alberta, Canada. *Mult Scler.* 2008;14(7):872–879.

32. Hirtz D, Thurman DJ, Gwinn-Hardy K, Mohamed M, Chaudhuri AR, Zalutsky R. How common are the 'common' neurologic disorders? *Neurology.* 2007;68(5): 326–337.

33. Simpson S, Jr., Pittas F, van der Mei I, Blizzard L, Ponsonby AL, Taylor B. Trends in the epidemiology of multiple sclerosis in Greater Hobart, Tasmania: 1951 to 2009. *J Neurol Neurosurg Psychiatry.* 2011;82(2):180–187.

34. Ebers G. Tasmania: state of MS in Australia. *J Neurol Neurosurg Psychiatry.* 2011; 82(2):119.

35. Marrie RA, Cohen J, Stuve O, et al. A systematic review of the incidence and prevalence of comorbidity in multiple sclerosis: overview. *Mult Scler.* 2015;21(3):263–281.

36. Marrie RA, Hanwell H. General health issues in multiple sclerosis: comorbidities, secondary conditions, and health behaviors. *Continuum.* 2013;19(4 Multiple Sclerosis):1046–1057.

37. Marrie RA, Horwitz R, Cutter G, Tyry T. Cumulative impact of comorbidity on quality of life in MS. *Acta Neurol Scand.* 2012;125(3):180–186.

38. Marrie RA, Horwitz R, Cutter G, Tyry T, Campagnolo D, Vollmer T. Comorbidity delays diagnosis and increases disability at diagnosis in MS. *Neurology.* 2009; 72(2):117–124.

39. Marrie RA, Horwitz R, Cutter G, Tyry T, Campagnolo D, Vollmer T. The burden of mental comorbidity in multiple sclerosis: frequent, underdiagnosed, and undertreated. *Mult Scler.* 2009;15(3):385–392.

40. Marrie RA, Reider N, Cohen J, et al. A systematic review of the incidence and prevalence of cardiac, cerebrovascular, and peripheral vascular disease in multiple sclerosis. *Mult Scler.* 2015;21(3):318–331.

41. Marrie RA, Yu BN, Leung S, et al. Prevalence and incidence of ischemic heart disease in multiple sclerosis: a population-based validation study. *Multiple Sclerosis and Related Disorders.* 2013;2(4):355–361.

42. Marrie RA, Rudick R, Horwitz R, et al. Vascular comorbidity is associated with more rapid disability progression in multiple sclerosis. *Neurology.* 2010;74(13):1041–1047.

43. Sadovnick AD, Ebers GC, Dyment DA, Risch NJ. Evidence for genetic basis of multiple sclerosis: the Canadian Collaborative Study Group. *Lancet.* 1996;347 (9017):1728–1730.

44. Dyment DA, Yee IM, Ebers GC, Sadovnick AD. Multiple sclerosis in stepsiblings: recurrence risk and ascertainment. *J Neurol Neurosurg Psychiatry.* 2006;77(2):258–259.

45. Ebers GC, Sadovnick AD, Risch NJ. A genetic basis for familial aggregation in multiple sclerosis. Canadian Collaborative Study Group. *Nature.* 1995;377(6545):150–151.

46. Sadovnick AD, Yee IM, Ebers GC, Risch NJ. Effect of age at onset and parental disease status on sibling risks for MS. *Neurology.* 1998;50(3):719–723.

47. Ebers GC, Sadovnick AD, Dyment DA, Yee IM, Willer CJ, Risch N. Parent-of-origin effect in multiple sclerosis: observations in half-siblings. *Lancet.* 2004;363(9423): 1773–1774.

48. Herrera BM, Ramagopalan SV, Lincoln MR, et al. Parent-of-origin effects in MS. Observations from avuncular pairs. *Neurology.* 2008;71(11):799–803.

49. Kantarci OH, Barcellos LF, Atkinson EJ, et al. Men transmit MS more often to their children vs women: the Carter effect. *Neurology.* 2006;67(2):305–310.

50. Ebers GC, Kukay K, Bulman DE, et al. A full genome search in multiple sclerosis. *Nat Genet.* 1996;13(4):472–476.

51. Olsson T, Hillert J. The genetics of multiple sclerosis and its experimental models. *Curr Opin Neurol.* 2008;21(3):255–260.

52. Svejgaard A. The immunogenetics of multiple sclerosis. *Immunogenetics.* 2008.

53. Goodin DS. The genetic and environmental bases of complex human-disease: extending the utility of twin-studies. *PLoS One.* 2012;7(12):e47875.

54. Ponsonby AL, van der Mei I, Dwyer T, et al. Exposure to infant siblings during early life and risk of multiple sclerosis. *JAMA.* 2005;293(4):463–469.

55. Sawcer S, Hellenthal G, Pirinen M, et al. Genetic risk and a primary role for cell-mediated immune mechanisms in multiple sclerosis. *Nature.* 2011;476(7359):214–219.

56. Amato MP, Zipoli V, Goretti B, et al. Benign multiple sclerosis: cognitive, psychological and social aspects in a clinical cohort. *J Neurol.* 2006;253(8):1054–1059.

57. Correale J, Ysrraelit MC, Fiol MP. Benign multiple sclerosis: does it exist? *Curr Neurol Neurosci Rep.* 2012;12(5):601–609.

58. Correale J, Peirano I, Romano L. Benign multiple sclerosis: a new definition of this entity is needed. *Mult Scler.* 2012;18(2):210–218.

59. Jenkins TM, Khaleeli Z, Thompson AJ. Diagnosis and management of primary progressive multiple sclerosis. *Minerva Med.* 2008;99(2):141–155.

60. Stefferl A, Schubart A, Storch M, et al. Butyrophilin, a milk protein, modulates the encephalitogenic T cell response to myelin oligodendrocyte glycoprotein in experimental auto-immune encephalomyelitis. *J Immunol.* 2000;165(5):2859–2865.

61. Poser CM. The multiple sclerosis trait and the development of multiple sclerosis: genetic vulnerability and environmental effect. *Clin Neurol Neurosurg.* 2006;108(3): 227–233.

62. Holmoy T. The immunology of multiple sclerosis: disease mechanisms and therapeutic targets. *Minerva Med.* 2008;99(2):119–140.

63. Chaudhuri A, Behan PO. Treatment of multiple sclerosis: beyond the NICE guidelines. *QJM.* 2005;98(5):373–378.

64. Filippi M, Rocca MA. MRI evidence for multiple sclerosis as a diffuse disease of the central nervous system. *J Neurol.* 2005;252 Suppl 5:v16–v24.

65. Filippi M, Rovaris M, Inglese M, et al. Interferon beta-1a for brain tissue loss in patients at presentation with syndromes suggestive of multiple sclerosis: a randomised, double-blind, placebo-controlled trial. *Lancet.* 2004;364(9444):1489–1496.

66. Bruck W. The pathology of multiple sclerosis is the result of focal inflammatory demyelination with axonal damage. *J Neurol.* 2005;252 Suppl 5:v3–v9.

67. Bruck W. Inflammatory demyelination is not central to the pathogenesis of multiple sclerosis. *J Neurol.* 2005;252 Suppl 5:v10–v15.

68. Zipp F, Aktas O. The brain as a target of inflammation: common pathways link inflammatory and neurodegenerative diseases. *Trends Neurosci.* 2006;29(9): 518–527.

69. Das UN, Vaddadi KS. Essential fatty acids in Huntington's disease. *Nutrition.* 2004; 20(10):942–947.

70. de Lau LM, Bornebroek M, Witteman JC, Hofman A, Koudstaal PJ, Breteler MM. Dietary fatty acids and the risk of Parkinson disease: the Rotterdam study. *Neurology*. 2005;64(12):2040–2045.

71. Das UN. Long-chain polyunsaturated fatty acids in memory formation and consolidation: further evidence and discussion. *Nutrition*. 2003;19(11–12):988–993.

72. Das UN. Can memory be improved? A discussion on the role of ras, GABA, acetylcholine, NO, insulin, TNF-alpha, and long-chain polyunsaturated fatty acids in memory formation and consolidation. *Brain Dev*. 2003;25(4):251–261.

73. Das UN, Fams. Long-chain polyunsaturated fatty acids in the growth and development of the brain and memory. *Nutrition*. 2003;19(1):62–65.

74. Zamaria N. Alteration of polyunsaturated fatty acid status and metabolism in health and disease. *Reprod Nutr Dev*. 2004;44(3):273–282.

75. Hogyes E, Nyakas C, Kiliaan A, Farkas T, Penke B, Luiten PG. Neuroprotective effect of developmental docosahexaenoic acid supplement against excitotoxic brain damage in infant rats. *Neuroscience*. 2003;119(4):999–1012.

76. Wang X, Zhao X, Mao ZY, Wang XM, Liu ZL. Neuroprotective effect of docosahexaenoic acid on glutamate-induced cytotoxicity in rat hippocampal cultures. *Neuroreport*. 2003;14(18):2457–2461.

77. Walford RL. The clinical promise of diet restriction. *Geriatrics*. 1990;45:81–83.

78. Johnson JB, Laub DR, John S. The effect on health of alternate day calorie restriction: eating less and more than needed on alternate days prolongs life. *Med Hypotheses*. 2006;67(2):209–211.

79. Sanna V, Di Giacomo A, La Cava A, et al. Leptin surge precedes onset of autoimmune encephalomyelitis and correlates with development of pathogenic T cell responses. *J Clin Invest*. 2003;111(2):241–250.

80. Simons LA, Simons J, McCallum J, Friedlander Y. Lifestyle factors and risk of dementia: Dubbo Study of the elderly. *Med J Aust*. 2006;184(2):68–70.

81. Ornish D, Scherwitz LW, Billings JH, et al. Intensive lifestyle changes for reversal of coronary heart disease. *JAMA*. 1998;280(23):2001–2007.

82. Casiraghi C, Dorovini-Zis K, Horwitz MS. Epstein-Barr virus infection of human brain microvessel endothelial cells: a novel role in multiple sclerosis. *J Neuroimmunol*. 2011;230(1–2):173–177.

83. Kang JH, Lin HC. Increased risk of multiple sclerosis after traumatic brain injury: a nationwide population-based study. *Journal of Neurotrauma*. 2012;29(1):90–95.

84. Lin CW, Huang YP, Pan SL. Spinal cord injury is related to an increased risk of multiple sclerosis: a population-based, propensity score-matched, longitudinal follow-up study. *Journal of neurotrauma*. 2015;32(9):655–659.

85. Damadian RV, Chu D. The possible role of cranio-cervical trauma and abnormal CSF hydrodynamics in the genesis of multiple sclerosis. *Physiological Chemistry and Physics and Medical NMR*. 2011;41:1–17.

86. De Stefano N, Cocco E, Lai M, et al. Imaging brain damage in first-degree relatives of sporadic and familial multiple sclerosis. *Ann Neurol*. 2006;59(4):634–639.

87. Patsopoulos NA, Bayer Pharma MSGWG, Steering Committees of Studies Evaluating I-b, et al. Genome-wide meta-analysis identifies novel multiple sclerosis susceptibility loci. *Ann Neurol*. 2011;70(6):897–912.

88. Oksenberg JR. Decoding multiple sclerosis: an update on genomics and future directions. *Expert Rev Neurother.* 2013;13(12 Suppl):11–19.

89. Winer S, Astsaturov I, Cheung RK, et al. T cells of multiple sclerosis patients target a common environmental peptide that causes encephalitis in mice. *J Immunol.* 2001;166(7):4751–4756.

90. Westall FC. Molecular mimicry revisited: gut bacteria and multiple sclerosis. *J Clin Microbiol.* 2006;44(6):2099–2104.

91. Corthals AP. Multiple sclerosis is not a disease of the immune system. *Q Rev Biol.* 2011;86(4):287–321.

92. Tettey P, Simpson S, Jr., Taylor BV, van der Mei IA. Vascular comorbidities in the onset and progression of multiple sclerosis. *J Neurol Sci.* 2014;347(1–2):23–33.

93. Moccia M, Lanzillo R, Palladino R, et al. The Framingham cardiovascular risk score in multiple sclerosis. *Eur J Neurol.* 2015;22(8):1176–1183.

94. Ben-Zacharia A. The relationship between Body Mass Index (BMI) and multiple sclerosis progression. 2015. Available at <www.abstracts2view.com/aan/view.php?nu=AAN15L1_P2.212&terms>, accessed 13 May 2015.

95. De Filippo C, Cavalieri D, Di Paola M, et al. Impact of diet in shaping gut microbiota revealed by a comparative study in children from Europe and rural Africa. *Proc Natl Acad Sci USA.* 2010;107(33):14691–14696.

96. Brown K, DeCoffe D, Molcan E, Gibson DL. Diet-induced dysbiosis of the intestinal microbiota and the effects on immunity and disease. *Nutrients.* 2012;4(8):1095–1119.

97. Berer K, Mues M, Koutrolos M, et al. Commensal microbiota and myelin autoantigen cooperate to trigger auto-immune demyelination. *Nature.* 2011;479(7374):538–541.

98. Riccio P, Rossano R. Nutrition facts in multiple sclerosis. *ASN Neuro.* 2015;7(1): 1759091414568183.

99. Haghikia A, Jorg S, Duscha A, et al. Dietary fatty acids directly impact central nervous system auto-immunity via the small intestine. *Immunity.* 2015;43:817–829.

100. Kurtzke JF. Epidemiologic evidence for multiple sclerosis as an infection. *Clin Microbiol Rev.* 1993;6:382–427.

101. Hammond SR, English DR, McLeod JG. The age-range of risk of developing multiple sclerosis: evidence from a migrant population in Australia. *Brain.* 2000;123(Pt 5): 968–974.

102. Ross RT, Cheang M. Geographic similarities between varicella and multiple sclerosis: an hypothesis on the environmental factor of multiple sclerosis. *J Clin Epidemiol.* 1995;48:731–737.

103. Sotelo J, Martinez-Palomo A, Ordonez G, Pineda B. Varicella-zoster virus in cerebrospinal fluid at relapses of multiple sclerosis. *Ann Neurol.* 2008;63(3):303–311.

104. Sotelo J, Ordonez G, Pineda B. Varicella-zoster virus at relapses of multiple sclerosis. *J Neurol.* 2007;254(4):493–500.

105. Perez-Cesari C, Saniger MM, Sotelo J. Frequent association of multiple sclerosis with varicella and zoster. *Acta Neurol Scand.* 2005;112(6):417–419.

106. Mancuso R, Delbue S, Borghi E, et al. Increased prevalence of varicella zoster virus DNA in cerebrospinal fluid from patients with multiple sclerosis. *J Med Virol.* 2007; 79(2):192–199.

107. Panitch HS. Influence of infection on exacerbations of multiple sclerosis. *Ann Neurol.* 1994;36:S25–S28.

108. Challoner PB, Smith KT, Parker JD, et al. Plaque-associated expression of human herpesvirus 6 in multiple sclerosis. *Proc Natl Acad Sci USA.* 1995;92(16):7440–7444.
109. Merelli E, Bedin R, Sola P, et al. Human herpes virus 6 and human herpes virus 8 DNA sequences in brains of multiple sclerosis patients, normal adults and children. *J Neurol.* 1997;244(7):450–454.
110. Soldan SS, Berti R, Salem N, et al. Association of human herpes virus 6 (HHV-6) with multiple sclerosis: increased IgM response to HHV-6 early antigen and detection of serum HHV-6 DNA. *Nat Med.* 1997;3(12):1394–1397.
111. Caselli E, Boni M, Bracci A, et al. Detection of antibodies directed against human herpesvirus 6 U94/REP in sera of patients affected by multiple sclerosis. *J Clin Microbiol.* 2002;40(11):4131–4137.
112. Chapenko S, Millers A, Nora Z, Logina I, Kukaine R, Murovska M. Correlation between HHV-6 reactivation and multiple sclerosis disease activity. *J Med Virol.* 2003;69(1):111–117.
113. Cermelli C, Berti R, Soldan SS, et al. High frequency of human herpesvirus 6 DNA in multiple sclerosis plaques isolated by laser microdissection. *J Infect Dis.* 2003;187(9):1377–1387.
114. Goodman AD, Mock DJ, Powers JM, Baker JV, Blumberg BM. Human herpesvirus 6 genome and antigen in acute multiple sclerosis lesions. *J Infect Dis.* 2003;187(9):1365–1376.
115. Opsahl ML, Kennedy PG. Early and late HHV-6 gene transcripts in multiple sclerosis lesions and normal appearing white matter. *Brain.* 2005;128:516–527.
116. Alvarez-Lafuente R, De Las Heras V, Bartolome M, Picazo JJ, Arroyo R. Beta-interferon treatment reduces human herpesvirus-6 viral load in multiple sclerosis relapses but not in remission. *Eur Neurol.* 2004;52(2):87–91.
117. Alvarez-Lafuente R, de Las Heras V, Garcia-Montojo M, Bartolome M, Arroyo R. Human herpesvirus-6 and multiple sclerosis: relapsing-remitting versus secondary progressive. *Mult Scler.* 2007;13(5):578–583.
118. Ascherio A, Munger KL, Lennette ET, et al. Epstein-Barr virus antibodies and risk of multiple sclerosis: a prospective study. *JAMA.* 2001;286(24):3083–3088.
119. Hollsberg P, Hansen HJ, Haahr S. Altered CD8+ T cell responses to selected Epstein-Barr virus immunodominant epitopes in patients with multiple sclerosis. *Clin Exp Immunol.* 2003;132(1):137–143.
120. Levin LI, Munger KL, Rubertone MV, et al. Multiple sclerosis and Epstein-Barr virus. *JAMA.* 2003;289(12):1533–1536.
121. Wagner HJ, Munger KL, Ascherio A. Plasma viral load of Epstein-Barr virus and risk of multiple sclerosis. *Eur J Neurol.* 2004;11(12):833–834.
122. Banwell B, Krupp L, Kennedy J, et al. Clinical features and viral serologies in children with multiple sclerosis: a multinational observational study. *Lancet Neurol.* 2007;6(9):773–781.
123. Sundstrom P, Juto P, Wadell G, et al. An altered immune response to Epstein-Barr virus in multiple sclerosis: a prospective study. *Neurology.* 2004;62(12):2277–2282.
124. Ramagopalan SV, Valdar W, Dyment DA, et al. Association of infectious mononucleosis with multiple sclerosis. A population-based study. *Neuroepidemiology.* 2009;32(4):257–262.

125. Thacker EL, Mirzaei F, Ascherio A. Infectious mononucleosis and risk for multiple sclerosis: a meta-analysis. *Ann Neurol*. 2006;59(3):499–503.

126. Posnett DN. Herpesviruses and auto-immunity. *Curr Opin Investig Drugs*. 2008; 9(5):505–514.

127. Ramagopalan SV, Handel AE, Giovannoni G, Rutherford Siegel S, Ebers GC, Chaplin G. Relationship of UV exposure to prevalence of multiple sclerosis in England. *Neurology*. 2011;76(16):1410–1414.

128. Paty DW, Oger JJF, Kastrukoff LF, et al. Magnetic resonance imaging in the diagnosis of multiple sclerosis (MS): a prospective study of comparison with clinical evaluation, evoked potentials, oligoclonal banding, and CT. *Neurology*. 1988;38:180–185.

129. Whiting P, Harbord R, Main C, et al. Accuracy of magnetic resonance imaging for the diagnosis of multiple sclerosis: systematic review. *BMJ*. 2006;332(7546):875–884.

130. Marrie RA, Yu N, Wei Y, Elliott L, Blanchard J. High rates of physician services utilization at least five years before multiple sclerosis diagnosis. *Mult Scler*. 2013; 19(8):1113–1119.

131. Runia TF, Jafari N, Hintzen RQ. Application of the 2010 revised criteria for the diagnosis of multiple sclerosis to patients with Clinically Isolated Syndromes. *Eur J Neurol*. 2013;20(12):1510–1516.

132. Rovira A, Leon A. MR in the diagnosis and monitoring of multiple sclerosis: an overview. *Eur J Radiol*. 2008;67(3):409–14.

133. Tedeschi G, Lavorgna L, Russo P, et al. Brain atrophy and lesion load in a large population of patients with multiple sclerosis. *Neurology*. 2005;65(2):280–285.

134. Mattarozzi K, Vignatelli L, Baldin E, et al. Effect of the disclosure of MS diagnosis on anxiety, mood and quality of life of patients: a prospective study. *International Journal of Clinical Practice*. 2012;66(5):504–514.

135. Fawcett TN, Lucas M. Multiple sclerosis: living the reality. *Br J Nurs*. 2006;15(1):46–51.

136. Elian M, Dean G. To tell or not to tell the diagnosis of multiple sclerosis. *Lancet*. 1985;6:27–28.

137. Papathanasopoulos PG, Nikolakopoulou A, Scolding NJ. Disclosing the diagnosis of multiple sclerosis. *J Neurol*. 2005;252:1307–1309.

138. National Institute for Health and Care Excellence. *Multiple Sclerosis: Management of Multiple Sclerosis in Primary and Secondary Care*. London: National Institute for Health and Care Excellence;2003.

139. National Institute for Health and Care Excellence. Multiple sclerosis: management of multiple sclerosis in primary and secondary care. 2014. Available at <www.nice. org.uk/guidance/cg186/chapter/1–recommendations>, accessed 20 April 2015.

140. Solari A, Acquarone N, Pucci E, et al. Communicating the diagnosis of multiple sclerosis—a qualitative study. *Mult Scler*. 2007;13(6):763–769.

141. Bogosian A, Moss-Morris R, Yardley L, Dennison L. Experiences of partners of people in the early stages of multiple sclerosis. *Mult Scler*. 2009;15(7);876–884.

142. Kirk-Brown AK, Van Dijk PA. An empowerment model of workplace support following disclosure, for people with MS. *Mult Scler*. 2014;20(12):1624–1632.

143. Kremenchutzky M, Rice GP, Baskerville J, Wingerchuk DM, Ebers GC. The natural history of multiple sclerosis: a geographically based study 9: Observations on the progressive phase of the disease. *Brain*. 2006;129:584–594.

144. Tremlett H, Paty D, Devonshire V. The natural history of primary progressive MS in British Columbia, Canada. *Neurology.* 2005;65(12):1919–1923.

145. Tremlett H, Paty D, Devonshire V. Disability progression in multiple sclerosis is slower than previously reported. *Neurology.* 2006;66(2):172–177.

146. Scott TF, Kassab SL, Singh S. Acute partial transverse myelitis with normal cerebral magnetic resonance imaging: transition rate to clinically definite multiple sclerosis. *Mult Scler.* 2005;11(4):373–377.

147. Pittock SJ, Mayr WT, McClelland RL, et al. Disability profile of MS did not change over 10 years in a population-based prevalence cohort. *Neurology.* 2004;62(4):601–606.

148. Confavreux C, Vukusic S. Age at disability milestones in multiple sclerosis. *Brain.* 2006;129:595–605.

149. Confavreux C, Vukusic S. Natural history of multiple sclerosis: a unifying concept. *Brain.* 2006;129:606–616.

150. Scalfari A, Neuhaus A, Daumer M, Muraro PA, Ebers GC. Onset of secondary progressive phase and long-term evolution of multiple sclerosis. *J Neurol Neurosurg Psychiatry.* 2014;85(1):67–75.

151. Bronnum-Hansen H, Koch-Henriksen N, Stenager E. Trends in survival and cause of death in Danish patients with multiple sclerosis. *Brain.* 2004;11:11.

152. Manouchehrinia A, Tanasescu R, Tench CR, Constantinescu CS. Mortality in multiple sclerosis: meta-analysis of standardised mortality ratios. *J Neurol Neurosurg Psychiatry.* 2015. doi: 10.1136/jnnp-2015-310361.

153. Hirst CL, Swingler R, Compston A, Ben-Shlomo Y, Robertson NP. Survival and cause of death in multiple sclerosis: a prospective population based study. *J Neurol Neurosurg Psychiatry.* 2008;79(9):1016–1021.

154. Hammond SR, McLeod JG, Macaskill P, English DR. Multiple sclerosis in Australia: prognostic factors. *J Clin Neurosci.* 2000;7(1):16–19.

155. Mowry EM, Pesic M, Grimes B, Deen S, Bacchetti P, Waubant E. Demyelinating events in early multiple sclerosis have inherent severity and recovery. *Neurology.* 2009;72(7):602–608.

156. Optic Neuritis Treatment Group. Neurologic impairment 10 years after optic neuritis. *Arch Neurol.* 2004;61(9):1386–1389.

157. Saidha S, Sotirchos ES, Ibrahim MA, et al. Microcystic macular oedema, thickness of the inner nuclear layer of the retina, and disease characteristics in multiple sclerosis: a retrospective study. *Lancet Neurol.* 2012;11(11):963–972.

158. Hellwig K, Schimrigk S, Beste C, Muller T, Gold R. Increase in relapse rate during assisted reproduction technique in patients with multiple sclerosis. *Eur Neurol.* 2009;61(2):65–68.

159. Michel L, Foucher Y, Vukusic S, et al. Increased risk of multiple sclerosis relapse after in vitro fertilisation. *J Neurol Neurosurg Psychiatry.* 2012;83(8):796–802.

160. Langer-Gould A, Huang SM, Gupta R, et al. Exclusive breastfeeding and the risk of postpartum relapses in women with multiple sclerosis. *Arch Neurol.* 2009;66(8):958–963.

161. Hellwig K, Rockhoff M, Herbstritt S, et al. Exclusive breastfeeding and the effect on postpartum multiple sclerosis relapses. *JAMA Neurology.* 2015;72(10):1132–1138.

162. Conradi S, Malzahn U, Paul F, et al. Breastfeeding is associated with lower risk for multiple sclerosis. *Mult Scler.* 2013;19(5):553–558.

Chapter 2

1. Paul JR. Clinical epidemiology. *J Clin Invest*. 1938;17:539–541.

2. Winslow C-EA. Preventive medicine and health promotion—ideals or realities? *Yale J Biol Med*. 1942;14:443–452.

3. American Board of Preventive Medicine. What is preventive medicine? 2015. Available at <www.theabpm.org/aboutus.cfm>, accessed 19 March 2015.

4. Doll R, Hill AB. Lung cancer and other causes of death in relation to smoking: a second report on the mortality of British doctors. *Br Med J*. 1956;2(5001):1071–1081.

5. Viseltear AJ. John R. Paul and the definition of preventive medicine. *Yale J Biol Med*. 1982; 55:167–172.

6. Suzuki D. *Letters to My Granchildren*. Vancouver: Newsouth; 2015.

7. Simon KC, Munger KL, Ascherio A. XVI European Charcot Foundation Lecture. Nutrition and environment: can MS be prevented? *J Neurol Sci*. 2011;311(1–2):1–8.

8. Corthals AP. Multiple sclerosis is not a disease of the immune system. *Q Rev Biol*. 2011;86(4):287–321.

9. Redfern J, Hyun K, Chew DP, et al. Prescription of secondary prevention medications, lifestyle advice, and referral to rehabilitation among acute coronary syndrome inpatients: results from a large prospective audit in Australia and New Zealand. *Heart*. 2014;100(16):1281–1288.

10. Sawcer S, Hellenthal G, Pirinen M, et al. Genetic risk and a primary role for cell-mediated immune mechanisms in multiple sclerosis. *Nature*. 2011;476(7359): 214–219.

11. Swank RL, Lerstad O, Strom A, Backer J. Multiple sclerosis in rural Norway: its geographic and occupational incidence in relation to nutrition. *N Engl J Med*. 1952;246(19):722–728.

12. Lauer K. Notes on the epidemiology of multiple sclerosis, with special reference to dietary habits. *Int J Mol Sci*. 2014;15(3):3533–3545.

13. Bjornevik K, Riise T, Casetta I, et al. Sun exposure and multiple sclerosis risk in Norway and Italy: the EnvIMS study. *Mult Scler*. 2014;20(8):1042–1049.

14. Lossius A, Riise T, Pugliatti M, et al. Season of infectious mononucleosis and risk of multiple sclerosis at different latitudes: the EnvIMS Study. *Mult Scler*. 2014;20(6): 669–674.

15. Lauer K. Environmental risk factors in multiple sclerosis. *Expert Rev Neurother*. 2010;10(3):421–440.

16. Ornish D, Scherwitz LW, Billings JH, et al. Intensive lifestyle changes for reversal of coronary heart disease. *JAMA*. 1998;280(23):2001–2007.

17. Pischke CR, Weidner G, Elliott-Eller M, Ornish D. Lifestyle changes and clinical profile in coronary heart disease patients with an ejection fraction of <or=40% or >40% in the Multicenter Lifestyle Demonstration Project. *Eur J Heart Fail*. 2007;9(9): 928–934.

18. Pischke CR, Scherwitz L, Weidner G, Ornish D. Long-term effects of lifestyle changes on well-being and cardiac variables among coronary heart disease patients. *Health Psychol*. 2008;27(5):584–592.

19. Pischke CR, Elliott-Eller M, Li M, Mendell N, Ornish D, Weidner G. Clinical events in coronary heart disease patients with an ejection fraction of 40% or less: 3-year follow-up results. *The Journal of Cardiovascular Nursing*. 2010;25(5):E8–E15.

20. Frattaroli J, Weidner G, Dnistrian AM, et al. Clinical events in prostate cancer lifestyle trial: results from two years of follow-up. *Urology.* 2008;72(6):1319–1323.
21. Daubenmier JJ, Weidner G, Marlin R, et al. Lifestyle and health-related quality of life of men with prostate cancer managed with active surveillance. *Urology.* 2006; 67(1):125–130.
22. Ornish D, Weidner G, Fair WR, et al. Intensive lifestyle changes may affect the progression of prostate cancer. *J Urol.* 2005;174(3):1065–1069; discussion 1069–1070.
23. Ornish D, Lin J, Chan JM, et al. Effect of comprehensive lifestyle changes on telomerase activity and telomere length in men with biopsy-proven low-risk prostate cancer: 5-year follow-up of a descriptive pilot study. *Lancet Oncol.* 2013;14(11):1112–1120.
24. Thomas LE. How evidence-based medicine biases physicians against nutrition. *Med Hypotheses.* 2013;81(6):1116–1119.
25. Swank RL. Multiple sclerosis: a correlation of its incidence with dietary fat. *Am J Med Sci.* 1950;220:421–430.
26. Swank RL, Dugan BB. Effect of low saturated fat diet in early and late cases of multiple sclerosis. *Lancet.* 1990;336(8706):37–39.
27. Jelinek GA, Hadgkiss E, Hassed C, et al. Difficulties in recruitment for a randomised controlled trial of lifestyle intervention for type 2 diabetes: implications for diabetes management. *OJEMD* 2012;2:53–57.
28. Jelinek GA, Hadgkiss EJ, Weiland TJ, Pereira NG, Marck CH, van der Meer DM. Association of fish consumption and omega-3 supplementation with quality of life, disability and disease activity in an international cohort of people with multiple sclerosis. *Int J Neurosci.* 2013;123(11):792–800.
29. Hadgkiss EJ, Jelinek GA, Weiland TJ, Pereira NG, Marck CH, van der Meer DM. The association of diet with quality of life, disability, and relapse rate in an international sample of people with multiple sclerosis. *Nutritional Neuroscience.* 2015;18(3):125–36.
30. Tettey P, Simpson S, Jr., Taylor B, et al. An adverse lipid profile is associated with disability and progression in disability, in people with MS. *Mult Scler.* 2014; 20(13):1737–1744.
31. Stefferl A, Schubart A, Storch M, et al. Butyrophilin, a milk protein, modulates the encephalitogenic T cell response to myelin oligodendrocyte glycoprotein in experimental auto-immune encephalomyelitis. *J Immunol.* 2000;165(5):2859–2865.
32. Winer S, Astsaturov I, Cheung RK, et al. T cells of multiple sclerosis patients target a common environmental peptide that causes encephalitis in mice. *J Immunol.* 2001;166(7):4751–4756.
33. Malosse D, Perron H, Sasco A, Seigneurin JM. Correlation between milk and dairy product consumption and multiple sclerosis prevalence: a worldwide study. *Neuroepidemiology.* 1992;11(4–6):304–312.
34. Jelinek G. *Taking Control of Multiple Sclerosis.* Melbourne: Hyland House; 2000.
35. Jelinek G. *Overcoming Multiple Sclerosis: An Evidence-based Guide to Recovery.* Sydney: Allen & Unwin; 2010.
36. Pierrot-Deseilligny C, Rivaud-Pechoux S, Clerson P, de Paz R, Souberbielle JC. Relationship between 25-OH-D serum level and relapse rate in multiple sclerosis patients before and after vitamin D supplementation. *Ther Adv Neurol Disord.* 2012; 5(4):187–198.

Chapter 3

1. Solari A, Filippini G, Mendozzi L, et al. Validation of Italian Multiple Sclerosis Quality of Life-54 questionnaire. *Journal of Neurology, Neurosurgery & Psychiatry.* 1999;67(2):158–162.

2. Yamamoto T, Ogata K, Katagishi M, et al. Validation of the Japanese-translated version Multiple Sclerosis Quality of Life-54 instrument. *Rinsho Shinkeigaku— Clinical Neurology.* 2004;44(7):417–421.

3. Acquadro C, Lafortune L, Mear I. Quality of life in multiple sclerosis: translation in French Canadian of the MSQoL-54. *Health Qual Life Outcomes.* 2003;1:70.

4. Amato MP, Ponziani G, Rossi F, Liedl CL, Stefanile C, Rossi L. Quality of life in multiple sclerosis: the impact of depression, fatigue and disability. *Mult Scler.* 2001;7(5): 340–344.

5. Wang JL, Reimer MA, Metz LM, Patten SB. Major depression and quality of life in individuals with multiple sclerosis. *Int J Psychiatry Med.* 2000;30(4):309–317.

6. Tepavcevic DK, Kostic J, Basuroski ID, Stojsavljevic N, Pekmezovic T, Drulovic J. The impact of sexual dysfunction on the quality of life measured by MSQoL-54 in patients with multiple sclerosis. *Mult Scler.* 2008;14(8):1131–1136.

7. Marrie RA. Demographic, genetic, and environmental factors that modify disease course. *Neurologic Clinics.* 2011;29(2):323–341.

8. Hohol MJ, Orav EJ, Weiner HL. Disease steps in multiple sclerosis: a longitudinal study comparing disease steps and EDSS to evaluate disease progression. *Mult Scler.* 1999;5(5):349.

9. Hohol MJ, Orav EJ, Weiner HL. Disease steps in multiple sclerosis: a simple approach to evaluate disease progression. *Neurology.* 1995;45(2):251–255.

10. Sangha O, Stucki G, Liang MH, Fossel AH, Katz JN. The Self-Administered Comorbidity Questionnaire: a new method to assess comorbidity for clinical and health services research. *Arthritis Rheum.* 2003;49(2):156–163.

11. Vickrey BG, Hays RD, Harooni R, Myers LW, Ellison GW. A health-related quality of life measure for multiple sclerosis. *Qual Life Res.* 1995;4(3):187–206.

12. McKellar S, Horsley P, Chambers R, et al. Development of the Diet Habits Questionnaire for use in cardiac rehabilitation. *Australian Journal of Primary Health.* 2008;14(3):43–47.

13. Craig CL, Marshall AL, Sjostrom M, et al. International physical activity questionnaire: 12-country reliability and validity. *Med Sci Sports Exerc.* 2003;35(8):1381–1395.

14. Blake R, McKay D. A single-item measure of social supports as a predictor of morbidity. *J Fam Pract.* 1986;22(1):82–84.

15. Krupp LB, LaRocca NG, Muir-Nash J, Steinberg AD. The fatigue severity scale. Application to patients with multiple sclerosis and systemic lupus erythematosus. *Archives of Neurology.* 1989;46(10):1121–1123.

16. Kroenke K, Spitzer RL, Williams JB. The Patient Health Questionnaire-2: validity of a two-item depression screener. *Med Care.* 2003;41(11):1284–1292.

17. Simpson S, Jr., Taylor BV, van der Mei I. The role of epidemiology in MS research: past successes, current challenges and future potential. *Mult Scler.* 2015;21(8): 969–977.

18. Zhang SM, Willett WC, Hernan MA, Olek MJ, Ascherio A. Dietary fat in relation to risk of multiple sclerosis among two large cohorts of women. *Am J Epidemiol.* 2000;152(11):1056–1064.
19. Hadgkiss EJ, Jelinek GA, Weiland TJ, Pereira NG, Marck CH, van der Meer DM. Methodology of an international study of people with multiple sclerosis recruited through Web 2.0 platforms: demographics, lifestyle, and disease characteristics. *Neurology Research International.* 2013:2013:580–596.

Step 1

1. Hedegaard CJ, Krakauer M, Bendtzen K, Lund H, Sellebjerg F, Nielsen CH. T helper cell type 1 (Th1), Th2 and Th17 responses to myelin basic protein and disease activity in multiple sclerosis. *Immunology.* 2008;125(2):161–169.
2. Calder PC. n-3 polyunsaturated fatty acids and cytokine production in health and disease. *Ann Nutr Metab.* 1997;41(4):203–234.
3. Calder PC. Immunoregulatory and anti-inflammatory effects of n-3 polyunsaturated fatty acids. *Braz J Med Biol Res.* 1998;31(4):467–490.
4. Calder PC. Omega–3 fatty acids and inflammatory processes. *Nutrients.* 2010;2(3): 355–374.
5. Harbige LS, Sharief MK. Polyunsaturated fatty acids in the pathogenesis and treatment of multiple sclerosis. *Br J Nutr.* 2007;98 Suppl 1:S46–53.
6. Gallai V, Sarchielli P, Trequattrini A, et al. Cytokine secretion and eicosanoid production in the peripheral blood mononuclear cells of MS patients undergoing dietary supplementation with n-3 polyunsaturated fatty acids. *J Neuroimmunol.* 1995;56:143–153.
7. Calabrese V, Bella R, Testa D, et al. Increased cerebrospinal fluid and plasma levels of ultraweak chemiluminescence are associated with changes in the thiol pool and lipid-soluble fluorescence in multiple sclerosis: the pathogenic role of oxidative stress. *Drugs Exp Clin Res.* 1998;24:125–131.
8. Toshniwal PK, Zarling EJ. Evidence for increased lipid peroxidation in multiple sclerosis. *Neurochem Res.* 1992;17:205–207.
9. Norris JM, Yin X, Lamb MM, et al. Omega-3 polyunsaturated fatty acid intake and islet auto-immunity in children at increased risk for type 1 diabetes. *JAMA.* 2007;298(12):1420–1428.
10. McCarty MF. Upregulation of lymphocyte apoptosis as a strategy for preventing and treating auto-immune disorders: a role for whole–food vegan diets, fish oil and dopamine agonists. *Med Hypotheses.* 2001;57(2):258–275.
11. McCarty MF. A moderately low phosphate intake may provide health benefits analogous to those conferred by UV light—a further advantage of vegan diets. *Med Hypotheses.* 2003;61(5–6):543–560.
12. Flower RJ, Perretti M. Controlling inflammation: a fat chance? *J Exp Med.* 2005; 201(5):671–674.
13. Chrysohoou C, Panagiotakos DB, Pitsavos C, Das UN, Stefanadis C. Adherence to the Mediterranean diet attenuates inflammation and coagulation process in healthy adults: The ATTICA Study. *J Am Coll Cardiol.* 2004;44(1):152–158.

14. Das UN, Ramos EJ, Meguid MM. Metabolic alterations during inflammation and its modulation by central actions of omega-3 fatty acids. *Curr Opin Clin Nutr Metab Care.* 2003;6(4):413–419.
15. Zampelas A, Panagiotakos DB, Pitsavos C, et al. Fish consumption among healthy adults is associated with decreased levels of inflammatory markers related to cardiovascular disease: the ATTICA study. *J Am Coll Cardiol.* 2005;46(1):120–124.
16. Holman RT, Johnson SB, Kokmen E. Deficiencies of polyunsaturated fatty acids and replacement by nonessential fatty acids in plasma lipids in multiple sclerosis. *Proc Natl Acad Sci USA.* 1989;86:4720–4724.
17. Cunnane SC, Ho SY, Dore-Duffy P, Ells KR, Horrobin DF. Essential fatty acid and lipid profiles in plasma and erythrocytes in patients with multiple sclerosis. *Am J Clin Nutr.* 1989;50(4):801–806.
18. Nightingale S, Woo E, Smith AD, et al. Red blood cell and adipose tissue fatty acids in mild inactive multiple sclerosis. *Acta Neurol Scand.* 1990;82(1):43–50.
19. Hon GM, Hassan MS, van Rensburg SJ, Abel S, Erasmus RT, Matsha T. Membrane saturated fatty acids and disease progression in multiple sclerosis patients. *Metab Brain Dis.* 2009;24(4):561–568.
20. Hon GM, Hassan MS, van Rensburg SJ, et al. Red blood cell membrane fluidity in the etiology of multiple sclerosis. *J Membr Biol.* 2009;232(1–3):25–34.
21. Weinstock-Guttman B, Zivadinov R, Mahfooz N, et al. Serum lipid profiles are associated with disability and MRI outcomes in multiple sclerosis. *Journal of neuroinflammation.* 2011;8:127.
22. Weinstock-Guttman B, Zivadinov R, Horakova D, et al. Lipid profiles are associated with lesion formation over 24 months in interferon-beta treated patients following the first demyelinating event. *J Neurol Neurosurg Psychiatry.* 2013;84(11):1186–1191.
23. Tettey P, Simpson S, Jr., Taylor B, et al. An adverse lipid profile is associated with disability and progression in disability, in people with MS. *Mult Scler.* 2014;20(13):1737–1744.
24. Sabate J, Haddad E, Tanzman JS, Jambazian P, Rajaram S. Serum lipid response to the graduated enrichment of a Step I diet with almonds: a randomized feeding trial. *Am J Clin Nutr.* 2003;77(6):1379–1384.
25. Jenkins DJ, Kendall CW, Marchie A, et al. Dose response of almonds on coronary heart disease risk factors: blood lipids, oxidized low-density lipoproteins, lipoprotein(a), homocysteine, and pulmonary nitric oxide: a randomized, controlled, crossover trial. *Circulation.* 2002;106(11):1327–1332.
26. Swank RL, Backer J. The geographic incidence of multiple sclerosis in Norway. *Trans Am Neurol Assoc.* 1950;51:274–275.
27. Knox EG. Foods and diseases. *Br J Prev Soc Med.* 1977;31(2):71–80.
28. Bernsohn J, Stephanides LM. Aetiology of multiple sclerosis. *Nature.* 1967;215(103):821–823.
29. Esparza ML, Sasaki S, Kesteloot H. Nutrition, latitude, and multiple sclerosis mortality: an ecologic study. *Am J Epidemiol.* 1995;142(7):733–737.
30. D'Hooghe MB, Haentjens P, Nagels G, De Keyser J. Alcohol, coffee, fish, smoking and disease progression in multiple sclerosis. *Eur J Neurol.* 2012;19(4):616–624.

31. Zhang SM, Willett WC, Hernan MA, Olek MJ, Ascherio A. Dietary fat in relation to risk of multiple sclerosis among two large cohorts of women. *Am J Epidemiol.* 2000;152(11):1056–1064.
32. Lauer K. Notes on the epidemiology of multiple sclerosis, with special reference to dietary habits. *Int J Mol Sci.* 2014;15(3):3533–3545.
33. Lauer K. Dietary exposures and multiple sclerosis: a review. *Rev Espanola de Esclerosis Multiple.* 2011;19:13–21.
34. Ghadirian P, Jain M, Ducic S, Shatenstein B, Morisset R. Nutritional factors in the aetiology of multiple sclerosis: a case-control study in Montreal, Canada. *Int J Epidemiol.* 1998;27(5):845–852.
35. Lauer K. The risk of multiple sclerosis in the U.S.A. in relation to sociogeographic features: a factor-analytic study. *J Clin Epidemiol.* 1994;47(1):43–48.
36. Gusev E, Boiko A, Lauer K, Riise T, Deomina T. Environmental risk factors in MS: a case-control study in Moscow. *Acta Neurol Scand.* 1996;94(6):386–394.
37. Swank RL, Dugan BB. Effect of low saturated fat diet in early and late cases of multiple sclerosis. *Lancet.* 1990;336(8706):37–39.
38. Swank RL, Dugan BB. *The Multiple Sclerosis Diet Book. A Low Fat Diet for the Treatment of MS.* New York: Doubleday; 1987.
39. Swank RL. Multiple sclerosis: fat–oil relationship. *Nutrition.* 1991;7(5):368–376.
40. Swank RL, Goodwin J. Review of MS patient survival on a Swank low saturated fat diet. *Nutrition.* 2003;19(2):161–162.
41. Das UN. Is there a role for saturated and long-chain fatty acids in multiple sclerosis? *Nutrition.* 2003;19(2):163–166.
42. Ben-Shlomo Y, Davey Smith G, Marmot MG. Dietary fat in the epidemiology of multiple sclerosis: has the situation been adequately assessed? *Neuroepidemiology.* 1992;11(4–6):214–225.
43. Anonymous. Lipids and multiple sclerosis. *Lancet.* 1990;336:25–26.
44. Weinstock-Guttman B, Baier M, Park Y, et al. Low fat dietary intervention with omega-3 fatty acid supplementation in multiple sclerosis patients. *Prostaglandins Leukot Essent Fatty Acids.* 2005;73:397–404.
45. McDougall J. Results of the diet and multiple sclerosis study. 2014. Available at <www.drmcdougall.com/2014/07/31/results-of-the-diet-multiple-sclerosis-study>, accessed 20 April 2015.
46. Bates D, Fawcett PR, Shaw DA, Weightman D. Polyunsaturated fatty acids in treatment of acute remitting multiple sclerosis. *Br Med J.* 1978;2(6149): 1390–1391.
47. Millar JH, Zilkha KJ, Langman MJ, et al. Double-blind trial of linoleate supplementation of the diet in multiple sclerosis. *Br Med J.* 1973;1(856):765–768.
48. Paty DW, Cousin HK, Read S, Adlakha K. Linoleic acid in multiple sclerosis: failure to show any therapeutic benefit. *Acta Neurol Scand.* 1978;58(1):53–58.
49. Meade CJ, Mertin J, Sheena J, Hunt R. Reduction by linoleic acid of the severity of experimental allergic encephalomyelitis in the guinea pig. *J Neurol Sci.* 1978; 35(2–3):291–308.
50. Dworkin RH, Bates D, Millar JH, Paty DW. Linoleic acid and multiple sclerosis: a reanalysis of three double-blind trials. *Neurology.* 1984;34(11):1441–1445.

51. Fitzgerald G, Harbige LS, Forti A, Crawford MA. The effect of nutritional counselling on diet and plasma EFA status in multiple sclerosis patients over 3 years. *Hum Nutr Appl Nutr.* 1987;41(5):297–310.

52. Graham J. *Multiple Sclerosis: A Self-help Guide to Its Management.* Northamptonshire: Thorsons; 1987.

53. Torkildsen O, Wergeland S, Bakke S, et al. Omega-3 fatty acid treatment in multiple sclerosis (OFAMS Study): a randomized, double-blind, placebo-controlled trial. *Arch Neurol.* 2012;69(8):1044–1051.

54. Bates D, Cartlidge NE, French JM, et al. A double-blind controlled trial of long chain n-3 polyunsaturated fatty acids in the treatment of multiple sclerosis. *J Neurol Neurosurg Psychiatry.* 1989;52(1):18–22.

55. van Meeteren ME, Teunissen CE, Dijkstra CD, van Tol EA. Antioxidants and polyunsaturated fatty acids in multiple sclerosis. *Eur J Clin Nutr.* 2005;59(12):1347–1361.

56. National Institute for Health and Care Excellence. *Multiple Sclerosis: Management of Multiple Sclerosis in Primary and Secondary Care.* London: National Institute for Health and Care Excellence;2003.

57. National Institute for Health and Care Excellence. Managing multiple sclerosis. 2014. Available at <http://pathways.nice.org.uk/pathways/multiple-sclerosis - path= view%3A/pathways/multiple-sclerosis/managing-multiple-sclerosis.xml&content =view-node%3Anodes-treatments-that-should-not-be-used>, accessed 10 October 2014.

58. Blondeau N, Widmann C, Lazdunski M, Heurteaux C. Polyunsaturated fatty acids induce ischemic and epileptic tolerance. *Neuroscience.* 2002;109(2):231–241.

59. Lauritzen I, Blondeau N, Heurteaux C, et al. Polyunsaturated fatty acids are potent neuroprotectors. *Eur Mol Biol Org J.* 2000;19:1784–1793.

60. Mayer M. Essential fatty acids and related molecular and cellular mechanisms in multiple sclerosis: a new look at old concepts. *Folia Biologica (Praha).* 1999;45:133–141.

61. McKellar S, Horsley P, Chambers R, et al. Development of the Diet Habits Questionnaire for use in cardiac rehabilitation. *Australian Journal of Primary Health.* 2008;14(3):43–47.

62. Hadgkiss EJ, Jelinek GA, Weiland TJ, Pereira NG, Marck CH, van der Meer DM. The association of diet with quality of life, disability, and relapse rate in an international sample of people with multiple sclerosis. *Nutritional Neuroscience.* 2015;18:125–36.

63. Jelinek GA, Hadgkiss EJ, Weiland TJ, Pereira NG, Marck CH, van der Meer DM. Association of fish consumption and omega-3 supplementation with quality of life, disability and disease activity in an international cohort of people with multiple sclerosis. *Int J Neurosci.* 2013;123(11):792–800.

64. Simopoulos A, Robinson J. *The Omega Plan.* Sydney: Hodder; 1998.

65. Cameron-Smith D, Sinclair AJ. Trans fats in Australian fast foods. *Med J Aust.* 2006;185(5):293.

66. Willett WC. Dietary fats and coronary heart disease. *Journal of Internal Medicine.* 2012;272(1):13–24.

67. Malosse D, Perron H. Correlation analysis between bovine populations, other farm animals, house pets, and multiple sclerosis prevalence. *Neuroepidemiology.* 1993; 12(1):15–27.

68. Malosse D, Perron H, Sasco A, Seigneurin JM. Correlation between milk and dairy product consumption and multiple sclerosis prevalence: a worldwide study. *Neuroepidemiology.* 1992;11(4–6):304–312.

69. Stefferl A, Schubart A, Storch M, et al. Butyrophilin, a milk protein, modulates the encephalitogenic T cell response to myelin oligodendrocyte glycoprotein in experimental auto-immune encephalomyelitis. *J Immunol.* 2000;165(5):2859–2865.

70. Winer S, Astsaturov I, Cheung RK, et al. T cells of multiple sclerosis patients target a common environmental peptide that causes encephalitis in mice. *J Immunol.* 2001;166(7):4751–4756.

71. Mana P, Goodyear M, Bernard C, Tomioka R, Freire-Garabal M, Linares D. Tolerance induction by molecular mimicry: prevention and suppression of experimental auto-immune encephalomyelitis with the milk protein butyrophilin. *Int Immunol.* 2004;16(3):489–499.

72. TRIGR Study Group. Study design of the trial to reduce IDDM in the genetically at risk (TRIGR). *Pediatr Diabetes.* 2007;8(3):117–137.

73. Knip M, Virtanen SM, Seppa K, et al. Dietary intervention in infancy and later signs of beta-cell auto-immunity. *N Engl J Med.* 2010;363(20):1900–1908.

74. Akerblom HK, Virtanen SM, Ilonen J, et al. Dietary manipulation of beta cell auto-immunity in infants at increased risk of type 1 diabetes: a pilot study. *Diabetologia.* 2005;48(5):829–837.

75. Chen H, Zhang SM, Hernan MA, Willett WC, Ascherio A. Diet and Parkinson's disease: a potential role of dairy products in men. *Ann Neurol.* 2002;52(6): 793–801.

76. Munger KL, Chitnis T, Frazier AL, Giovannucci E, Spiegelman D, Ascherio A. Dietary intake of vitamin D during adolescence and risk of multiple sclerosis. *Journal of Neurology.* 2011;258(3):479–485.

77. Farez MF, Fiol MP, Gaitan MI, Quintana FJ, Correale J. Sodium intake is associated with increased disease activity in multiple sclerosis. *J Neurol Neurosurg Psychiatry.* 2015;86(1):26–31.

78. Kleinewietfeld M, Manzel A, Titze J, et al. Sodium chloride drives auto-immune disease by the induction of pathogenic TH17 cells. *Nature.* 2013;496(7446):518–522.

79. Krementsov DN, Case LK, Hickey WF, Teuscher C. Exacerbation of auto-immune neuroinflammation by dietary sodium is genetically controlled and sex specific. *FASEB J.* 2015;29(8):3446–3457.

80. Hawkes CH. Are multiple sclerosis patients risk-takers? *QJM.* 2005;98(12):895–911.

81. Nortvedt MW, Riise T, Maeland JG. Multiple sclerosis and lifestyle factors: the Hordaland Health Study. *Neurol Sci.* 2005;26(5):334–339.

82. Goodin DS. Survey of multiple sclerosis in Northern California. Northern California MS Study Group. *Mult Scler.* 1999;5(2):78–88.

83. Foster M, Zivadinov R, Weinstock-Guttman B, et al. Associations of moderate alcohol consumption with clinical and MRI measures in multiple sclerosis. *J Neuroimmunol.* 2012;243(1–2):61–68.

84. Scott IC, Tan R, Stahl D, Steer S, Lewis CM, Cope AP. The protective effect of alcohol on developing rheumatoid arthritis: a systematic review and meta-analysis. *Rheumatology (Oxford).* 2013;52(5):856–867.

85. Weiland TJ, Hadgkiss EJ, Jelinek GA, Pereira NG, Marck CH, van der Meer DM. The association of alcohol consumption and smoking with quality of life, disability and disease activity in an international sample of people with multiple sclerosis. *J Neurol Sci.* 2014;336(1–2):211–219.

86. Ludvigsson JF, Olsson T, Ekbom A, Montgomery SM. A population-based study of coeliac disease, neurodegenerative and neuroinflammatory diseases. *Aliment Pharmacol Ther.* 2007;25(11):1317–1327.

87. Salvatore S, Finazzi S, Ghezzi A, et al. Multiple sclerosis and celiac disease: is there an increased risk? *Mult Scler.* 2004;10(6):711–712.

88. Pengiran Tengah CD, Lock RJ, Unsworth DJ, Wills AJ. Multiple sclerosis and occult gluten sensitivity. *Neurology.* 2004;62(12):2326–2327.

89. Borhani Haghighi A, Ansari N, Mokhtari M, Geramizadeh B, Lankarani KB. Multiple sclerosis and gluten sensitivity. *Clin Neurol Neurosurg.* 2007;109:651–3.

90. Nicoletti A, Patti F, Lo Fermo S, et al. Frequency of celiac disease is not increased among multiple sclerosis patients. *Mult Scler.* 2008;14(5):698–700.

91. Rodrigo L, Hernandez-Lahoz C, Fuentes D, Alvarez N, Lopez-Vazquez A, Gonzalez S. Prevalence of celiac disease in multiple sclerosis. *BMC Neurol.* 2011;11:31.

92. Di Marco R, Mangano K, Quattrocchi C, Amato F, Nicoletti F, Buschard K. Exacerbation of protracted-relapsing experimental allergic encephalomyelitis in DA rats by gluten-free diet. *Apmis.* 2004;112(10):651–655.

93. Bjelakovic G, Nikolova D, Gluud LL, Simonetti RG, Gluud C. Mortality in randomized trials of antioxidant supplements for primary and secondary prevention: systematic review and meta-analysis. *JAMA.* 2007;297(8):842–857.

94. Bjelakovic G, Nikolova D, Simonetti RG, Gluud C. Antioxidant supplements for preventing gastrointestinal cancers. *Cochrane Database Syst Rev.* 2004(4):CD004183.

95. Bjelakovic G, Nikolova D, Simonetti RG, Gluud C. Antioxidant supplements for prevention of gastrointestinal cancers: a systematic review and meta-analysis. *Lancet.* 2004;364(9441):1219–1228.

96. Bleys J, Miller ER, 3rd, Pastor-Barriuso R, Appel LJ, Guallar E. Vitamin-mineral supplementation and the progression of atherosclerosis: a meta-analysis of randomized controlled trials. *Am J Clin Nutr.* 2006;84(4):880–887.

97. Lawson KA, Wright ME, Subar A, et al. Multivitamin use and risk of prostate cancer in the National Institutes of Health-AARP Diet and Health Study. *J Natl Cancer Inst.* 2007;99(10):754–764.

98. Miller ER, 3rd, Pastor-Barriuso R, Dalal D, Riemersma RA, Appel LJ, Guallar E. Meta-analysis: high-dosage vitamin E supplementation may increase all-cause mortality. *Ann Intern Med.* 2005;142(1):37–46.

99. Vivekananthan DP, Penn MS, Sapp SK, Hsu A, Topol EJ. Use of antioxidant vitamins for the prevention of cardiovascular disease: meta-analysis of randomised trials. *Lancet.* 2003;361(9374):2017–2023.

100. Millen AE, Dodd KW, Subar AF. Use of vitamin, mineral, nonvitamin, and nonmineral supplements in the United States: The 1987, 1992, and 2000 National Health Interview Survey results. *J Am Diet Assoc.* 2004;104(6):942–950.

101. Bjelakovic G, Gluud C. Surviving antioxidant supplements. *J Natl Cancer Inst.* 2007;99(10):742–743.

102. Marik PE, Flemmer M. Do dietary supplements have beneficial health effects in industrialized nations: what is the evidence? *JPEN. Journal of Parenteral and Enteral Nutrition.* 2012;36(2):159–168.

103. Zhang SM, Hernan MA, Olek MJ, Spiegelman D, Willett WC, Ascherio A. Intakes of carotenoids, vitamin C, and vitamin E and MS risk among two large cohorts of women. *Neurology.* 2001;57(1):75–80.

104. Bolland MJ, Barber PA, Doughty RN, et al. Vascular events in healthy older women receiving calcium supplementation: randomised controlled trial. *BMJ.* 2008; 336(7638):262–266.

105. Reid IR, Bolland MJ, Grey A. Effect of calcium supplementation on hip fractures. *Osteoporos Int.* 2008;19(8):1119–1123.

106. Bischoff-Ferrari HA, Dawson-Hughes B, Baron JA, et al. Calcium intake and hip fracture risk in men and women: a meta-analysis of prospective cohort studies and randomized controlled trials. *Am J Clin Nutr.* 2007;86(6):1780–1790.

107. Bolland MJ, Avenell A, Baron JA, et al. Effect of calcium supplements on risk of myo-cardial infarction and cardiovascular events: meta-analysis. *BMJ.* 2010;341:c3691.

108. Holick MF. Vitamin D: A millenium perspective. *J Cell Biochem.* 2003;88(2):296–307.

109. Bischoff-Ferrari HA, Dawson-Hughes B. Where do we stand on vitamin D? *Bone.* 2007;41(1 Suppl 1):S13–19.

110. Munger KL, Levin LI, Hollis BW, Howard NS, Ascherio A. Serum 25–hydroxy vitamin D levels and risk of multiple sclerosis. *JAMA.* 2006;296:2832–2838.

111. Miller A, Korem M, Almog R, Galboiz Y. Vitamin B12, demyelination, remyelination and repair in multiple sclerosis. *J Neurol Sci.* 2005;233(1–2):93–97.

112. Flood VM, Smith WT, Webb KL, Rochtchina E, Anderson VE, Mitchell P. Prevalence of low serum folate and vitamin B12 in an older Australian population. *Aust N Z J Public Health.* 2006;30(1):38–41.

113. Bial AK. Review: Limited evidence from 2 randomised controlled trials suggests that oral and intramuscular vitamin B12 have similar effectiveness for vitamin B12 deficiency. *Evid Based Med.* 2006;11(1):9.

114. Butler CC, Vidal-Alaball J, Cannings-John R, et al. Oral vitamin B12 versus intra-muscular vitamin B12 for vitamin B12 deficiency: a systematic review of randomized controlled trials. *Fam Pract.* 2006;23(3):279–285.

115. Rabunal Rey R, Monte Secades R, Pena Zemsch M, Bal Alvaredo M, Gomez Gigirey A. Should we use oral replacement for vitamin B12 deficiency as the first option of treatment?. *Rev Clin Esp.* 2007;207(4):179–182.

116. Pitkin RM. Folate and neural tube defects. *Am J Clin Nutr.* 2007;85(1):285S–288S.

117. Huo Y, Li J, Qin X, et al. Efficacy of folic acid therapy in primary prevention of stroke among adults with hypertension in China: The CSPPT Randomized Clinical Trial. *JAMA.* 2015;313(13):1325–1335.

118. Stampfer M, Willett W. Folate supplements for stroke prevention: Targeted trial trumps the rest. *JAMA.* 2015; 313(13):1321–1322.

119. Kaneko S, Wang J, Kaneko M, et al. Protecting axonal degeneration by increasing nicotinamide adenine dinucleotide levels in experimental auto-immune encephalo-myelitis models. *J Neurosci.* 2006;26(38):9794–9804.

120. Serafini M. Red wine, tea and antioxidants. *Lancet.* 1994;344:626.

121. Zhang X, Haaf M, Todorich B, et al. Cytokine toxicity to oligodendrocyte precursors is mediated by iron. *Glia*. 2005;52(3):199–208.

122. Abo-Krysha N, Rashed L. The role of iron dysregulation in the pathogenesis of multiple sclerosis: an Egyptian study. *Mult Scler*. 2008;14(5):602–608.

123. Zhang GX, Yu S, Gran B, Rostami A. Glucosamine abrogates the acute phase of experimental auto-immune encephalomyelitis by induction of th2 response. *J Immunol*. 2005;175(11):7202–7208.

124. Grigorian A, Araujo L, Naidu NN, Place DJ, Choudhury B, Demetriou M. N-acetylglucosamine inhibits T-helper 1 (Th1)/T-helper 17 (Th17) cell responses and treats experimental auto-immune encephalomyelitis. *The Journal of Biological Chemistry*. 2011;286(46):40133–40141.

125. Sanoobar M, Eghtesadi S, Azimi A, Khalili M, Jazayeri S, Reza Gohari M. Coenzyme Q10 supplementation reduces oxidative stress and increases antioxidant enzyme activity in patients with relapsing-remitting multiple sclerosis. *Int J Neurosci*. 2013;123(11):776–782.

126. Sanoobar M, Dehghan P, Khalili M, Azimi A, Seifar F. Coenzyme Q10 as a treatment for fatigue and depression in multiple sclerosis patients: A double blind randomized clinical trial. *Nutritional Neuroscience*. 2016;19:138–43.

127. Barbato JC. Have no fear, MitoQ10 is here. *Hypertension*. 2009;54(2):222–223.

128. Ghosh A, Chandran K, Kalivendi SV, et al. Neuroprotection by a mitochondria-targeted drug in a Parkinson's disease model. *Free Radical Biology & Medicine*. 2010; 49(11):1674–1684.

129. Schwingshackl L, Missbach B, Konig J, Hoffmann G. Adherence to a Mediterranean diet and risk of diabetes: a systematic review and meta-analysis. *Public Health Nutr*. 2015;18(7):1292–1299.

130. Sofi F, Macchi C, Abbate R, Gensini GF, Casini A. Mediterranean diet and health status: an updated meta-analysis and a proposal for a literature-based adherence score. *Public Health Nutr*. 2014;17(12):2769–2782.

131. Schwingshackl L, Hoffmann G. Adherence to Mediterranean diet and risk of cancer: a systematic review and meta-analysis of observational studies. *Int J Cancer*. 2014; 135(8):1884–1897.

132. Schwingshackl L, Hoffmann G. Mediterranean dietary pattern, inflammation and endothelial function: a systematic review and meta-analysis of intervention trials. *Nutr Metab Cardiovasc Dis*. 2014;24(9):929–939.

133. Huo R, Du T, Xu Y, et al. Effects of Mediterranean-style diet on glycemic control, weight loss and cardiovascular risk factors among type 2 diabetes individuals: a meta-analysis. *Eur J Clin Nutr*. 2014;69(11):1200–1208.

134. Esposito K, Chiodini P, Maiorino MI, Bellastella G, Panagiotakos D, Giugliano D. Which diet for prevention of type 2 diabetes? A meta-analysis of prospective studies. *Endocrine*. 2014;47(1):107–116.

135. Psaltopoulou T, Sergentanis TN, Panagiotakos DB, Sergentanis IN, Kosti R, Scarmeas N. Mediterranean diet, stroke, cognitive impairment, and depression: a meta-analysis. *Ann Neurol*. 2013;74(4):580–591.

136. Campbell TC, Campbell TM. *The China Study: The Most Comprehensive Study of Nutrition Ever Conducted and the Startling Implications for Diet, Weight Loss, and Long-term Health.* New York: Benbella Books; 2006.

137. Esselstyn CB. *Prevent and Reverse Heart Disease: The Revolutionary, Scientifically Proven, Nutrition-Based Cure.* New York: Avery; 2008.

138. Ornish D. Can lifestyle changes reverse coronary heart disease? *World Review of Nutrition and Dietetics.* 1993;72:38–48.

139. Ornish D, Brown SE, Scherwitz LW, et al. Lifestyle changes and heart disease. *Lancet.* 1990;336(8717):741–742.

140. Ornish D, Brown SE, Scherwitz LW, et al. Can lifestyle changes reverse coronary heart disease? The Lifestyle Heart Trial. *Lancet.* 1990;336(8708):129–133.

141. Ornish D, Scherwitz LW, Billings JH, et al. Intensive lifestyle changes for reversal of coronary heart disease. *JAMA.* 1998;280(23):2001–2007.

142. Ornish D, Magbanua MJ, Weidner G, et al. Changes in prostate gene expression in men undergoing an intensive nutrition and lifestyle intervention. *Proc Natl Acad Sci USA.* 2008;105(24):8369–8374.

143. Ornish D, Weidner G, Fair WR, et al. Intensive lifestyle changes may affect the progression of prostate cancer. *J Urol.* 2005;174(3):1065–1069; discussion 1069–1070.

144. Ornish DM, Lee KL, Fair WR, Pettengill EB, Carroll PR. Dietary trial in prostate cancer: early experience and implications for clinical trial design. *Urology.* 2001;57 (4 Suppl 1):200–201.

145. Ornish D. Intensive lifestyle changes and health reform. *Lancet Oncol.* 2009;10(7): 638–639.

146. Ornish D, Lin J, Daubenmier J, et al. Increased telomerase activity and comprehensive lifestyle changes: a pilot study. *Lancet Oncol.* 2008;9(11):1048–1057.

147. Radd S, Marsh KA. Practical tips for preparing healthy and delicious plant-based meals. *Med J Aust.* 2013;199(4 Suppl):S41–45.

148. Albert BB, Derraik JGB, Cameron-Smith D, et al. Fish oil supplements in New Zealand are highly oxidised and do not meet label content of n-3 PUFA. Available at <www.nature.com/srep/2015/150121/srep07928/full/srep07928.html>, accessed 23 April 2015.

149. Erasmus U. *Fats that Heal, Fats that Kill: The Complete Guide to Fats, Oils, Cholesterol and Human Health.* 3rd ed. Summertown, TN: Alive Books; 2010.

150. Lauer K. Environmental risk factors in multiple sclerosis. *Expert Review of Neurotherapeutics.* 2010;10(3):421–440.

Step 2

1. Berg SZ. UV Radiation, auto-immunity, and questions galore. *The Scientist.* Available at <www.the-scientist.com/?articles.view/articleNo/14729/title/UV-Radiation--Auto-immunity--and-Questions-Galore>, accessed 21 April 2015.

2. Garland FC, White MR, Garland CF, Shaw E, Gorham ED. Occupational sunlight exposure and melanoma in the U.S. Navy. *Arch Environ Health.* 1990;45(5):261–267.

3. Diamond TH, Ho KW, Rohl PG, Meerkin M. Annual intramuscular injection of a megadose of cholecalciferol for treatment of vitamin D deficiency: efficacy and safety data. *Med J Aust.* 2005;183(1):10–12.

4. Garcion E, Wion-Barbot N, Montero-Menei CN, Berger F, Wion D. New clues about vitamin D functions in the nervous system. *Trends Endocrin Metab.* 2002;13:100–105.

5. May E, Asadullah K, Zugel U. Immunoregulation through 1,25-dihydroxy-vitamin D3 and its analogs. *Curr Drug Targets Inflamm Allergy.* 2004;3(4):377–393.

6. Ashtari F, Toghianifar N, Zarkesh-Esfahani SH, Mansourian M. Short-term effect of high-dose vitamin D on the level of interleukin 10 in patients with multiple sclerosis: a randomized, double-blind, placebo-controlled clinical trial. *Neuro-immunomodulation.* 2015;22(6):200–204.

7. Hart PH, Gorman S. Exposure to UV wavelengths in sunlight suppresses immunity: to what extent is UV-induced vitamin D3 the mediator responsible? *The Clinical biochemist. Reviews / Australian Association of Clinical Biochemists.* 2013;34(1):3–13.

8. Dumas AM, Jauberteau-Marchan MO. The protective role of Langerhans' cells and sunlight in multiple sclerosis. *Med Hypotheses.* 2000;55:517–520.

9. Baarnhielm M, Hedstrom AK, Kockum I, et al. Sunlight is associated with decreased multiple sclerosis risk: no interaction with human leukocyte antigen-DRB1*15. *Eur J Neurol.* 2012;19(7):955–962.

10. Grant WB, Strange RC, Garland CF. Sunshine is good medicine: the health benefits of ultraviolet-B induced vitamin D production. *J Cosmet Dermatol.* 2003;2(2):86–98.

11. Holick MF. Sunlight and vitamin D for bone health and prevention of auto-immune diseases, cancers, and cardiovascular disease. *Am J Clin Nutr.* 2004;80(6):1678S-1688S.

12. Holick MF. The vitamin D epidemic and its health consequences. *J Nutr.* 2005;135(11):2739S-2748S.

13. Ebeling PR. Megadose therapy for vitamin D deficiency. *Med J Aust.* 2005;183(1):4–5.

14. Holick MF, Chen TC. Vitamin D deficiency: a worldwide problem with health consequences. *Am J Clin Nutr.* 2008;87(4):1080S–1086S.

15. Grant WB, Garland CF, Holick MF. Comparisons of estimated economic burdens due to insufficient solar ultraviolet irradiance and vitamin D and excess solar UV irradiance for the United States. *Photochem Photobiol.* 2005;81(6):1276–1286.

16. Grant WB, Holick MF. Benefits and requirements of vitamin D for optimal health: a review. *Altern Med Rev.* 2005;10(2):94–111.

17. Flicker L, Mead K, MacInnis RJ, et al. Serum vitamin D and falls in older women in residential care in Australia. *J Am Geriatr Soc.* 2003;51(11):1533–1538.

18. Pasco JA, Henry MJ, Kotowicz MA, et al. Seasonal periodicity of serum vitamin D and parathyroid hormone, bone resorption, and fractures: the Geelong Osteoporosis Study. *J Bone Miner Res.* 2004;19(5):752–758.

19. Bischoff HA, Stahelin HB, Dick W, et al. Effects of vitamin D and calcium supple-mentation on falls: a randomized controlled trial. *J Bone Miner Res.* 2003;18(2):343–351.

20. Zittermann A. Vitamin D in preventive medicine: are we ignoring the evidence? *Br J Nutr.* 2003;89(5):552–572.

21. Grimes DS, Hindle E, Dyer T. Sunlight, cholesterol and coronary heart disease. *QJM*. 1996;89(8):579–589.

22. Arnson Y, Amital H, Shoenfeld Y. Vitamin D and auto-immunity: new aetiological and therapeutic considerations. *Ann Rheum Dis*. 2007;66(9):1137–1142.

23. Ponsonby AL, Lucas RM, van der Mei IA. UVR, vitamin D and three auto-immune diseases—multiple sclerosis, type 1 diabetes, rheumatoid arthritis. *Photochem Photobiol*. 2005;81(6):1267–1275.

24. Ponsonby AL, McMichael A, van der Mei I. Ultraviolet radiation and auto-immune disease: insights from epidemiological research. *Toxicology*. 2002;181–182:71–78.

25. Mohr SB, Garland CF, Gorham ED, Garland FC. The association between ultraviolet B irradiance, vitamin D status and incidence rates of type 1 diabetes in 51 regions worldwide. *Diabetologia*. 2008;51(8):1391–1398.

26. Zipitis CS, Akobeng AK. Vitamin D supplementation in early childhood and risk of type 1 diabetes: a systematic review and meta-analysis. *Arch Dis Child*. 2008; 93(6):512–517.

27. Grant WB. Ecologic studies of solar UV-B radiation and cancer mortality rates. *Recent Results Cancer Res*. 2003;164:371–377.

28. Autier P, Gandini S. Vitamin D supplementation and total mortality: a meta-analysis of randomized controlled trials. *Arch Intern Med*. 2007;167(16):1730–1737.

29. Melamed ML, Michos ED, Post W, Astor B. 25–hydroxyvitamin D levels and the risk of mortality in the general population. *Arch Intern Med*. 2008;168(15):1629–1637.

30. Wei MY, Giovannucci EL. Vitamin D and multiple health outcomes in the Harvard cohorts. *Molecular nutrition & food research*. 2010;54(8):1114–1126.

31. Cannell JJ, Vieth R, Umhau JC, et al. Epidemic influenza and vitamin D. *Epidemiology and infection*. 2006;134(6):1129–1140.

32. Sabetta JR, DePetrillo P, Cipriani RJ, Smardin J, Burns LA, Landry ML. Serum 25–hydroxyvitamin D and the incidence of acute viral respiratory tract infections in healthy adults. *PLoS One*. 2010;5(6):e11088.

33. Lucas RM, Ponsonby AL. Ultraviolet radiation and health: friend and foe. *Med J Aust*. 2002;177(11–12):594–598.

34. Holick MF. Vitamin D: A millenium perspective. *J Cell Biochem*. 2003;88(2):296–307.

35. Esparza ML, Sasaki S, Kesteloot H. Nutrition, latitude, and multiple sclerosis mortality: an ecologic study. *Am J Epidemiol*. 1995;142(7):733–737.

36. Llorca J, Guerrero P, Prieto-Salceda D, Dierssen-Sotos T. Mortality of multiple sclerosis in Spain: Demonstration of a north–south gradient. *Neuroepidemiology*. 2005;24(3):135–140.

37. Kampman MT, Wilsgaard T, Mellgren SI. Outdoor activities and diet in childhood and adolescence relate to MS risk above the Arctic Circle. *J Neurol*. 2007;254(4):471–477.

38. Hutter C. On the causes of multiple sclerosis. *Med Hypotheses*. 1993;41(2):93–96.

39. Hutter CD, Laing P. Multiple sclerosis: sunlight, diet, immunology and aetiology. *Med Hypotheses*. 1996;46(2):67–74.

40. Kampman MT, Brustad M. Vitamin D: A candidate for the environmental effect in multiple sclerosis: observations from Norway. *Neuroepidemiology*. 2008;30(3):140–146.

41. Deluca HF, Cantorna MT. Vitamin D: its role and uses in immunology. *Faseb J*. 2001;15(14):2579–2585.

42. Nataf S, Garcion E, Darcy F, Chabannes D, Muller JY, Brachet P. 1,25 Dihydroxy-vitamin D3 exerts regional effects in the central nervous system during experimental allergic encephalomyelitis. *J Neuropathol Exp Neurol.* 1996;55(8):904–914.

43. Wang Y, Marling SJ, McKnight SM, Danielson AL, Severson KS, Deluca HF. Suppression of experimental auto-immune encephalomyelitis by 300–315nm ultra-violet light. *Arch Biochem Biophys.* 2013;536(1):81–86.

44. Freedman DM, Dosemeci M, Alavanja MC. Mortality from multiple sclerosis and exposure to residential and occupational solar radiation: a case-control study based on death certificates. *Occup Environ Med.* 2000;57(6):418–421.

45. Westberg M, Feychting M, Jonsson F, Nise G, Gustavsson P. Occupational exposure to UV light and mortality from multiple sclerosis. *Am J Ind Med.* 2009.

46. Bjornevik K, Riise T, Casetta I, et al. Sun exposure and multiple sclerosis risk in Norway and Italy: The EnvIMS study. *Mult Scler.* 2014;20(8):1042–1049.

47. Goldacre MJ, Seagroatt V, Yeates D, Acheson ED. Skin cancer in people with multiple sclerosis: a record linkage study. *J Epidemiol Community Health.* 2004;58(2):142–144.

48. van der Mei IA, Ponsonby AL, Blizzard L, Dwyer T. Regional variation in multiple sclerosis prevalence in Australia and its association with ambient ultraviolet radiation. *Neuroepidemiology.* 2001;20(3):168–174.

49. Staples J, Ponsonby AL, Lim L. Low maternal exposure to ultraviolet radiation in pregnancy, month of birth, and risk of multiple sclerosis in offspring: longitudinal analysis. *BMJ.* 2010;340:c1640.

50. van der Mei IA, Ponsonby AL, Dwyer T, et al. Past exposure to sun, skin phenotype, and risk of multiple sclerosis: case-control study. *BMJ.* 2003;327(7410):316.

51. Islam T, Gauderman WJ, Cozen W, Mack TM. Childhood sun exposure influences risk of multiple sclerosis in monozygotic twins. *Neurology.* 2007;69(4):381–388.

52. Munger KL, Levin LI, Hollis BW, Howard NS, Ascherio A. Serum 25–hydroxy-vitamin D levels and risk of multiple sclerosis. *JAMA.* 2006;296:2832–2838.

53. Banwell B, Bar-Or A, Arnold DL, et al. Clinical, environmental, and genetic determinants of multiple sclerosis in children with acute demyelination: a prospective national cohort study. *Lancet Neurol.* 2011;10(5):436–445.

54. Ozgocmen S, Bulut S, Ilhan N, Gulkesen A, Ardicoglu O, Ozkan Y. Vitamin D deficiency and reduced bone mineral density in multiple sclerosis: effect of ambulatory status and functional capacity. *J Bone Miner Metab.* 2005;23(4):309–313.

55. Munger KL, Zhang SM, O'Reilly E, et al. Vitamin D intake and incidence of multiple sclerosis. *Neurology.* 2004;62(1):60–65.

56. Cortese M, Riise T, Bjornevik K, et al. Timing of use of cod liver oil, a vitamin D source, and multiple sclerosis risk: The EnvIMS study. *Mult Scler.* 2015;21(14):1856–1864.

57. Ascherio A, Munger KL, Simon KC. Vitamin D and multiple sclerosis. *Lancet neurology.* 2010;9(6):599–612.

58. Vitamin D: hope on the horizon for MS prevention? *Lancet Neurol.* 2010;9(6):555.

59. Goldberg P. Multiple sclerosis: vitamin D and calcium as environmental determinants of prevalence (a viewpoint). Part 1: sunlight, dietary factors and epidemiology. *Int J Environ Studies.* 1974;6:19–27.

60. Heaney RP, Davies KM, Chen TC, Holick MF, Barger-Lux MJ. Human serum 25–hydroxycholecalciferol response to extended oral dosing with cholecalciferol. *Am J Clin Nutr.* 2003;77(1):204–210.

61. Hayes CE, Cantorna MT, DeLuca HF. Vitamin D and multiple sclerosis. *Proc Soc Exp Biol Med.* 1997;216(1):21–27.

62. Goldberg P, Fleming MC, Picard EH. Multiple sclerosis: decreased relapse rate through dietary supplementation with calcium, magnesium and vitamin D. *Med Hypotheses.* 1986;21(2):193–200.

63. Embry AF, Snowdon LR, Vieth R. Vitamin D and seasonal fluctuations of gadolinium-enhancing magnetic resonance imaging lesions in multiple sclerosis. *Ann Neurol.* 2000;48(2):271–272.

64. Soilu-Hanninen M, Airas L, Mononen I, Heikkila A, Viljanen M, Hanninen A. 25-hydroxyvitamin D levels in serum at the onset of multiple sclerosis. *Mult Scler.* 2005;11(3):266–271.

65. Soilu-Hanninen M, Laaksonen M, Laitinen I, Eralinna JP, Lilius EM, Mononen I. A longitudinal study of serum 25–hydroxyvitamin D and intact PTH levels indicate the importance of vitamin D and calcium homeostasis regulation in multiple sclerosis. *J Neurol Neurosurg Psychiatry.* 2007;79(2):152–157.

66. Correale J, Ysrraelit MC, Gaitan MI. Immunomodulatory effects of vitamin D in multiple sclerosis. *Brain.* 2009;132(Part 5):1146–1160.

67. Faulkner MA, Ryan-Haddad AM, Lenz TL, Degner K. Osteoporosis in long-term care residents with multiple sclerosis. *Consult Pharm.* 2005;20(2):128–136.

68. VanAmerongen BM, Dijkstra CD, Lips P, Polman CH. Multiple sclerosis and vitamin D: an update. *Eur J Clin Nutr.* 2004;58(8):1095–1109.

69. McDowell TY, Amr S, Culpepper WJ, et al. Sun exposure, vitamin D and age at disease onset in relapsing multiple sclerosis. *Neuroepidemiology.* 2011;36(1):39–45.

70. Ascherio A, Munger KL, White R, et al. Vitamin D as an early predictor of multiple sclerosis activity and progression. *JAMA neurology.* 2014;71(3):306–314.

71. Tremlett H, van der Mei IA, Pittas F, et al. Monthly ambient sunlight, infections and relapse rates in multiple sclerosis. *Neuroepidemiology.* 2008;31(4):271–279.

72. Runia TF, Hop WC, de Rijke YB, Buljevac D, Hintzen RQ. Lower serum vitamin D levels are associated with a higher relapse risk in multiple sclerosis. *Neurology.* 2012;79(3):261–266.

73. Karczmarewicz E, Czekuc-Kryskiewicz E, Pludowski P. Effect of vitamin D status on pharmacological treatment efficiency: Impact on cost-effective management in medicine. *Dermato-endocrinology.* 2013;5(1):1–6.

74. Rodda CP, Benson JE, Vincent AJ, Whitehead CL, Polykov A, Vollenhoven B. Maternal vitamin D supplementation during pregnancy prevents vitamin D deficiency in the newborn: an open-label randomized controlled trial. *Clinical endocrinology.* 2015;83(3):3363–3368.

75. Chaudhuri A. Why we should offer routine vitamin D supplementation in pregnancy and childhood to prevent multiple sclerosis. *Med Hypotheses.* 2005;64(3):608–618.

76. Etemadifar M, Janghorbani M. Efficacy of high-dose vitamin D3 supplementation in vitamin D deficient pregnant women with multiple sclerosis: Preliminary findings of a randomized-controlled trial. *Iranian Journal of Neurology.* 2015;14(2):67–73.

77. Simpson S, Jr., Taylor B, Blizzard L, et al. Higher 25–hydroxyvitamin D is associated with lower relapse risk in multiple sclerosis. *Annals of neurology.* 2010;68(2):193–203.

78. Spelman T, Gray O, Trojano M, et al. Seasonal variation of relapse rate in multiple sclerosis is latitude-dependent. *Ann Neurol.* 2014;76(6):880–890.

79. Pierrot-Deseilligny C, Rivaud-Pechoux S, Clerson P, de Paz R, Souberbielle JC. Relationship between 25-OH-D serum level and relapse rate in multiple sclerosis patients before and after vitamin D supplementation. *Ther Adv Neurol Disord.* 2012;5(4):187–198.

80. Kimball SM, Ursell MR, O'Connor P, Vieth R. Safety of vitamin D3 in adults with multiple sclerosis. *Am J Clin Nutr.* 2007;86(3):645–651.

81. Soilu-Hanninen M, Aivo J, Lindstrom BM, et al. A randomised, double blind, placebo controlled trial with vitamin D3 as an add on treatment to interferon beta-1b in patients with multiple sclerosis. *J Neurol Neurosurg Psychiatry.* 2012;83(5): 565–571.

82. Allen AC, Kelly S, Basdeo SA, et al. A pilot study of the immunological effects of high-dose vitamin D in healthy volunteers. *Mult Scler.* 2012;18(12):1797–1800.

83. Hayes CE, Hubler SL, Moore JR, Barta LE, Praska CE, Nashold FE. Vitamin D actions on CD4(+) T cells in auto-immune disease. *Frontiers in Immunology.* 2015;6:100.

84. Working Group of the Australian and New Zealand Bone and Mineral Society Endocrine Society of Australia Osteoporosis Australia. Vitamin D and adult bone health in Australia and New Zealand: a position statement. *Med J Aust.* 2005;182(6): 281–285.

85. Vieth R. Why the optimal requirement for Vitamin D(3) is probably much higher than what is officially recommended for adults. *J Steroid Biochem Mol Biol.* 2004;89–90:575–579.

86. Pasco JA, Henry MJ, Nicholson GC, Sanders KM, Kotowicz MA. Vitamin D status of women in the Geelong Osteoporosis Study: association with diet and casual exposure to sunlight. *Med J Aust.* 2001;175(8):401–405.

87. Nowson CA, McGrath JJ, Ebeling PR, et al. Vitamin D and health in adults in Australia and New Zealand: a position statement. *Med J Aust.* 2012;196(11):686–687.

88. Moan J, Porojnicu AC. The photobiology of vitamin D, a topic of renewed focus. *Tidsskr Nor Laegeforen.* 2006;126(8):1048–1052.

89. Sanders KM, Stuart AL, Williamson EJ, et al. Annual high-dose oral vitamin D and falls and fractures in older women: a randomized controlled trial. *JAMA.* 2010; 303(18):1815–1822.

90. Sanders KM, Stuart AL, Williamson EJ, et al. Annual high-dose vitamin D3 and mental well-being: randomised controlled trial. *The British Journal of Psychiatry: The Journal of Mental Science.* 2011;198(5):357–364.

91. Vieth R. Vitamin D supplementation, 25–hydroxyvitamin D concentrations, and safety. *Am J Clin Nutr.* 1999;69(5):842–856.

92. Hathcock JN, Shao A, Vieth R, Heaney R. Risk assessment for vitamin D. *Am J Clin Nutr.* 2007;85(1):6–18.

93. Kolata G. Report questions need for 2 diet supplements. *New York Times,* 29 November 2010. Available at <www.nytimes.com/2010/11/30/health/30vitamin. html?_r=4&hp&. 2010>, accessed 10 October 2014.

94. Holick MF, Binkley NC, Bischoff-Ferrari HA, et al. Evaluation, treatment, and pre-vention of vitamin D deficiency: an Endocrine Society clinical practice guideline. *J Clin Endocrinol Metab.* 2011;96(7):1911–1930.

95. Kimball S, Vieth R. Self-prescribed high-dose vitamin D(3): effects on biochemical parameters in two men. *Ann Clin Biochem.* 2008;45(Pt 1):106–110.

96. Dudenkov DV, Yawn BP, Oberhelman SS, et al. Changing incidence of serum 25-hydroxyvitamin D values above 50 ng/mL: A 10–Year population-based study. *Mayo Clin Proc.* 2015;90(5):577–586.

97. Wingerchuk DM, Lesaux J, Rice GP, Kremenchutzky M, Ebers GC. A pilot study of oral calcitriol (1,25–dihydroxyvitamin D3) for relapsing-remitting multiple sclero-sis. *J Neurol Neurosurg Psychiatry.* 2005;76(9):1294–1296.

98. Bjelakovic G, Gluud LL, Nikolova D, et al. Vitamin D supplementation for pre-vention of mortality in adults. *Cochrane Database Syst Rev.* 2014;1:CD007470.

99. Stein MS, Liu Y, Gray OM, et al. A randomized trial of high-dose vitamin D2 in relapsing-remitting multiple sclerosis. *Neurology.* 2011;77(17):1611–1618.

100. van der Mei IA, Ponsonby AL, Dwyer T, et al. Vitamin D levels in people with multiple sclerosis and community controls in Tasmania, Australia. *J Neurol.* 2007;254(5): 581–590.

101. Menzies Research Institute. Information on vitamin D levels for people with multiple sclerosis. *MS Research Australia Newsletter.* Available at <www.menzies.utas.edu.au/pdf/Vitamin_D_A4_Brochure_VanderMei.pdf. 2009>, accessed 21 July 2014.

102. Barnes MS, Bonham MP, Robson PJ, et al. Assessment of 25–hydroxyvitamin D and 1,25-dihydroxyvitamin D3 concentrations in male and female multiple sclerosis patients and control volunteers. *Mult Scler.* 2007;13(5):670–672.

103. Hollis BW. Vitamin D requirement during pregnancy and lactation. *J Bone Miner Res.* 2007;22 Suppl 2:V39–44.

104. Airas L, Jalkanen A, Alanen A, Pirttila T, Marttila RJ. Breast-feeding, postpartum and prepregnancy disease activity in multiple sclerosis. *Neurology.* 2010;75(5):474–476.

105. Langer-Gould A, Huang SM, Gupta R, et al. Exclusive breastfeeding and the risk of postpartum relapses in women with multiple sclerosis. *Arch Neurol.* 2009;66(8): 958–963.

106. Hutchinson M. If I had CIS with MRI diagnostic of MS, I would take vitamin D 10,000 IU daily: Commentary. *Mult Scler.* 2013;19(2):143–144.

107. Brum DG, Comini-Frota ER, Vasconcelos CC, Dias-Tosta E. Supplementation and therapeutic use of vitamin D in patients with multiple sclerosis: consensus of the Scientific Department of Neuroimmunology of the Brazilian Academy of Neurology. *Arq Neuropsiquiatr.* 2014;72(2):152–156.

108. Michaelsson K, Wolk A, Langenskiold S, et al. Milk intake and risk of mortality and fractures in women and men: cohort studies. *BMJ.* 2014;349:g6015.

109. Owusu W, Willett WC, Feskanich D, Ascherio A, Spiegelman D, Colditz GA. Calcium intake and the incidence of forearm and hip fractures among men. *J Nutr.* 1997;127(9):1782–1787.

110. Feskanich D, Willett WC, Stampfer MJ, Colditz GA. Milk, dietary calcium, and bone fractures in women: a 12–year prospective study. *Am J Public Health.* 1997;87(6): 992–997.

111. Lanou AJ, Berkow SE, Barnard ND. Calcium, dairy products, and bone health in children and young adults: a reevaluation of the evidence. *Pediatrics.* 2005;115(3): 736–743.
112. New SA. Nutrition Society Medal lecture. The role of the skeleton in acid–base homeostasis. *The Proceedings of the Nutrition Society.* 2002;61(2):151–164.
113. Heaney RP, Dowell MS, Hale CA, Bendich A. Calcium absorption varies within the reference range for serum 25–hydroxyvitamin D. *J Am Coll Nutr.* 2003;22(2):142–146.
114. Taylor BV. Sunshine and multiple sclerosis. *J Neurol Neurosurg Psychiatry.* 2013; 84(10):1066.

Step 3

1. Woodcock J, Franco OH, Orsini N, Roberts I. Non-vigorous physical activity and all-cause mortality: systematic review and meta-analysis of cohort studies. *Int J Epidemiol.* 2011;40(1):121–138.
2. Warburton DE, Nicol CW, Bredin SS. Health benefits of physical activity: the evidence. *CMAJ.* 2006;174(6):801–809.
3. Warburton DE, Nicol CW, Bredin SS. Prescribing exercise as preventive therapy. *CMAJ.* 2006;174(7):961–974.
4. Naci H, Ioannidis JP. Comparative effectiveness of exercise and drug interventions on mortality outcomes: metaepidemiological study. *BMJ.* 2013;347:f5577.
5. Erikssen G. Physical fitness and changes in mortality: the survival of the fittest. *Sports Med.* 2001;31(8):571–576.
6. Erikssen G, Liestol K, Bjornholt J, Thaulow E, Sandvik L, Erikssen J. Changes in physical fitness and changes in mortality. *Lancet.* 1998;352(9130):759–762.
7. Faselis C, Doumas M, Pittaras A, et al. Exercise capacity and all-cause mortality in male veterans with hypertension aged >/=70 years. *Hypertension.* 2014;64(1):30–35.
8. Leeper NJ, Myers J, Zhou M, et al. Exercise capacity is the strongest predictor of mortality in patients with peripheral arterial disease. *J Vasc Surg.* 2013;57(3):728–733.
9. Nylen ES, Kokkinos P, Myers J, Faselis C. Prognostic effect of exercise capacity on mortality in older adults with diabetes mellitus. *J Am Geriatr Soc.* 2010;58(10): 1850–1854.
10. Kokkinos P, Myers J, Faselis C, et al. Exercise capacity and mortality in older men: a 20-year follow-up study. *Circulation.* 2010;122(8):790–797.
11. Kokkinos P, Doumas M, Myers J, et al. A graded association of exercise capacity and all-cause mortality in males with high-normal blood pressure. *Blood pressure.* 2009;18(5):261–267.
12. Myers J, Prakash M, Froelicher V, Do D, Partington S, Atwood JE. Exercise capacity and mortality among men referred for exercise testing. *N Engl J Med.* 2002;346(11): 793–801.
13. Blair SN, Kohl HW, 3rd, Barlow CE, Paffenbarger RS, Jr., Gibbons LW, Macera CA. Changes in physical fitness and all-cause mortality. A prospective study of healthy and unhealthy men. *JAMA.* 1995;273(14):1093–1098.
14. Arem H, Moore SC, Patel A, et al. Leisure time physical activity and mortality: a detailed pooled analysis of the dose–response relationship. *JAMA Internal Medicine.* 2015;175(6):959–967.

15. Gebel K, Ding D, Chey T, Stamatakis E, Brown WJ, Bauman AE. Effect of moderate to vigorous physical activity on all-cause mortality in middle-aged and older Australians. *JAMA Internal Medicine.* 2015;175(6):970–977.
16. Adamson BC, Ensari I, Motl RW. Effect of exercise on depressive symptoms in adults with neurologic disorders: a systematic review and meta-analysis. *Arch Phys Med Rehabil.* 2015;96(7):1329–1338.
17. Haydon AM, Macinnis RJ, English DR, Giles GG. Effect of physical activity and body size on survival after diagnosis with colorectal cancer. *Gut.* 2006;55(1):62–67.
18. Holmes MD, Chen WY, Feskanich D, Kroenke CH, Colditz GA. Physical activity and survival after breast cancer diagnosis. *JAMA.* 2005;293(20):2479–2486.
19. Liu-Ambrose TY, Khan KM, Eng JJ, Heinonen A, McKay HA. Both resistance and agility training increase cortical bone density in 75- to 85-year-old women with low bone mass: a 6-month randomized controlled trial. *Journal of Clinical Densitometry: The Official Journal of the International Society for Clinical Densitometry.* 2004;7(4):390–398.
20. Warburton DE, Gledhill N, Quinney A. Musculoskeletal fitness and health. *Canadian Journal of Applied Physiology = Revue Canadienne de physiologie appliquee.* 2001;26(2):217–237.
21. Warburton DE, Glendhill N, Quinney A. The effects of changes in musculoskeletal fitness on health. *Canadian Journal of Applied Physiology = Revue Canadienne de physiologie appliquee.* 2001;26(2):161–216.
22. Brill PA, Macera CA, Davis DR, Blair SN, Gordon N. Muscular strength and physical function. *Med Sci Sports Exerc.* 2000;32(2):412–416.
23. Blair SN, LaMonte MJ, Nichaman MZ. The evolution of physical activity recommendations: how much is enough? *Am J Clin Nutr.* 2004;79(5):913S-920S.
24. Russell WR. *Multiple Sclerosis: Control of the Disease.* Oxford: Pergamon Press; 1976.
25. Motl RW, Gosney JL. Effect of exercise training on quality of life in multiple sclerosis: a meta-analysis. *Mult Scler.* 2008;14(1):129–135.
26. Heine M, van de Port I, Rietberg MB, van Wegen EE, Kwakkel G. Exercise therapy for fatigue in multiple sclerosis. *Cochrane Database Syst Rev.* 2015;9:CD009956.
27. Marrie R, Horwitz R, Cutter G, Tyry T, Campagnolo D, Vollmer T. High frequency of adverse health behaviors in multiple sclerosis. *Mult Scler.* 2009;15(1):105–113.
28. Motl RW, Arnett PA, Smith MM, Barwick FH, Ahlstrom B, Stover EJ. Worsening of symptoms is associated with lower physical activity levels in individuals with multiple sclerosis. *Mult Scler.* 2008;14(1):140–142.
29. Marrie RA, Rudick R, Horwitz R, et al. Vascular comorbidity is associated with more rapid disability progression in multiple sclerosis. *Neurology.* 2010;74(13):1041–1047.
30. Gallien P, Nicolas B, Robineau S, Petrilli S, Houedakor J, Durufle A. Physical training and multiple sclerosis. *Ann Readapt Med Phys.* 2007;50(6):373–376.
31. Brown TR, Kraft GH. Exercise and rehabilitation for individuals with multiple sclerosis. *Phys Med Rehabil Clin N Am.* 2005;16(2):513–555.
32. Bjarnadottir OH, Konradsdottir AD, Reynisdottir K, Olafsson E. Multiple sclerosis and brief moderate exercise: a randomised study. *Mult Scler.* 2007;13(6):776–782.

33. Gutierrez GM, Chow JW, Tillman MD, McCoy SC, Castellano V, White LJ. Resistance training improves gait kinematics in persons with multiple sclerosis. *Arch Phys Med Rehabil.* 2005;86(9):1824–1829.

34. Kileff J, Ashburn A. A pilot study of the effect of aerobic exercise on people with moderate disability multiple sclerosis. *Clin Rehabil.* 2005;19(2):165–169.

35. Rietberg M, Brooks D, Uitdehaag B, Kwakkel G. Exercise therapy for multiple sclerosis. *Cochrane Database Syst Rev.* 2005(1):CD003980.

36. Langeskov-Christensen M, Heine M, Kwakkel G, Dalqas U. Aerobic capacity in persons with multiple sclerosis: a systemic review and meta-analysis, *Sports Med.* 2015;45:905–23.

37. Romberg A, Virtanen A, Ruutiainen J. Long-term exercise improves functional impairment but not quality of life in multiple sclerosis. *J Neurol.* 2005;252(7):839–845.

38. Romberg A, Virtanen A, Ruutiainen J, et al. Effects of a 6-month exercise program on patients with multiple sclerosis: a randomized study. *Neurology.* 2004;63(11):2034–2038.

39. White LJ, Dressendorfer RH. Exercise and multiple sclerosis. *Sports Med.* 2004;34(15):1077–1100.

40. White LJ, McCoy SC, Castellano V, et al. Resistance training improves strength and functional capacity in persons with multiple sclerosis. *Mult Scler.* 2004;10(6):668–674.

41. Taylor KT, Hadgkiss EJ, Jelinek GA, et al. Lifestyle and demographic factors and medications associated with depression risk in an international sample of people with multiple sclerosis. *BMC Psychiatry; in press.* 2014;14:327.

42. Kerdoncuff V, Durufle A, Le Tallec H, et al. Multiple sclerosis and physical activities (In French). *Ann Readapt Med Phys.* 2005;49(1):32–36.

43. Sutherland G, Andersen MB. Exercise and multiple sclerosis: physiological, psychological, and quality of life issues. *J Sports Med Phys Fitness.* 2001;41(4):421–432.

44. Fragoso YD, Santana DL, Pinto RC. The positive effects of a physical activity program for multiple sclerosis patients with fatigue. *NeuroRehabilitation.* 2008;23(2):153–157.

45. McCullagh R, Fitzgerald AP, Murphy RP, Cooke G. Long-term benefits of exercising on quality of life and fatigue in multiple sclerosis patients with mild disability: a pilot study. *Clin Rehabil.* 2008;22(3):206–214.

46. Weiland TJ, Jelinek GA, Hadgkiss EJ, et al. Clinically significant fatigue: Prevalence and associated factors in an international sample of adults with multiple sclerosis. *PLOS One.* 2015;10(2):e0115541.

47. Marck CH, Hadgkiss E, Weiland TJ, van der Meer DM, Pereira N, Jelinek GA. Physical activity and associated levels of disability and quality of life in people with multiple sclerosis: a large international survey. *BMC neurology.* 2014;14:143.

48. Motl RW, McAuley E. Pathways between physical activity and quality of life in adults with multiple sclerosis. *Health Psychol.* 2009;28(6):682–689.

49. van den Berg M, Dawes H, Wade DT, et al. Treadmill training for individuals with multiple sclerosis: a pilot randomised trial. *J Neurol Neurosurg Psychiatry.* 2006;77(4):531–533.

50. Surakka J, Romberg A, Ruutiainen J, et al. Effects of aerobic and strength exercise on motor fatigue in men and women with multiple sclerosis: a randomized controlled trial. *Clin Rehabil.* 2004;18(7):737–746.

51. Rampello A, Franceschini M, Piepoli M, et al. Effect of aerobic training on walking capacity and maximal exercise tolerance in patients with multiple sclerosis: a randomized crossover controlled study. *Phys Ther.* 2007;87(5):545–555; discussion 555–549.

52. Kuspinar A, Rodriguez AM, Mayo NE. The effects of clinical interventions on health-related quality of life in multiple sclerosis: a meta-analysis. *Mult Scler.* 2012;18(12): 1686–1704.

53. Motl RW, Gosney JL. Effect of exercise training on quality of life in multiple sclerosis: a meta-analysis. *Mult Scler.* 2008;14(1):129–135.

54. Dalgas U, Stenager E, Jakobsen J, et al. Fatigue, mood and quality of life improve in MS patients after progressive resistance training. *Mult Scler.* 2010;16(4):480–490.

55. Taylor NF, Dodd KJ, Prasad D, Denisenko S. Progressive resistance exercise for people with multiple sclerosis. *Disabil Rehabil.* 2006;28(18):1119–1126.

56. Dodd KJ, Taylor NF, Denisenko S, Prasad D. A qualitative analysis of a progressive resistance exercise programme for people with multiple sclerosis. *Disabil Rehabil.* 2006;28(18):1127–1134.

57. Taylor NF, Dodd KJ, Damiano DL. Progressive resistance exercise in physical therapy: a summary of systematic reviews. *Phys Ther.* 2005;85(11):1208–1223.

58. Braendvik SM, Koret T, Helbostad JL, et al. Treadmill training or progressive strength training to improve walking in people with multiple sclerosis? A randomized parallel group trial. *Physiotherapy Research International: The Journal for Researchers and Clinicians in Physical Therapy.* 2015;doi: 10.1002/pri.1636.

59. Dalgas U, Stenager E. Progressive resistance therapy is not the best way to rehabilitate deficits due to multiple sclerosis: no. *Mult Scler.* 2014;20(2):141–142.

60. Kjolhede T, Vissing K, de Place L, et al. Neuromuscular adaptations to long-term progressive resistance training translates to improved functional capacity for people with multiple sclerosis and is maintained at follow-up. *Mult Scler.* 2014;21(5):599–611.

61. Dalgas U, Stenager E, Ingemann-Hansen T. Multiple sclerosis and physical exercise: recommendations for the application of resistance-, endurance- and combined training. *Mult Scler.* 2008;14(1):35–53.

62. Brown RF, Valpiani EM, Tennant CC, et al. Longitudinal assessment of anxiety, depression, and fatigue in people with multiple sclerosis. *Psychol Psychother.* 2008; 82(Part 1):41–56.

63. Hassanpour Dehkordi A. Influence of yoga and aerobics exercise on fatigue, pain and psychosocial status in patients with multiple sclerosis: a randomized trial. *J Sports Med Phys Fitness.* 2015. Available at <www.ncbi.nlm.nih.gov/pubmed/?term= Hassanpour+Dehkordi+A.+Influence+of+yoga+and+aerobics+exercise+on+fatigue %2C+pain+and+psychosocial+status+in+patients+with+multiple+sclerosis%3A+a+ randomized+trial>, accessed 12 December 2015.

64. Leavitt VM, Cirnigliaro C, Cohen A, et al. Aerobic exercise increases hippocampal volume and improves memory in multiple sclerosis: preliminary findings. *Neurocase.* 2014;20(6):695–697.

65. Ten Brinke LF, Bolandzadeh N, Nagamatsu LS, et al. Aerobic exercise increases hippocampal volume in older women with probable mild cognitive impairment: a 6-month randomised controlled trial. *Br J Sports Med.* 2014;49(4):248–254.

66. Fiatarone Singh MA, Gates N, Saigal N, et al. The Study of Mental and Resistance Training (SMART) Study: resistance training and/or cognitive training in mild cognitive impairment—a randomized, double-blind, double-sham controlled trial. *J Am Med Directors Ass.* 2014;15(12):873–880.

67. Baker LD, Frank LL, Foster-Schubert K, et al. Effects of aerobic exercise on mild cognitive impairment: a controlled trial. *Arch Neurol.* 2010;67(1):71–79.

68. Gold SM, Schulz KH, Hartmann S, et al. Basal serum levels and reactivity of nerve growth factor and brain-derived neurotrophic factor to standardized acute exercise in multiple sclerosis and controls. *J Neuroimmunol.* 2003;138(1–2):99–105.

69. Schulz KH, Heesen C. Effects of exercise in chronically ill patients: examples from oncology and neurology. *Bundesgesundheitsblatt Gesundheitsforschung Gesundheitsschutz.* 2005;48(8):906–913.

70. Dalgas U, Stenager E. Exercise and disease progression in multiple sclerosis: can exercise slow down the progression of multiple sclerosis? *Ther Adv Neurol Disord.* 2012;5(2):81–95.

71. Heesen C, Romberg A, Gold S, Schulz KH. Physical exercise in multiple sclerosis: supportive care or a putative disease-modifying treatment. *Expert Rev Neurother.* 2006;6(3):347–355.

72. White LJ, Castellano V. Exercise and brain health: implications for multiple sclerosis: Part 1—neuronal growth factors. *Sports Med.* 2008;38(2):91–100.

73. White LJ, Castellano V. Exercise and brain health: implications for multiple sclerosis. Part II: immune factors and stress hormones. *Sports Med.* 2008;38(3):179–186.

74. Das UN. Anti-inflammatory nature of exercise. *Nutrition.* 2004;20(3):323–326.

75. Stuifbergen AK, Blozis SA, Harrison TC, Becker HA. Exercise, functional limitations, and quality of life: a longitudinal study of persons with multiple sclerosis. *Archives of Physical Medicine & Rehabilitation.* 2006;87(7):935–943.

76. Rietberg MB, Brooks D, Uitdehaag BM, Kwakkel G. Exercise therapy for multiple sclerosis. *Cochrane Database Syst Rev.* 2005(1):CD003980.

77. Tallner A, Waschbisch A, Wenny I, et al. Multiple sclerosis relapses are not associated with exercise. *Mult Scler.* 2012;18(2):232–235.

78. Stuifbergen AK, Blozis SA, Harrison TC, Becker HA. Exercise, functional limitations, and quality of life: a longitudinal study of persons with multiple sclerosis. *Arch Phys Med Rehabil.* 2006;87(7):935–943.

79. Motl RW. Physical activity and its measurement and determinants in multiple sclerosis. *Minerva Med.* 2008;99(2):157–165.

80. Nortvedt MW, Riise T, Maeland JG. Multiple sclerosis and lifestyle factors: the Hordaland Health Study. *Neurol Sci.* 2005;26(5):334–339.

81. Sandroff BM, Dlugonski D, Weikert M, Suh Y, Balantrapu S, Motl RW. Physical activity and multiple sclerosis: new insights regarding inactivity. *Acta Neurol Scand.* 2012;126(4):256–262.

82. Turner AP, Kivlahan DR, Haselkorn JK. Exercise and quality of life among people with multiple sclerosis: looking beyond physical functioning to mental health and participation in life. *Arch Phys Med Rehabil.* 2009;90(3):420–428.

83. Filipi ML, Kucera DL, Filipi EO, Ridpath AC, Leuschen MP. Improvement in strength following resistance training in MS patients despite varied disability levels. *NeuroRehabilitation.* 2011;28(4):373–382.

84. Pilutti LA, Lelli DA, Paulseth JE, et al. Effects of 12 weeks of supported treadmill training on functional ability and quality of life in progressive multiple sclerosis: a pilot study. *Arch Phys Med Rehabil.* 2011;92(1):31–36.

85. Motl RW, McAuley E, Snook EM, Gliottoni RC. Physical activity and quality of life in multiple sclerosis: intermediary roles of disability, fatigue, mood, pain, self-efficacy and social support. *Psychol Health Med.* 2009;14(1):111–124.

86. Motl RW, Snook EM. Physical activity, self-efficacy, and quality of life in multiple sclerosis. *Ann Behav Med.* 2008;35(1):111–115.

87. Motl RW, Pilutti LA. The benefits of exercise training in multiple sclerosis. *Nat Rev Neurol.* 2012;8(9):487–497.

88. Suh Y, Weikert M, Dlugonski D, Sandroff B, Motl RW. Physical activity, social support, and depression: possible independent and indirect associations in persons with multiple sclerosis. *Psychol Health Med.* 2012;17(2):196–206.

89. Andreasen AK, Stenager E, Dalgas U. The effect of exercise therapy on fatigue in multiple sclerosis. *Mult Scler.* 2011;17(9):1041–1054.

90. McCullagh R, Fitzgerald AP, Murphy RP, Cooke G. Long-term benefits of exercising on quality of life and fatigue in multiple sclerosis patients with mild disability: a pilot study. *Clinical Rehabilitation.* 2008;22(3):206–214.

91. Dodd KJ, Taylor NF, Shields N, Prasad D, McDonald E, Gillon A. Progressive resistance training did not improve walking but can improve muscle performance, quality of life and fatigue in adults with multiple sclerosis: a randomized controlled trial. *Mult Scler.* 2011;17(11):1362–1374.

92. Huisinga JM, Filipi ML, Stergiou N. Elliptical exercise improves fatigue ratings and quality of life in patients with multiple sclerosis. *J Rehabil Res Dev.* 2011;48(7): 881–890.

93. Pilutti LA. Adapted exercise interventions for persons with progressive multiple sclerosis. *Appl Physiol Nutr Metab.* 2013;38(3):357.

94. Stroud NM, Minahan CL. The impact of regular physical activity on fatigue, depression and quality of life in persons with multiple sclerosis. *Health & Quality of Life Outcomes.* 2009;7:68.

95. MS Australia. Strength and cardiorespiratory exercise for people with multiple sclerosis (MS). *Practice for Health Professionals.* 2009. Available at <www.ms.org.au/attachments/documents/ms_practice/strength.aspx>, accessed 15 November 2015.

96. Harmon M. *Exercise as Part of Everyday Life.* Sydney: National MS Society; 2011. Available at <www.nationalmssociety.org/NationalMSSociety/media/MSNationalFiles/Brochures/Brochure-Exercise-as-Part-of-Everyday-Life.pdf>, accessed 15 November 2015.

97. Tremblay MS, Warburton DE, Janssen I, et al. New Canadian physical activity guidelines. *Applied physiology, nutrition, and metabolism = Physiologie appliquee, nutrition et metabolisme.* 2011;36(1):36–46; 47–58.

98. Canadian Society for Exercise Physiology. *MS Get Fit Toolkit: A resource to help adults living with multiple sclerosis (MS) meet the Canadian Physical Activity Guidelines;*

2013. Available at http://mssociety.ca/physicalactivity/MS_GetFit_toolkit_ENG.
pdf>, accessed 15 November 2015.

99. Giesser BS. Exercise in the management of persons with multiple sclerosis. *Ther Adv
Neurol Disord.* 2015;8(3):123–130.

Step 4

1. Benson H, Greenwood MM, Klemchuk H. The relaxation response: psychophysio-
logic aspects and clinical applications. *Int J Psychiatry Med.* 1975;6(1–2):87–98.

2. Hedstrom AK, Akerstedt T, Hillert J, Olsson T, Alfredsson L. Shift work at young
age is associated with increased risk for multiple sclerosis. *Ann Neurol.* 2011;70(5):
733–741.

3. Gold SM, Mohr DC, Huitinga I, Flachenecker P, Sternberg EM, Heesen C. The
role of stress–response systems for the pathogenesis and progression of MS. *Trends
Immunol.* 2005; 26(12):644–652.

4. Lalive PH, Burkhard PR, Chofflon M. TNF-alpha and psychologically stressful
events in healthy subjects: potential relevance for multiple sclerosis relapse. *Behav
Neurosci.* 2002;116(6):1093–1097.

5. Mohr DC, Pelletier D. A temporal framework for understanding the effects of
stressful life events on inflammation in patients with multiple sclerosis. *Brain Behav
Immun.* 2006;20(1):27–36.

6. Strenge H. The relationship between psychological stress and the clinical course
of multiple sclerosis. An update. *Psychother Psychosom Med Psychol.* 2001;51(3–4):
166–175.

7. Ackerman KD, Stover A, Heyman R, et al. Relationship of cardiovascular reactivity, stressful life events, and multiple sclerosis disease activity. *Brain Behav Immun.*
2003;17(3):141–151.

8. Buljevac D, Hop WC, Reedeker W, et al. Self reported stressful life events and
exacerbations in multiple sclerosis: prospective study. *BMJ.* 2003;327(7416):646.

9. Golan D, Somer E, Dishon S, Cuzin-Disegni L, Miller A. Impact of exposure to war
stress on exacerbations of multiple sclerosis. *Ann Neurol.* 2008;64(2):143–148.

10. Mitsonis CI, Zervas IM, Mitropoulos PA, et al. The impact of stressful life events on
risk of relapse in women with multiple sclerosis: a prospective study. *Eur Psychiatry.*
2008;23(7):497–504.

11. Mohr DC, Goodkin DE, Bacchetti P, et al. Psychological stress and the subsequent
appearance of new brain MRI lesions in MS. *Neurology.* 2000;55(1):55–61.

12. Mohr DC, Goodkin DE, Nelson S, Cox D, Weiner M. Moderating effects of coping
on the relationship between stress and the development of new brain lesions in
multiple sclerosis. *Psychosom Med.* 2002;64(5):803–809.

13. Burns MN, Nawacki E, Kwasny MJ, Pelletier D, Mohr DC. Do positive or negative
stressful events predict the development of new brain lesions in people with multiple
sclerosis? *Psychol Med.* 2014;44(2):349–359.

14. Anderson RM, Funnell MM. Patient empowerment: myths and misconceptions.
Patient Educ Couns. 2010;79(3):277–282.

15. Hibbard JH, Stockard J, Mahoney ER, Tusler M. Development of the Patient Activation Measure (PAM): conceptualizing and measuring activation in patients and consumers. *Health Serv Res.* 2004;39(1):1005–1026.

16. Mosen DM, Schmittdiel J, Hibbard J, Sobel D, Remmers C, Bellows J. Is patient activation associated with outcomes of care for adults with chronic conditions? *J Ambul Care Manage.* 2007;30(1):21–29.

17. Magnezi R, Glasser S, Shalev H, Sheiber A, Reuveni H. Patient activation, depression and quality of life. *Patient Educ Couns.* 2014;94(3):432–437.

18. Riazi A, Thompson AJ, Hobart JC. Self-efficacy predicts self-reported health status in multiple sclerosis. *Mult Scler.* 2004;10(1):61–66.

19. Stepleman L, Rutter MC, Hibbard J, Johns L, Wright D, Hughes M. Validation of the patient activation measure in a multiple sclerosis clinic sample and implications for care. *Disability & Rehabilitation.* 2010;32(19):1558–1567.

20. Jongen PJ, Wesnes K, van Geel B, et al. Does self-efficacy affect cognitive performance in persons with Clinically Isolated Syndrome and early relapsing-remitting multiple sclerosis? *Mult Scler Int.* 2015;2015:960282.

21. Costa DC, Sa MJ, Calheiros JM. The effect of social support on the quality of life of patients with multiple sclerosis. *Arq Neuropsiquiatr.* 2012;70(2):108–113.

22. Phillips LJ, Stuifbergen AK. The influence of positive experiences on depression and quality of life in persons with multiple sclerosis. *Journal of Holistic Nursing.* 2008;26(1):41–48.

23. Madan S, Pakenham KI. The stress-buffering effects of hope on adjustment to multiple sclerosis. *International Journal of Behavioral Medicine.* 2014;21(6):877–890.

24. Isaksson A-K, Ahlstrom G. From symptom to diagnosis: illness experiences of multiple sclerosis patients. *Journal of Neuroscience Nursing.* 2006;38(4):229–237.

25. Jelinek GA, Neate SL. The influence of the pharmaceutical industry in medicine. *Journal of Law and Medicine.* 2009;17(2):216–223.

26. Madan S, Pakenham KI. The stress-buffering effects of hope on changes in adjustment to caregiving in multiple sclerosis. *Journal of Health Psychology.* 2013;20(9): 1207–1221.

27. Siegel BS. *Love, Medicine and Miracles.* New York: HarperCollins; 1990.

28. Dyer W. Becoming a waking dreamer. In R Carlson, B Shield eds, *Handbook for the Soul.* Sydney: Transworld; 1995.

29. Mackereth PA, Booth K, Hillier VF, Caress AL. Reflexology and progressive muscle relaxation training for people with multiple sclerosis: a crossover trial. *Complement Ther Clin Pract.* 2009;15(1):14–21.

30. Kern S, Ziemssen T. Review: brain–immune communication psychoneuroimmunology of multiple sclerosis. *Mult Scler.* 2007;14:6–21.

31. Levin AB, Hadgkiss EJ, Weiland TJ, Jelinek GA. Meditation as an adjunct to the management of multiple sclerosis. *Neurol Res Int.* 2014:704691.

32. Arias AJ, Steinberg K, Banga A, Trestman RL. Systematic review of the efficacy of meditation techniques as treatments for medical illness. *J Altern Complement Med.* 2006;12(8):817–832.

33. Ostermann T, Schmid W. Music therapy in the treatment of multiple sclerosis: a comprehensive literature review. *Expert Rev Neurother.* 2006;6(4):469–477.

34. Brown CA, Jones AK. Meditation experience predicts less negative appraisal of pain: electrophysiological evidence for the involvement of anticipatory neural responses. *Pain*. 2010;150(3):428–438.

35. Grossman P, Kappos L, Gensicke H, et al. MS quality of life, depression, and fatigue improve after mindfulness training: a randomized trial. *Neurology*. 2010;75(13): 1141–1149.

36. Bogosian A, Chadwick P, Windgassen S, et al. Distress improves after mindfulness training for progressive MS: a pilot randomised trial. *Mult Scler.* 2015;21:434–94.

37. Kuspinar A, Rodriguez A, Mayo NE. The effects of clinical interventions of health-related quality of life in multiple sclerosis: a meta-analysis. *Multiple Sclerosis Journal*. 2012;18(12):1686–1704.

38. Senders A, Wahbeh H, Spain R, Shinto L. Mind–body medicine for multiple sclerosis: a systematic review. *Auto-immune Dis*. 2012;2012:567324.

39. Levin AB, Hadgkiss EJ, Weiland TJ, et al. Can meditation influence quality of life, depression, and disease outcome in multiple sclerosis? Findings from a large international web-based study. *Behavioural Neurology*. 2014;2014:916519.

40. Marrie RA, Reingold S, Cohen J, et al. The incidence and prevalence of psychiatric disorders in multiple sclerosis: a systematic review. *Mult Scler.* 2015;21(3): 305–317.

41. Smyth JM, Stone AA, Hurewitz A, Kaell A. Effects of writing about stressful experiences on symptom reduction in patients with asthma or rheumatoid arthritis: a randomized trial. *JAMA*. 1999;281(14):1304–1309.

42. Spiegel D. Healing words: emotional expression and disease outcome. *JAMA*. 1999;281:1328–1329.

43. Phillips DP, Ruth TE, Wagner LM. Psychology and survival. *Lancet* 1993;342:1142–5

44. Kabat-Zinn J, Wheeler E, Light T, et al. Influence of a mindfulness meditation-based stress reduction intervention on rates of skin clearing in patients with moderate to severe psoriasis undergoing phototherapy (UVB) and photochemotherapy (PUVA). *Psychosom Med* 1998;60:625–32.

45. Derogatis LR, Abeloff MD, Meliseratos N. Psychological coping mechanisms and survival time in metastatic breast cancer. *JAMA* 1979;242:1504–1508.

46. Greer S. Psychological response to cancer and survival, *Psychol Med* 1991;21:43–9.

47. Sadovnick AD, Remick RA, Allen J, et al. Depression and multiple sclerosis. *Neurology*. 1996;46(3):628–632.

48. Galeazzi GM, Ferrari S, Giaroli G, et al. Psychiatric disorders and depression in multiple sclerosis outpatients: impact of disability and interferon beta therapy. *Neurol Sci*. 2005;26(4):255–262.

49. Figved N, Klevan G, Myhr KM, et al. Neuropsychiatric symptoms in patients with multiple sclerosis. *Acta Psychiatr Scand*. 2005;112(6):463–468.

50. Khan F, McPhail T, Brand C, Turner-Stokes L, Kilpatrick T. Multiple sclerosis: disability profile and quality of life in an Australian community cohort. *Int J Rehabil Res*. 2006;29(2):87–96.

51. McGuigan C, Hutchinson M. Unrecognised symptoms of depression in a community-based population with multiple sclerosis. *J Neurol*. 2005;253(2):219–223.

52. Sollom AC, Kneebone, II. Treatment of depression in people who have multiple sclerosis. *Mult Scler.* 2007;13(5):632–635.

53. Patten SB, Williams JV, Metz L. Anti-depressant use in association with interferon and glatiramer acetate treatment in multiple sclerosis. *Mult Scler.* 2007;14(3):406–411.

54. Jose Sa M. Psychological aspects of multiple sclerosis. *Clin Neurol Neurosurg.* 2008; 110(9):868–877.

55. D'Alisa S, Miscio G, Baudo S, Simone A, Tesio L, Mauro A. Depression is the main determinant of quality of life in multiple sclerosis: a classification-regression (CART) study. *Disabil Rehabil.* 2006;28(5):307–314.

56. Benedict RH, Wahlig E, Bakshi R, et al. Predicting quality of life in multiple sclerosis: accounting for physical disability, fatigue, cognition, mood disorder, personality, and behavior change. *J Neurol Sci.* 2005;231(1–2):29–34.

57. Goldman Consensus Group. The Goldman Consensus statement on depression in multiple sclerosis. *Mult Scler.* 2005;11(3):328–337.

58. Arnett PA, Barwick FH, Beeney JE. Depression in multiple sclerosis: review and theoretical proposal. *J Int Neuropsychol Soc.* 2008;14(5):691–724.

59. Sutcigil L, Oktenli C, Musabak U, et al. Pro- and anti-inflammatory cytokine balance in major depression: effect of sertraline therapy. *Clin Dev Immunol.* 2007;2007:76396.

60. Gold SM, Irwin MR. Depression and immunity: inflammation and depressive symptoms in multiple sclerosis. *Neurol Clin.* 2006;24(3):507–519.

61. Mohr DC, Goodkin DE, Islar J, Hauser SL, Genain CP. Treatment of depression is associated with suppression of nonspecific and antigen-specific T(H)1 responses in multiple sclerosis. *Arch Neurol.* 2001;58(7):1081–1086.

62. Ytterberg C, Johansson S, Holmqvist LW, Koch LV. Longitudinal variations and pre-dictors of increased perceived impact of multiple sclerosis, a two-year study. *J Neurol Sci.* 2008;270:53–9.

63. Even C, Friedman S, Dardennes R, Zuber M, Guelfi JD. Prevalence of depression in multiple sclerosis: a review and meta-analysis. *Rev Neurol (Paris).* 2004;160(10): 917–925.

64. White CP, White MB, Russell CS. Invisible and visible symptoms of multiple scler-osis: which are more predictive of health distress? *J Neurosci Nurs.* 2008;40(2): 85–95, 102.

65. Koch MW, Glazenborg A, Uyttenboogaart M, Mostert J, De Keyser J. Pharmacologic treatment of depression in multiple sclerosis. *Cochrane Database Syst Rev.* 2011(2): CD007295.

66. Sarris J, O'Neil A, Coulson CE, Schweitzer I, Berk M. Lifestyle medicine for depres-sion. *BMC psychiatry.* 2014;14(1):107.

67. García-Toro M, Ibarra O, Gili M, et al. Four hygienic-dietary recommendations as add-on treatment in depression: A randomized-controlled trial. *Journal of Affective Disorders.* 2012;140(2):200–203.

68. Jacka FN, Mykletun A, Berk M. Moving towards a population health approach to the primary prevention of common mental disorders. *BMC Medicine.* 2012;10:149.

69. Jensen MP, Smith AE, Bombardier CH, Yorkston KM, Miro J, Molton IR. Social support, depression, and physical disability: Age and diagnostic group effects. *Disabil Health J.* 2014;7(2):164–172.

70. Vargas GA, Arnett PA. Positive everyday experiences interact with social support to predict depression in multiple sclerosis. *J Int Neuropsychol Soc.* 2010;16(6): 1039–1046.

71. Stuifbergen AK, Becker H. Health promotion practices in women with multiple sclerosis: increasing quality and years of healthy life. *Physical Medicine and Rehabilitation Clinics of North America.* 2001;12(1):9–22.

72. Dinan T, Siggins L, Scully P, O'Brien S, Ross P, Stanton C. Investigating the inflammatory phenotype of major depression: focus on cytokines and polyunsaturated fatty acids. *J Psychiatr Res.* 2008;43(4):471–476.

73. Morgan AJ, Jorm AF. Self-help interventions for depressive disorders and depressive symptoms: a systematic review. *Ann Gen Psychiatry.* 2008;7(1):13.

74. Su KP. Mind–body interface: the role of n-3 fatty acids in psychoneuroimmunology, somatic presentation, and medical illness comorbidity of depression. *Asia Pac J Clin Nutr.* 2008;17 Suppl 1:151–157.

75. Adams PB, Lawson S, Sanigorski A, et al. Arachidonic acid to eicosapentanoic acid ration in blood correlates positively with clinical symptoms of depression. *Lipids.* 1996;31:S157–S161.

76. Li F, Liu X, Zhang D. Fish consumption and risk of depression: a meta-analysis. *J Epidemiol Community Health.* 2015. doi: 10.1136/jech-2015-206278.

77. da Silva TM, Munhoz RP, Alvarez C, et al. Depression in Parkinson's disease: a double-blind, randomized, placebo-controlled pilot study of omega-3 fatty-acid supplementation. *J Affect Disord.* 2008;111(2–3):351–359.

78. Gloth FM, III, Alam W, Hollis B. Vitamin D vs broad spectrum phototherapy in the treatment of seasonal affective disorder. *J Nutr Health Aging.* 1999;3(1):5–7.

79. Jorde R, Waterloo K, Saleh F, Haug E, Svartberg J. Neuropsychological function in relation to serum parathyroid hormone and serum 25–hydroxyvitamin D levels: The Tromso study. *J Neurol.* 2005;253(4):464–470.

80. Lansdowne AT, Provost SC. Vitamin D3 enhances mood in healthy subjects during Chapterwinter. *Psychopharmacology (Berl).* 1998;135(4):319–323.

81. Stumpf WE, Privette TH. Light, vitamin D and psychiatry. Role of 1,25 dihydroxy-vitamin D3 (soltriol) in etiology and therapy of seasonal affective disorder and other mental processes. *Psychopharmacology (Berl).* 1989;97(3):285–294.

82. Sjonnesen K, Berzins S, Fiest KM, et al. Evaluation of the 9-item Patient Health Questionnaire (PHQ-9) as an assessment instrument for symptoms of depression in patients with multiple sclerosis. *Postgrad Med.* 2012;124(5):69–77.

83. Kroenke K, Spitzer RL, Williams JB. The Patient Health Questionnaire-2: validity of a two-item depression screener. *Med Care.* 2003;41(11):1284–1292.

84. Taylor KT, Hadgkiss EJ, Jelinek GA, et al. Lifestyle factors, demographics and medications associated with depression risk in an international sample of people with multiple sclerosis. *BMC Psychiatry.* 2014;14: 327.

85. Weiland TJ, Jelinek GA, Hadgkiss EJ, et al. Clinically significant fatigue: prevalence and associated factors in an international sample of adults with multiple sclerosis. *PLOS One.* 2015;10(2);e0115541

86. Monash University. Mindfulness at Monash. 2012. Available at <http://monash.edu/counselling/mindfulness.html>, accessed 10 November 2014.

87. Faculty of Medical and Health Sciences. CALM—Computer Assisted Learning for the Mind. 2012. Available at <www.calm.auckland.ac.nz/18.html>, accessed 10 November 2014.

Step 5

1. Wandinger KP, Wessel K, Trillenberg P, Heindl N, Kirchner H. Effect of high-dose methylprednisolone administration on immune functions in multiple sclerosis patients. *Acta Neurol Scand.* 1998;97(6):359–365.

2. Filipovic SR, Drulovic J, Stojsavljevic N, Levic Z. The effects of high-dose intravenous methylprednisolone on event-related potentials in patients with multiple sclerosis. *J Neurol Sci.* 1997;152(2):147–153.

3. Milligan NM, Newcombe R, Compston DA. A double-blind controlled trial of high dose methylprednisolone in patients with multiple sclerosis: 1. Clinical effects. *J Neurol Neurosurg Psychiatry.* 1987;50(5):511–516.

4. Beck RW, Cleary PA, Trobe JD, et al. The effect of corticosteroids for acute optic neuritis on the subsequent development of multiple sclerosis. The Optic Neuritis Study Group. *N Engl J Med.* 1993;329(24):1764–1769.

5. Alam SM, Kyriakides T, Lawden M, Newman PK. Methylprednisolone in multiple sclerosis: a comparison of oral with intravenous therapy at equivalent high dose. *J Neurol Neurosurg Psychiatry.* 1993;56(11):1219–1220.

6. Barnes D, Hughes RA, Morris RW, et al. Randomised trial of oral and intravenous methylprednisolone in acute relapses of multiple sclerosis. *Lancet.* 1997;349(9056): 902–906.

7. Sellebjerg F, Frederiksen JL, Nielsen PM, Olesen J. Double-blind, randomized, placebo-controlled study of oral, high-dose methylprednisolone in attacks of MS. *Neurology.* 1998;51(2):529–534.

8. Le Page E, Veillard D, Laplaud DA, et al. Oral versus intravenous high-dose methylprednisolone for treatment of relapses in patients with multiple sclerosis (COPOUSEP): a randomised, controlled, double-blind, non-inferiority trial. *Lancet.* 2015;386(9997):974–981.

9. Tremlett HL, Luscombe DK, Wiles CM. Use of corticosteroids in multiple sclerosis by consultant neurologists in the United Kingdom. *J Neurol Neurosurg Psychiatry.* 1998;65:362–365.

10. Morrow SA, Stoian CA, Dmitrovic J, Chan SC, Metz LM. The bioavailability of IV methylprednisolone and oral prednisone in multiple sclerosis. *Neurology.* 2004; 63(6):1079–1080.

11. National Institute for Health and Care Excellence. Multiple sclerosis: management of multiple sclerosis in primary and secondary care. 2014. Available at <www.nice. org.uk/guidance/cg186/chapter/1–recommendations>, accessed 20 April 2015.

12. Perumal JS, Caon C, Hreha S, et al. Oral prednisone taper following intravenous steroids fails to improve disability or recovery from relapses in multiple sclerosis. *Eur J Neurol.* 2008;15(7):677–680.

13. Glass-Marmor L, Paperna T, Ben-Yosef Y, Miller A. Chronotherapy using cortico-steroids for multiple sclerosis relapses. *J Neurol Neurosurg Psychiatry.* 2006;78(8): 886–888.

14. Fog T. The long-term treatment of multiple sclerosis with corticoids. *Acta Neurol Scand.* 1965;41:S473–S484.

15. Then Bergh F, Kumpfel T, Schumann E, et al. Monthly intravenous methylpredniso-lone in relapsing-remitting multiple sclerosis—reduction of enhancing lesions, T2 lesion volume and plasma prolactin concentrations. *BMC Neurol.* 2006;6:19.

16. Goodkin DE, Kinkel RP, Weinstock-Guttman B, et al. A phase II study of IV methyl-prednisolone in secondary-progressive multiple sclerosis. *Neurology.* 1998;51(1): 239–245.

17. Hoffmann V, Kuhn W, Schimrigk S, et al. Repeat intrathecal triamcinolone acetonide application is beneficial in progressive MS patients. *Eur J Neurol.* 2006;13(1):72–76.

18. Hoffmann V, Schimrigk S, Islamova S, et al. Efficacy and safety of repeated intra-thecal triamcinolone acetonide application in progressive multiple sclerosis patients. *J Neurol Sci.* 2003;211(1–2):81–84.

19. Wingerchuk DM, Carter JL. Multiple sclerosis: current and emerging disease-modifying therapies and treatment strategies. *Mayo Clin Proc.* 2014;89(2):225–240.

20. Kavaliunas A, Stawiarz L, Hedbom J, Glaser A, Hillert J. The influence of immu-nomodulatory treatment on the clinical course of multiple sclerosis. *Advances in Experimental Medicine and Biology.* 2015;822:19–24.

21. Khan O, Rieckmann P, Boyko A, Selmaj K, Zivadinov R. Three times weekly glatiramer acetate in relapsing-remitting multiple sclerosis. *Ann Neurol.* 2013;73(6): 705–713.

22. McKeage K. Glatiramer Acetate 40 mg/mL in relapsing-remitting multiple sclerosis: a review. *CNS Drugs.* 2015;29(5):425–432.

23. Wiendl H, Meuth SG. Pharmacological Approaches to delaying disability progres-sion in patients with multiple sclerosis. *Drugs.* 2015;75(9):947–977.

24. Tramacere I, Del Giovane C, Salanti G, D'Amico R, Filippini G. Immunomodulators and immunosuppressants for relapsing-remitting multiple sclerosis: a network meta-analysis. *Cochrane Database Syst Rev.* 2015;9:CD011381.

25. Martinelli Boneschi F, Vacchi L, Rovaris M, Capra R, Comi G. Mitoxantrone for multiple sclerosis. *Cochrane Database Syst Rev.* 2013;5:CD002127.

26. Cree BA. 2014 multiple sclerosis therapeutic update. *The Neurohospitalist.* 2014;4(2): 63–65.

27. Raftery JP. Paying for costly pharmaceuticals: regulation of new drugs in Australia, England and New Zealand. *Med J Aust.* 2008;188(1):26–28.

28. Hartung DM, Bourdette DN, Ahmed SM, Whitham RH. The cost of multiple scler-osis drugs in the US and the pharmaceutical industry: Too big to fail? *Neurology.* 2015;84(21):2185–2192.

29. The IFNB Multiple Sclerosis Study Group. Interferon beta-1b is effective in relapsing-remitting multiple sclerosis. 1. Clinical results of a multicenter, random-ized, double-blind, placebo-controlled trial. *Neurology.* 1993;43:655–661.

30. The IFNB Multiple Sclerosis Study Group and the University of British Columbia MS/MRI Analysis Group. Interferon beta-1b in the treatment of multiple sclerosis: final outcome of the randomized controlled trial. *Neurology.* 1995;45:1277–1285.

31. Ebers GC, Traboulsee A, Li D, et al. Analysis of clinical outcomes according to original treatment groups 16 years after the pivotal IFNB-1b trial. *J Neurol Neurosurg Psychiatry.* 2010;81(8):907–912.

32. European Study Group on Interferon beta-1b in secondary progressive MS. Placebo-controlled multicentre randomised trial of interferon beta-1b in secondary progressive multiple sclerosis. *Lancet.* 1998;352: 1491–1497.

33. D'Amico D, La Mantia L, Rigamonti A, et al. Prevalence of primary headaches in people with multiple sclerosis. *Cephalalgia.* 2004;24(11):980–984.

34. Loftis JM, Hauser P. The phenomenology and treatment of interferon-induced depression. *J Affect Disord.* 2004;82(2):175–190.

35. Taylor KT, Hadgkiss EJ, Jelinek GA, et al. Lifestyle and demographic factors and medications associated with depression risk in an international sample of people with multiple sclerosis. *BMC Psychiatry.* 2014;14:327. doi: 10.1186/s12888-014-0327-3.

36. Durelli L, Clerico M. The importance of maintaining effective therapy in multiple sclerosis. *J Neurol.* 2005;252 Suppl 3:iii38–iii43.

37. Myhr KM, Riise T, Green Lilleas FE, et al. Interferon-alpha2a reduces MRI disease activity in relapsing-remitting multiple sclerosis. *Neurology.* 1999;52:1049–1056.

38. Tremlett HL, Yoshida EM, Oger J. Liver injury associated with the beta-interferons for MS: a comparison between the three products. *Neurology.* 2004;62(4):628–631.

39. Caraccio N, Dardano A, Manfredonia F, et al. Long-term follow-up of 106 multiple sclerosis patients undergoing IFN-{beta} 1a or 1b therapy: predictive factors of thyroid disease development and duration. *J Clin Endocrinol Metab.* 2005;90(7):4133–4137.

40. Monzani F, Caraccio N, Dardano A, Ferrannini E. Thyroid auto-immunity and dysfunction associated with type I interferon therapy. *Clin Exp Med.* 2004;3(4):199–210.

41. Midgard R, Ag KE, Trondsen E, Spigset O. Life-threatening acute pancreatitis associated with interferon beta-1a treatment in multiple sclerosis. *Neurology.* 2005;65(1): 170–171.

42. Tai YJ, Tam M. Fixed drug eruption with interferon-beta-1b. *Australas J Dermatol.* 2005;46(3):154–157.

43. Ekstein D, Linetsky E, Abramsky O, Karussis D. Polyneuropathy associated with interferon beta treatment in patients with multiple sclerosis. *Neurology.* 2005;65(3): 456–458.

44. O'Rourke KE, Hutchinson M. Stopping beta-interferon therapy in multiple sclerosis: an analysis of stopping patterns. *Mult Scler.* 2005;11(1):46–50.

45. Boskovic R, Wide R, Wolpin J, Bauer DJ, Koren G. The reproductive effects of beta interferon therapy in pregnancy: a longitudinal cohort. *Neurology.* 2005;65(6):807–811.

46. Filippini G, Munari L, Incorvaia B, et al. Interferons in relapsing-remitting multiple sclerosis: a systematic review. *Lancet.* 2003;361:545–552.

47. Trojano M, Paolicelli D, Zimatore GB, et al. The IFNbeta treatment of multiple sclerosis (MS) in clinical practice: the experience at the MS Center of Bari, Italy. *Neurol Sci.* 2005;26 Suppl 4:s179–182.

48. Pozzilli C, Prosperini L, Sbardella E, De Giglio L, Onesti E, Tomassini V. Post-marketing survey on clinical response to interferon beta in relapsing multiple sclerosis: the Roman experience. *Neurol Sci.* 2005;26(Supplement 4):s174–s178.

49. Shirani A, Zhao Y, Karim ME, et al. Association between use of interferon beta and progression of disability in patients with relapsing-remitting multiple sclerosis. *JAMA.* 2012;308(3):247–256.

50. Derfuss T, Kappos L. Evaluating the potential benefit of interferon treatment in multiple sclerosis. *JAMA.* 2012;308(3):290–291.

51. Boggild M, Palace J, Barton P, et al. Multiple sclerosis risk sharing scheme: two year results of clinical cohort study with historical comparator. *BMJ.* 2009;339:b4677.

52. Nortvedt MW, Riise T, Myhr KM, et al. Type 1 interferons and the quality of life of multiple sclerosis patients. Results from a clinical trial of interferon alfa-2a. *Mult Scler.* 1999;5:317–322.

53. Simone IL, Ceccarelli A, Tortorella C, et al. Influence of Interferon beta treatment on quality of life in multiple sclerosis patients. *Health Qual Life Outcomes.* 2006; 4:96.

54. Schrempf W, Ziemssen T. Glatiramer acetate: mechanisms of action in multiple sclerosis. *Auto-immun Rev.* 2007;6(7):469–475.

55. Aharoni R, Herschkovitz A, Eilam R, et al. Demyelination arrest and remyelination induced by glatiramer acetate treatment of experimental auto-immune encephalo-myelitis. *Proc Natl Acad Sci USA.* 2008;105(32):11358–11363.

56. Hestvik A, Skorstad G, Price D, Vartdal F, Holmoy T. Multiple sclerosis: glatiramer acetate induces anti-inflammatory T cells in the cerebrospinal fluid. *Mult Scler.* 2008;14(6):749–758.

57. Iarlori C, Gambi D, Lugaresi A, et al. Reduction of free radicals in multiple sclerosis: effect of glatiramer acetate (Copaxone(R)). *Mult Scler.* 2008;14(6):739–748.

58. Blanchette F, Neuhaus O. Glatiramer acetate: evidence for a dual mechanism of action. *J Neurol.* 2008;255 Suppl 1:26–36.

59. Kreitman RR, Blanchette F. On the horizon: possible neuroprotective role for glatiramer acetate. *Mult Scler.* 2004;10 Suppl 1:S81–86; discussion S86–89.

60. Khan O, Shen Y, Caon C, et al. Axonal metabolic recovery and potential neuro-protective effect of glatiramer acetate in relapsing-remitting multiple sclerosis. *Mult Scler.* 2005;11(6):646–651.

61. Bornstein MB, Miller A, Slagle S, et al. A pilot trial of Cop 1 in exacerbating-remitting multiple sclerosis. *N Engl J Med.* 1987;317(7):408–414.

62. Johnson KP, Brooks BR, Cohen JA, et al. Extended use of glatiramer acetate (Copaxone) is well tolerated and maintains its clinical effect on multiple sclerosis relapse rate and degree of disability. Copolymer 1 Multiple Sclerosis Study Group. *Neurology.* 1998;50(3):701–708.

63. Comi G, Filippi M, Wolinsky JS. European/Canadian multicenter, double-blind, ran-domized, placebo-controlled study of the effects of glatiramer acetate on magnetic resonance imaging—measured disease activity and burden in patients with relaps-ing multiple sclerosis. European/Canadian Glatiramer Acetate Study Group. *Ann Neurol.* 2001;49(3):290–297.

64. Johnson KP, Brooks BR, Ford CC, et al. Sustained clinical benefits of glatiramer acetate in relapsing multiple sclerosis patients observed for 6 years. Copolymer 1 Multiple Sclerosis Study Group. *Mult Scler.* 2000;6(4):255–266.

65. Baumhackl U. The search for a balance between short and long-term treatment outcomes in multiple sclerosis. *J Neurol.* 2008;255 Suppl 1:75–83.

66. Brochet B. Long-term effects of glatiramer acetate in multiple sclerosis. *Rev Neurol (Paris).* 2008;164(11):917–926.

67. Johnson KP, Ford CC, Lisak RP, Wolinsky JS. Neurologic consequence of delaying glatiramer acetate therapy for multiple sclerosis: 8-year data. *Acta Neurol Scand.* 2005;111(1):42–47.

68. Rovaris M, Comi G, Rocca M, et al. Long-term follow-up of patients treated with glatiramer acetate: a multicentre, multinational extension of the European/ Canadian double-blind, placebo-controlled, MRI-monitored trial. *Mult Scler.* 2007; 13(4):502–508.

69. La Mantia L, Milanese C, D'Amico R. Meta-analysis of clinical trials with copolymer 1 in multiple sclerosis. *Eur Neurol.* 2000;43(4):189–193.

70. Sormani MP, Bruzzi P, Comi G, Filippi M. The distribution of the magnetic resonance imaging response to glatiramer acetate in multiple sclerosis. *Mult Scler.* 2005;11(4):447–449.

71. Munari L, Lovati R, Boiko A. Therapy with glatiramer acetate for multiple sclerosis. *Cochrane Database Syst Rev.* 2004(1):CD004678.

72. Wolinsky JS. The use of glatiramer acetate in the treatment of multiple sclerosis. *Adv Neurol.* 2006;98:273–292.

73. Bell C, Graham J, Earnshaw S, Oleen-Burkey M, Castelli-Haley J, Johnson K. Cost-effectiveness of four immunomodulatory therapies for relapsing-remitting multiple sclerosis: A Markov model based on long-term clinical data. *J Manag Care Pharm.* 2007;13(3):245–261.

74. MS Society of Canada. MS therapy may help delay conversion from CIS to clinically definite MS. Available at <www.mssociety.ca/en/research/medmmo_20080116. htm>, accessed 20 February 2014.

75. Fazekas F, Baumhackl U, Berger T, et al. Decision-making for and impact of early immunomodulatory treatment: the Austrian Clinically Isolated Syndrome Study (ACISS). *Eur J Neurol.* 2010;17(6):852–860.

76. Argyriou AA, Makris N. Multiple sclerosis and reproductive risks in women. *Reprod Sci.* 2008;15(8):755–764.

77. Madray MM, Greene JF, Jr., Butler DF. Glatiramer acetate-associated, CD30+, primary, cutaneous, anaplastic large-cell lymphoma. *Arch Neurol.* 2008;65(10):1378–1379.

78. Flechter S, Kott E, Steiner-Birmanns B, Nisipeanu P, Korczyn AD. Copolymer 1 (glatiramer acetate) in relapsing forms of multiple sclerosis: open multicenter study of alternate-day administration. *Clin Neuropharmacol.* 2002;25(1):11–15.

79. Vollmer T, Panitch H, Bar-Or A, et al. Glatiramer acetate after induction therapy with mitoxantrone in relapsing multiple sclerosis. *Mult Scler.* 2008;14(5):663–670.

80. Fridkis-Hareli M, Santambrogio L, Stern JN, Fugger L, Brosnan C, Strominger JL. Novel synthetic amino acid copolymers that inhibit autoantigen-specific T cell

responses and suppress experimental auto-immune encephalomyelitis. *J Clin Invest.* 2002;109(12):1635–1643.

81. Matsoukas J, Apostolopoulos V, Kalbacher H, et al. Design and synthesis of a novel potent myelin basic protein epitope 87–99 cyclic analogue: enhanced stability and biological properties of mimics render them a potentially new class of immuno-modulators. *J Med Chem.* 2005;48(5):1470–1480.

82. De Stefano N, Filippi M, Confavreux C, et al. The results of two multicenter, open-label studies assessing efficacy, tolerability and safety of protiramer, a high molecular weight synthetic copolymeric mixture, in patients with relapsing-remitting multiple sclerosis. *Mult Scler.* 2009;15(2):238–243.

83. Cohen J, Belova A, Selmaj K, et al. Equivalence of generic glatiramer acetate in multiple sclerosis: a randomized clinical trial. *JAMA Neurology.* 2015:1–9. doi: 10.1001/jamaneurol.2015.2154.

84. Kalincik T, Jokubaitis V, Izquierdo G, et al. Comparative effectiveness of glatiramer acetate and interferon beta formulations in relapsing-remitting multiple sclerosis. *Mult Scler.* 2014;21(9):1159–1171.

85. Miller DH, Khan OA, Sheremata WA, et al. A controlled trial of natalizumab for relapsing multiple sclerosis. *N Engl J Med.* 2003;348(1):15–23.

86. Polman CH, O'Connor PW, Havrdova E, et al. A randomized, placebo-controlled trial of natalizumab for relapsing multiple sclerosis. *N Engl J Med.* 2006;354(9):899–910.

87. Rudick RA, Stuart WH, Calabresi PA, et al. Natalizumab plus interferon beta-1a for relapsing multiple sclerosis. *N Engl J Med.* 2006;354(9):911–923.

88. Miller DH, Soon D, Fernando KT, et al. MRI outcomes in a placebo-controlled trial of natalizumab in relapsing MS. *Neurology.* 2007;68(17):1390–1401.

89. Yousry TA, Major EO, Ryschkewitsch C, et al. Evaluation of patients treated with natalizumab for progressive multifocal leukoencephalopathy. *N Engl J Med.* 2006;354(9):924–933.

90. Mullen JT, Vartanian TK, Atkins MB. Melanoma complicating treatment with natalizumab for multiple sclerosis. *N Engl J Med.* 2008;358(6):647–648.

91. Baker TE, Cooper SD, Kessler L, Hale TW. Transfer of natalizumab into breast milk in a mother with multiple sclerosis. *J Hum Lact.* 2015;31(2):233–236.

92. Melis M, Cocco E, Frau J, et al. Post-natalizumab clinical and radiological findings in a cohort of multiple sclerosis patients: 12–month follow-up. *Neurol Sci.* 2014;35(3):401–408.

93. Maqraner MJ, Coret F, Navarré A, et al. Pulsed steroids followed by glatiramer acetate to prevent inflammatory activity after cessation of natalizumab therapy: a prospective, 6-month observational study. *J Neurol* 2011;258:1805–11.

94. Sangalli F, Moiola L, Ferre L, et al. Long-term management of natalizumab discontinuation in a large monocentric cohort of multiple sclerosis patients. *Multiple Sclerosis and Related Disorders.* 2014;3(4):520–526.

95. Rinaldi F, Seppi D, Calabrese M, Perini P, Gallo P. Switching therapy from natalizumab to fingolimod in relapsing-remitting multiple sclerosis: clinical and magnetic resonance imaging findings. *Mult Scler.* 2012;18(11):1640–1643.

96. Sempere AP, Martin-Medina P, Berenguer-Ruiz L, et al. Switching from natalizumab to fingolimod: an observational study. *Acta Neurol Scand.* 2013;128(2):e6–e10.

97. Kappos L, Radue EW, Comi G, et al. Switching from natalizumab to fingolimod: a randomized, placebo-controlled study in RRMS. *Neurology.* 2015;85(1):29–39.

98. Havla J, Kleiter I, Kumpfel T. Bridging, switching or drug holidays: how to treat a patient who stops natalizumab? *Ther Clin Risk Manag.* 2013;9:361–369.

99. Doggrell SA. Oral fingolimod for relapsing-remitting multiple sclerosis: evaluation of Kappos L, Radue EW, O'Connor P, et al. A placebo-controlled trial of oral fingolimod in relapsing multiple sclerosis. *N Engl J Med* 2010;362:387–401; and Cohen JA, Barkhof F, Comi G, et al. Oral fingolimod or intramuscular interferon for relapsing multiple sclerosis. *N Engl J Med* 2010;362:402–15. *Expert Opin Pharmacother.* 2010;11(10):1777–1781.

100. Kappos L, Radue EW, O'Connor P, et al. A placebo-controlled trial of oral fingolimod in relapsing multiple sclerosis. *N Engl J Med.* 2010;362(5):387–401.

101. Cohen JA, Barkhof F, Comi G, et al. Oral fingolimod or intramuscular interferon for relapsing multiple sclerosis. *N Engl J Med.* 2010;362(5):402–415.

102. Calabresi PA, Radue EW, Goodin D, et al. Safety and efficacy of fingolimod in patients with relapsing-remitting multiple sclerosis (FREEDOMS II): a double-blind, randomised, placebo-controlled, phase 3 trial. *Lancet Neurol.* 2014;13(6):545–556.

103. Racca V, Di Rienzo M, Cavarretta R, et al. Fingolimod effects on left ventricular function in multiple sclerosis. *Mult Scler.* 2015. Available at <www.ncbi.nlm.nih.gov/pubmed/26041795>, accessed 20 November 2015.

104. Havla JB, Pellkofer HL, Meinl I, Gerdes LA, Hohlfeld R, Kumpfel T. Rebound of disease activity after withdrawal of fingolimod (FTY720) treatment. *Arch Neurol.* 2012;69(2):262–264.

105. Hakiki B, Portaccio E, Giannini M, Razzolini L, Pasto L, Amato MP. Withdrawal of fingolimod treatment for relapsing-remitting multiple sclerosis: report of six cases. *Mult Scler.* 2012;18(11):1636–1639.

106. Karlsson G, Francis G, Koren G, et al. Pregnancy outcomes in the clinical development program of fingolimod in multiple sclerosis. *Neurology.* 2014;82(8):674–680.

107. Chikura B, Lane S, Dawson JK. Clinical expression of leflunomide-induced pneumonitis. *Rheumatology (Oxford).* 2009;48(9):1065–1068.

108. Inokuma S. Leflunomide-induced interstitial pneumonitis might be a representative of disease-modifying antirheumatic drug-induced lung injury. *Expert Opin Drug Saf.* 2011;10(4):603–611.

109. O'Connor P, Wolinsky JS, Confavreux C, et al. Randomized trial of oral teriflunomide for relapsing multiple sclerosis. *N Engl J Med.* 2011;365(14):1293–1303.

110. Freedman MS, Wolinsky JS, Wamil B, et al. Teriflunomide added to interferon-beta in relapsing multiple sclerosis: a randomized phase II trial. *Neurology.* 2012;78(23): 1877–1885.

111. He D, Xu Z, Dong S, et al. Teriflunomide for multiple sclerosis. *Cochrane Database Syst Rev.* 2012;12:CD009882.

112. Bomprezzi R. Dimethyl fumarate in the treatment of relapsing-remitting multiple sclerosis: an overview. *Ther Adv Neurol Disord.* 2015;8(1):20–30.

113. Gold R, Kappos L, Arnold DL, et al. Placebo-controlled phase 3 study of oral BG-12 for relapsing multiple sclerosis. *N Engl J Med.* 2012;367(12):1098–1107.

114. Fox RJ, Miller DH, Phillips JT, et al. Placebo-controlled phase 3 study of oral BG-12 or glatiramer in multiple sclerosis. *N Engl J Med.* 2012;367(12):1087–1097.

115. Balasubramaniam P, Stevenson O, Berth-Jones J. Fumaric acid esters in severe psoriasis, including experience of use in combination with other systemic modalities. *The British Journal of Dermatology.* 2004;150(4):741–746.

116. Hoefnagel JJ, Thio HB, Willemze R, Bouwes Bavinck JN. Long-term safety aspects of systemic therapy with fumaric acid esters in severe psoriasis. *The British Journal of Dermatology.* 2003;149(2):363–369.

117. Reich K, Thaci D, Mrowietz U, Kamps A, Neureither M, Luger T. Efficacy and safety of fumaric acid esters in the long-term treatment of psoriasis: a retrospective study (FUTURE). *Journal der Deutschen Dermatologischen Gesellschaft = Journal of the German Society of Dermatology : JDDG.* 2009;7(7):603–611.

118. van Oosten BW, Killestein J, Barkhof F, Polman CH, Wattjes MP. PML in a patient treated with dimethyl fumarate from a compounding pharmacy. *N Engl J Med.* 2013;368(17):1658–1659.

119. Kappos L, Giovannoni G, Gold R, et al. Time course of clinical and neuroradiological effects of delayed-release dimethyl fumarate in multiple sclerosis. *Eur J Neurol.* 2015;22(4):664–671.

120. Cohen JA, Coles AJ, Arnold DL, et al. Alemtuzumab versus interferon beta 1a as first-line treatment for patients with relapsing-remitting multiple sclerosis: a randomised controlled phase 3 trial. *Lancet.* 2012;380(9856):1819–1828.

121. Coles AJ, Twyman CL, Arnold DL, et al. Alemtuzumab for patients with relapsing multiple sclerosis after disease-modifying therapy: a randomised controlled phase 3 trial. *Lancet.* 2012;380(9856):1829–1839.

122. Tuohy O, Costelloe L, Hill-Cawthorne G, et al. Alemtuzumab treatment of multiple sclerosis: long-term safety and efficacy. *J Neurol Neurosurg Psychiatry.* 2015;86(2):208–215.

123. Havrdova E, Horakova D, Kovarova I. Alemtuzumab in the treatment of multiple sclerosis: key clinical trial results and considerations for use. *Ther Adv Neurol Disord.* 2015;8(1):31–45.

124. Wynn D, Kaufman M, Montalban X, et al. Daclizumab in active relapsing multiple sclerosis (CHOICE study): a phase 2, randomised, double-blind, placebo-controlled, add-on trial with interferon beta. *Lancet Neurol.* 2010;9(4):381–390.

125. Kappos L, Wiendl H, Selmaj K, et al. Daclizumab HYP versus Interferon Beta-1a in Relapsing Multiple Sclerosis. *N Engl J Med.* 2015;373(15):1418–1428.

126. Kappos L, Li D, Calabresi PA, et al. Ocrelizumab in relapsing-remitting multiple sclerosis: a phase 2, randomised, placebo-controlled, multicentre trial. *Lancet.* 2011;378(9805):1779–1787.

127. Filippi M, Rocca MA, Pagani E, et al. Placebo-controlled trial of oral laquinimod in multiple sclerosis: MRI evidence of an effect on brain tissue damage. *J Neurol Neurosurg Psychiatry.* 2014;85(8):851–858.

128. Comi G, Jeffery D, Kappos L, et al. Placebo-controlled trial of oral laquinimod for multiple sclerosis. *N Engl J Med.* 2012;366(11):1000–1009.

129. Vollmer TL, Sorensen PS, Selmaj K, et al. A randomized placebo-controlled phase III trial of oral laquinimod for multiple sclerosis. *J Neurol.* 2014;261(4): 773–783.

130. Millefiorini E, Gasperini C, Pozzilli C, et al. Randomized placebo-controlled trial of mitoxantrone in relapsing-remitting multiple sclerosis: 24-month clinical and MRI outcome. *J Neurol.* 1997;244(3):153–159.

131. Edan G, Miller D, Clanet M, et al. Therapeutic effect of mitoxantrone combined with methylprednisolone in multiple sclerosis: a randomised multicentre study of active disease using MRI and clinical criteria. *J Neurol Neurosurg Psychiatry.* 1997;62(2):112–118.

132. Hartung HP, Gonsette R, Konig N, et al. Mitoxantrone in progressive multiple sclerosis: a placebo-controlled, double-blind, randomised, multicentre trial. *Lancet.* 2002;360(9350):2018–2025.

133. Debouverie M, Taillandier L, Pittion-Vouyovitch S, Louis S, Vespignani H. Clinical follow-up of 304 patients with multiple sclerosis three years after mitoxantrone treatment. *Mult Scler.* 2007;13(5):626–631.

134. Correale J, Rush C, Amengual A, Goicochea MT. Mitoxantrone as rescue therapy in worsening relapsing-remitting MS patients receiving IFN-beta. *J Neuroimmunol.* 2005;162(1–2):173–183.

135. Cocco E, Marchi P, Sardu C, et al. Mitoxantrone treatment in patients with early relapsing-remitting multiple sclerosis. *Mult Scler.* 2007.

136. Martinelli BF, Rovaris M, Capra R, Comi G, Martinelli Boneschi F. Mitoxantrone for multiple sclerosis. *Cochrane Database Syst Rev.* 2005(4):CD002127.

137. Murray TJ. The cardiac effects of mitoxantrone: do the benefits in multiple sclerosis outweigh the risks? *Expert Opin Drug Saf.* 2006;5(2):265–274.

138. Gonsette RE. New immunosuppressants with potential implication in multiple sclerosis. *J Neurol Sci.* 2004;223(1):87–93.

139. Gonsette RE. Pixantrone (BBR2778): a new immunosuppressant in multiple sclerosis with a low cardiotoxicity. *J Neurol Sci.* 2004;223(1):81–86.

140. Pascual AM, Tellez N, Bosca I, et al. Revision of the risk of secondary leukemia after mitoxantrone in multiple sclerosis populations is required. *Mult Scler.* 2009;15: 1303–10.

141. Giovannoni G, Comi G, Cook S, et al. A placebo-controlled trial of oral cladribine for relapsing multiple sclerosis. *N Engl J Med.* 2010;362(5):416–426.

142. Likosky WH, Fireman B, Elmore R, et al. Intense immunosuppression in chronic progressive multiple sclerosis: the Kaiser study. *J Neurol Neurosurg Psychiatry.* 1991; 54:1055–1060.

143. The Canadian Cooperative Multiple Sclerosis Study Group. The Canadian Cooperative trial of cyclophosphamide and plasma exchange in progressive multiple sclerosis. *Lancet.* 1991;337:441–446.

144. Weiner HL, Mackin GA, Orav EJ, et al. Intermittent cyclophosphamide pulse therapy in progressive multiple sclerosis: final report of the Northeast Cooperative Multiple Sclerosis Treatment Group. *Neurology.* 1993;43:910–918.

145. Smith DR, Weinstock-Guttman B, Cohen JA, et al. A randomized blinded trial of combination therapy with cyclophosphamide in patients with active multiple sclerosis on interferon beta. *Mult Scler.* 2005;11(5):573–582.

146. Patti F, Reggio E, Palermo F, et al. Stabilization of rapidly worsening multiple sclerosis for 36 months in patients treated with interferon beta plus cyclophosphamide followed by interferon beta. *J Neurol.* 2004;251(12):1502–1506.

147. Bittencourt PR, Gomes-da-Silva MM. Multiple sclerosis: long-term remission after a high dose of cyclophosphamide. *Acta Neurol Scand.* 2005;111(3):195–198.

148. Fazekas F, Deisenhammer F, Strasser-Fuchs S, Nahler G, Mamoli B. Randomised placebo-controlled trial of monthly intravenous immunoglobulin therapy in relapsing-remitting multiple sclerosis. Austrian Immunoglobulin in Multiple Sclerosis Study Group. *Lancet.* 1997;349(9052):589–593.

149. Sorensen PS, Wanscher B, Jensen CV, et al. Intravenous immunoglobulin G reduces MRI activity in relapsing multiple sclerosis. *Neurology.* 1998;50(5):1273–1281.

150. Achiron A, Kishner I, Sarova-Pinhas I, et al. Intravenous immunoglobulin treatment following the first demyelinating event suggestive of multiple sclerosis: a randomized, double-blind, placebo-controlled trial. *Arch Neurol.* 2004;61(10): 1515–1520.

151. Kalanie H, Tabatabaii SS. Combined immunoglobulin and azathioprine in multiple sclerosis. *Eur Neurol.* 1998;39:178–181.

152. Fazekas F, Sorensen PS, Filippi M, et al. MRI results from the European Study on Intravenous Immunoglobulin in Secondary Progressive Multiple Sclerosis (ESIMS). *Mult Scler.* 2005;11(4):433–440.

153. Hommes OR, Sorensen PS, Fazekas F, et al. Intravenous immunoglobulin in secondary progressive multiple sclerosis: randomised placebo-controlled trial. *Lancet.* 2004;364(9440):1149–1156.

154. Stangel M, Gold R. High-dose intravenous immunoglobulins in the treatment of multiple sclerosis: an update. *Nervenarzt.* 2005.

155. Katz U, Kishner I, Magalashvili D, Shoenfeld Y, Achiron A. Long term safety of IVIg therapy in multiple sclerosis: 10 years experience. *Auto-immunity.* 2006;39(6): 513–517.

156. Pohlau D, Przuntek H, Sailer M, et al. Intravenous immunoglobulin in primary and secondary chronic progressive multiple sclerosis: a randomized placebo controlled multicentre study. *Mult Scler.* 2007;13(9):1107–1117.

157. Massacesi L, Parigi A, Barilaro A, et al. Efficacy of azathioprine on multiple sclerosis new brain lesions evaluated using magnetic resonance imaging. *Arch Neurol.* 2005;62(12):1843–1847.

158. Massacesi L, Tramacere I, Amoroso S, et al. Azathioprine versus beta interferons for relapsing-remitting multiple sclerosis: a multicentre randomized non-inferiority trial. *PLoS One.* 2014;9(11):e113371.

159. Milder DG. Partial and significant reversal of progressive visual and neurological deficits in multiple sclerosis: a possible therapeutic effect. *Clin Experiment Ophthalmol.* 2002;30(5):363–366.

160. Fernandez O, Guerrero M, Mayorga C, et al. Combination therapy with interferon beta-1b and azathioprine in secondary progressive multiple sclerosis. A two-year pilot study. *J Neurol.* 2002;249(8):1058–1062.

161. Pulicken M, Bash CN, Costello K, et al. Optimization of the safety and efficacy of interferon beta 1b and azathioprine combination therapy in multiple sclerosis. *Mult Scler.* 2005;11(2):169–174.

162. Goodkin DE, Rudick RA, VanderBrug Medendorp S, et al. Low-dose (7.5 mg) oral methotrexate reduces the rate of progression in chronic progressive multiple sclerosis. *Ann Neurol.* 1995;37(1):30–40.

163. Lang TJ. Estrogen as an immunomodulator. *Clin Immunol.* 2004;113(3):224–230.

164. Salemi G, Callari G, Gammino M, et al. The relapse rate of multiple sclerosis changes during pregnancy: a study. *Acta Neurol Scand.* 2004;110(1):23–26.

165. Subramanian S, Matejuk A, Zamora A, Vandenbark AA, Offner H. Oral feeding with ethinyl estradiol suppresses and treats experimental auto-immune encephalomyelitis in SJL mice and inhibits the recruitment of inflammatory cells into the central nervous system. *J Immunol.* 2003;170(3):1548–1555.

166. Offner H. Neuroimmunoprotective effects of estrogen and derivatives in experimental auto-immune encephalomyelitis: therapeutic implications for multiple sclerosis. *J Neurosci Res.* 2004;78(5):603–624.

167. Hernan MA, Hohol MJ, Olek MJ, Spiegelman D, Ascherio A. Oral contraceptives and the incidence of multiple sclerosis. *Neurology.* 2000;55(6):848–854.

168. Alonso A, Jick SS, Olek MJ, Ascherio A, Jick H, Hernan MA. Recent use of oral contraceptives and the risk of multiple sclerosis. *Arch Neurol.* 2005;62(9):1362–1365.

169. Pozzilli C, De Giglio L, Barletta VT, et al. Oral contraceptives combined with interferon beta in multiple sclerosis. *Neurology(R) neuroimmunology & neuroinflammation.* 2015;2(4):e120.

170. Sicotte NL, Giesser BS, Tandon V, et al. Testosterone treatment in multiple sclerosis: a pilot study. *Arch Neurol.* 2007;64(5):683–688.

171. Kwiatkowska-Patzer B, Walski M, Frontczak-Baniewicz M, Zalewska T, Baranowska B, Lipkowski AW. Matrix metalloproteases activity and ultrastructural changes in the early phase of experimental allergic encephalomyelitis. The effect of oral treatment with spinal cord hydrolisate proteins in Lewis rat. The pilot study. *Folia Neuropathol.* 2004;42(2):107–111.

172. Brundula V, Rewcastle NB, Metz LM, Bernard CC, Yong VW. Targeting leukocyte MMPs and transmigration: minocycline as a potential therapy for multiple sclerosis. *Brain.* 2002;125(Pt 6):1297–1308.

173. Metz LM, Zhang Y, Yeung M, et al. Minocycline reduces gadolinium-enhancing magnetic resonance imaging lesions in multiple sclerosis. *Ann Neurol.* 2004;55(5):756.

174. Zabad RK, Metz LM, Todoruk TR, et al. The clinical response to minocycline in multiple sclerosis is accompanied by beneficial immune changes: a pilot study. *Mult Scler.* 2007;13(4):517–526.

175. Zhang Y, Metz LM, Yong VW, et al. Pilot study of minocycline in relapsing-remitting multiple sclerosis. *Can J Neurol Sci.* 2008;35(2):185–191.

176. Giuliani F, Fu SA, Metz LM, Yong VW. Effective combination of minocycline and interferon-beta in a model of multiple sclerosis. *J Neuroimmunol.* 2005;165(1–2): 83–91.

177. Luccarini I, Ballerini C, Biagioli T, et al. Combined treatment with atorvastatin and minocycline suppresses severity of EAE. *Exp Neurol.* 2008;211(1):214–226.

178. Agrawal YP. Low dose naltrexone therapy in multiple sclerosis. *Med Hypotheses.* 2005;64(4):721–724.

179. Rahn KA, McLaughlin PJ, Zagon IS. Prevention and diminished expression of experimental auto-immune encephalomyelitis by low dose naltrexone (LDN) or opioid growth factor (OGF) for an extended period: therapeutic implications for multiple sclerosis. *Brain Res.* 2011;1381:243–253.

180. Gironi M, Martinelli-Boneschi F, Sacerdote P, et al. A pilot trial of low-dose naltrexone in primary progressive multiple sclerosis. *Mult Scler.* 2008;14(8):1076–1083.

181. Sharafaddinzadeh N, Moghtaderi A, Kashipazha D, Majdinasab N, Shalbafan B. The effect of low-dose naltrexone on quality of life of patients with multiple sclerosis: a randomized placebo-controlled trial. *Mult Scler.* 2010;16(8):964–969.

182. Cree BA, Kornyeyeva E, Goodin DS. Pilot trial of low-dose naltrexone and quality of life in multiple sclerosis. *Ann Neurol.* 2010;68(2):145–150.

183. Youssef S, Stuve O, Patarroyo JC, et al. The HMG-CoA reductase inhibitor, atorvastatin, promotes a Th2 bias and reverses paralysis in central nervous system auto-immune disease. *Nature.* 2002;420(6911):78–84.

184. Ifergan I, Wosik K, Cayrol R, et al. Statins reduce human blood–brain barrier permeability and restrict leukocyte migration: relevance to multiple sclerosis. *Ann Neurol.* 2006;60(1):45–55.

185. Tsakiri A, Kallenbach K, Fuglo D, Wanscher B, Larsson H, Frederiksen J. Simvastatin improves final visual outcome in acute optic neuritis: a randomized study. *Mult Scler.* 2012;18(1):72–81.

186. Chataway J, Schuerer N, Alsanousi A, et al. Effect of high-dose simvastatin on brain atrophy and disability in secondary progressive multiple sclerosis (MS-STAT): a randomised, placebo-controlled, phase 2 trial. *Lancet.* 2014;383(9936): 2213–2221.

187. Perras C. Sativex for the management of multiple sclerosis symptoms. *Issues Emerg Health Technol.* 2005(72):1–4.

188. Zajicek JP, Sanders HP, Wright DE, et al. Cannabinoids in multiple sclerosis (CAMS) study: safety and efficacy data for 12 months follow up. *J Neurol Neurosurg Psychiatry.* 2005;76(12):1664–1669.

189. Jackson SJ, Diemel LT, Pryce G, Baker D. Cannabinoids and neuroprotection in CNS inflammatory disease. *J Neurol Sci.* 2005;233:21–5.

190. Malfitano AM, Matarese G, Bifulco M. From cannabis to endocannabinoids in multiple sclerosis: a paradigm of central nervous system auto-immune diseases. *Curr Drug Targets CNS Neurol Disord.* 2005;4(6):667–675.

191. Capello E, Saccardi R, Murialdo A, et al. Intense immunosuppression followed by autologous stem cell transplantation in severe multiple sclerosis. *Neurol Sci.* 2005;26(Supplement 4):s200–s203.

192. ABC News. Man walks again after MS stem cell treatment. Available at <www.abc.net. au/news/2009–12–14/man-walks-again-after-ms-stem-cell-treatment/2597864>, accessed 9 April 2015.

193. Fassas A, Kimiskidis VK, Sakellari I, et al. Long-term results of stem cell transplantation for MS: a single-center experience. *Neurology.* 2011;76(12):1066–1070.

194. Nash RA, Hutton GJ, Racke MK, et al. High-dose immunosuppressive therapy and autologous hematopoietic cell transplantation for relapsing-remitting multiple sclerosis (HALT-MS): a 3-year interim report. *JAMA neurology.* 2015;72(2):159–169.

195. Achiron A, Lavie G, Kishner I, et al. T cell vaccination in multiple sclerosis relapsing-remitting nonresponders patients. *Clin Immunol.* 2004;113(2):155–160.

196. Loftus B, Newsom B, Montgomery M, et al. Autologous attenuated T-cell vaccine (Tovaxin®) dose escalation in multiple sclerosis relapsing-remitting and secondary progressive patients nonresponsive to approved immunomodulatory therapies. *Clin Immunol.* 2009;131(2)202–215.

197. Karussis D, Shor H, Yachnin J, et al. T cell vaccination benefits relapsing progressive multiple sclerosis patients: a randomized, double-blind clinical trial. *PLoS One.* 2012;7(12):e50478.

198. Jurynczyk M, Walczak A, Jurewicz A, Jesionek-Kupnicka D, Szczepanik M, Selmaj K. Immune regulation of multiple sclerosis by transdermally applied myelin peptides. *Ann Neurol.* 2010;68(5):593–601.

199. Steinman L, Zamvil SS. Delivery of myelin peptides through the first line of defense, skin, to counter auto-immunity in multiple sclerosis. *Ann Neurol.* 2010;68(5): 567–569.

200. Stuve O, Cravens PD, Eagar TN. DNA-based vaccines: the future of multiple sclerosis therapy? *Expert Rev Neurother.* 2008;8(3):351–360.

201. Garren H, Robinson WH, Krasulova E, et al. Phase 2 trial of a DNA vaccine encoding myelin basic protein for multiple sclerosis. *Ann Neurol.* 2008;63(5):611–620.

202. Warren KG, Catz I, Ferenczi LZ, Krantz MJ. Intravenous synthetic peptide MBP8298 delayed disease progression in an HLA Class II-defined cohort of patients with progressive multiple sclerosis: results of a 24-month double-blind placebo-controlled clinical trial and 5 years of follow-up treatment. *Eur J Neurol.* 2006;13(8): 887–895.

203. Fleming JO, Isaak A, Lee JE, et al. Probiotic helminth administration in relapsing-remitting multiple sclerosis: a phase 1 study. *Mult Scler.* 2011;17(6):743–754.

204. Vermersch P, Benrabah R, Schmidt N, et al. Masitinib treatment in patients with progressive multiple sclerosis: a randomized pilot study. *BMC Neurol.* 2012;12:36.

205. Lycke J, Svennerholm B, Hjelmquist E, et al. Acyclovir treatment of relapsing-remitting multiple sclerosis. A randomized, placebo-controlled, double-blind study. *J Neurol.* 1996;243:214–224.

206. Friedman JE, Zabriskie JB, Plank C, et al. A randomized clinical trial of valacyclovir in multiple sclerosis. *Mult Scler.* 2005;11(3):286–295.

207. Scalfari A, Neuhaus A, Daumer M, Muraro PA, Ebers GC. Onset of secondary progressive phase and long-term evolution of multiple sclerosis. *J Neurol Neurosurg Psychiatry.* 2014;85(1):67–75.

208. Menzin J, Caon C, Nichols C, White LA, Friedman M, Pill MW. Narrative review of the literature on adherence to disease-modifying therapies among patients with multiple sclerosis. *J Manag Care Pharm.* 2013;19(1 Suppl A):S24–40.
209. Sheng P, Hou L, Wang X, et al. Efficacy of modafinil on fatigue and excessive daytime sleepiness associated with neurological disorders: a systematic review and meta-analysis. *PLoS One.* 2013;8(12):e81802.
210. Weiland TJ, Jelinek GA, Hadgkiss EJ, et al. Clinically significant fatigue: Prevalence and associated factors in an international sample of adults with multiple sclerosis. *PLOS One.* 2015;10(2):e0115541. doi: 10.1371/journal.pone.0115541.
211. Thelen JM, Lynch SG, Bruce AS, Hancock LM, Bruce JM. Polypharmacy in multiple sclerosis: Relationship with fatigue, perceived cognition, and objective cognitive performance. *J Psychosom Res.* 2014;76(5):400–404.
212. Zwibel HL, Smrtka J. Improving quality of life in multiple sclerosis: an unmet need. *Am J Manag Care.* 2011;17 Suppl 5 Improving:S139–145.
213. Berger JR. Functional improvement and symptom management in multiple sclerosis: clinical efficacy of current therapies. *Am J Manag Care.* 2011;17 Suppl 5 Improving:S146–153.
214. Johnson KP, Due DL. Benefits of glatiramer acetate in the treatment of relapsing-remitting multiple sclerosis. *Expert review of pharmacoeconomics & outcomes research.* 2009;9(3):205–214.
215. Ziemssen T, Bajenaru OA, Carra A, et al. A 2-year observational study of patients with relapsing-remitting multiple sclerosis converting to glatiramer acetate from other disease-modifying therapies: the COPTIMIZE trial. *J Neurol.* 2014;261(11):2101–2111.
216. Alkhawajah M, Oger J. When to initiate disease-modifying drugs for relapsing remitting multiple sclerosis in adults? *Mult Scler Int.* 2011;2011:724871.
217. Marrie RA, Salter AR, Tyry T, Fox RJ, Cutter GR. Preferred sources of health information in persons with multiple sclerosis: degree of trust and information sought. *J Med Internet Res.* 2013;15(4):e67.
218. Mayo Clinic. Personalised therapy for multiple sclerosis (MS). 2015. Available at <www.mayoclinic.org/diseases-conditions/multiple-sclerosis/in-depth/personalized-therapy-for-multiple-sclerosis/art-20095758?pg=2>, accessed 28 April 2015.
219. Soilu-Hanninen M, Aivo J, Lindstrom BM, et al. A randomised, double blind, placebo controlled trial with vitamin D3 as an add on treatment to interferon beta-1b in patients with multiple sclerosis. *J Neurol Neurosurg Psychiatry.* 2012;83(5):565–571.
220. Milo R. Effectiveness of multiple sclerosis treatment with current immunomodulatory drugs. *Expert Opin Pharmacother.* 2015;16(5):659–673.
221. Castelli-Haley J, Oleen-Burkey MK, Lage MJ, Johnson KP. Glatiramer acetate versus interferon beta-1a for subcutaneous administration: comparison of outcomes among multiple sclerosis patients. *Adv Ther.* 2008;25(7):658–673.
222. La Mantia L, Di Pietrantonj C, Rovaris M, et al. Comparative efficacy of interferon beta versus glatiramer acetate for relapsing-remitting multiple sclerosis. *J Neurol Neurosurg Psychiatry.* 2014;86(9):1016–1020.
223. Milanese C, Beghi E, Giordano L, La Mantia L, Mascoli N, Confalonieri P. A post-marketing study on immunomodulating treatments for relapsing-remitting multiple sclerosis in Lombardia: preliminary results. *Neurol Sci.* 2005;26 Suppl 4:s171–173.

224. Caon C, Din M, Ching W, Tselis A, Lisak R, Khan O. Clinical course after change of immunomodulating therapy in relapsing-remitting multiple sclerosis. *Eur J Neurol.* 2006;13(5):471–474.
225. Carra A, Onaha P, Luetic G, et al. Therapeutic outcome 3 years after switching of immunomodulatory therapies in patients with relapsing-remitting multiple sclerosis in Argentina. *Eur J Neurol.* 2008;15(4):386–393.
226. Gajofatto A, Bacchetti P, Grimes B, High A, Waubant E. Switching first-line disease-modifying therapy after failure: impact on the course of relapsing-remitting multiple sclerosis. *Mult Scler.* 2008;15(1):50–58.
227. Coyle PK. Switching algorithms: from one immunomodulatory agent to another. *J Neurol.* 2008;255 Suppl 1:44–50.

Step 6

1. Andersen O. Conclusion: National incidence and risk factor assessments may become a basis for the evaluation of prevention trials—prospects from the Third Nordic MS Symposium. *Acta Neurol Scand Suppl.* 2015;132(199):71–75.
2. Hernan MA, Oleky MJ, Ascherio A. Cigarette smoking and incidence of multiple sclerosis. *Am J Epidemiol.* 2001;154(1):69–74.
3. Riise T, Nortvedt MW, Ascherio A. Smoking is a risk factor for multiple sclerosis. *Neurology.* 2003;61(8):1122–1124.
4. Di Pauli F, Reindl M, Ehling R, et al. Smoking is a risk factor for early conversion to clinically definite multiple sclerosis. *Mult Scler.* 2008.
5. Hawkes CH. Smoking is a risk factor for multiple sclerosis: a metanalysis. *Mult Scler.* 2007;13(5):610–615.
6. Hernan MA, Jick SS, Logroscino G, Olek MJ, Ascherio A, Jick H. Cigarette smoking and the progression of multiple sclerosis. *Brain.* 2005;128:1461–1465.
7. Sundstrom P, Nystrom L. Smoking worsens the prognosis in multiple sclerosis. *Mult Scler.* 2008;14:1031–5.
8. Marrie RA, Horwitz RI, Cutter G, Tyry T, Vollmer T. Smokers with multiple sclerosis are more likely to report comorbid autoimmune diseases. *Neuroepidemiology.* 2011;36(2):85–90.
9. Ramanujam R, Hedstrom AK, Manouchehrinia A, et al. Effect of Smoking Cessation on Multiple Sclerosis Prognosis. *JAMA neurology.* 2015:1–7.
10. Ebers GC, Heigenhauser L, Daumer M, Lederer C, Noseworthy JH. Disability as an outcome in MS clinical trials. *Neurology.* 2008;71:624–31.
11. Mikaeloff Y, Caridade G, Tardieu M, Suissa S. Parental smoking at home and the risk of childhood-onset multiple sclerosis in children. *Brain.* 2007;130(Pt 10):2589–2595.
12. Hedstrom AK, Baarnhielm M, Olsson T, Alfredsson L. Exposure to environmental tobacco smoke is associated with increased risk for multiple sclerosis. *Mult Scler.* 2011;17(7):788–793.
13. van der Mei IA, Ponsonby AL, Dwyer T, et al. Past exposure to sun, skin phenotype, and risk of multiple sclerosis: case-control study. *BMJ.* 2003;327(7410):316.
14. Munger KL, Zhang SM, O'Reilly E, et al. Vitamin D intake and incidence of multiple sclerosis. *Neurology.* 2004;62(1):60–65.

15. Brown SJ. The role of vitamin D in multiple sclerosis. *Ann Pharmacother.* 2006;40(6): 1158–1161.

16. Ramagopalan SV, Maugeri NJ, Handunnetthi L, et al. Expression of the multiple sclerosis-associated MHC class II Allele HLA-DRB1*1501 is regulated by vitamin D. *PLoS Genet.* 2009;5(2):e1000369.

17. Salzer J, Hallmans G, Nystrom M, Stenlund H, Wadell G, Sundstrom P. Vitamin D as a protective factor in multiple sclerosis. *Neurology.* 2012;79(21):2140–2145.

18. Derakhshandi H, Etemadifar M, Feizi A, et al. Preventive effect of vitamin D3 supplementation on conversion of optic neuritis to clinically definite multiple sclerosis: a double blind, randomized, placebo-controlled pilot clinical trial. *Acta Neurol Belg.* 2013;113(3):257–263.

19. Sundstrom P, Salzer J. Vitamin D and multiple sclerosis—from epidemiology to prevention. *Acta Neurol Scand Suppl.* 2015;132(199):56–61.

20. Chapman S, MacKenzie R. The global research neglect of unassisted smoking cessation: causes and consequences. *PLoS medicine.* 2010;7(2):e1000216.

21. Etter JF, Burri M, Stapleton J. The impact of pharmaceutical company funding on results of randomized trials of nicotine replacement therapy for smoking cessation: a meta-analysis. *Addiction.* 2007;102(5):815–822.

22. Parry O, Thomson C, Fowkes FG. Dependent behaviours and beliefs: a qualitative study of older long-term smokers with arterial disease. *Addiction.* 2001;96(9): 1337–1347.

23. Chaudhuri A. Why we should offer routine vitamin D supplementation in pregnancy and childhood to prevent multiple sclerosis. *Med Hypothesis* 2005;64:608–18.

24. Torkildsen O, Grytten N, Aarseth J, Myhr KM, Kampman MT. Month of birth as a risk factor for multiple sclerosis: an update. *Acta Neurol Scand Suppl* 2012;195: 58–62.

Step 7

1. Hadgkiss EJ, Jelinek GA, Taylor KL, et al. Engagement in a program promoting lifestyle modification is associated with better patient-reported outcomes for people with MS. *Neurol Sci.* 2015;36(6):845–52. doi: 10.1007/s10072–015–2089–1.

2. Ornish D, Scherwitz LW, Billings JH, et al. Intensive lifestyle changes for reversal of coronary heart disease. *JAMA.* 1998;280(23):2001–2007.

3. Ornish D, Weidner G, Fair WR, et al. Intensive lifestyle changes may affect the progression of prostate cancer. *J Urol.* 2005;174(3):1065–1069; discussion 1069–1070.

4. Swank RL, Dugan BB. Effect of low saturated fat diet in early and late cases of multiple sclerosis. *Lancet.* 1990;336(8706):37–39.

5. Li MP, Jelinek GA, Weiland TJ, Mackinlay CA, Dye S, Gawler I. Effect of a residential retreat promoting lifestyle modifications on health-related quality of life in people with multiple sclerosis. *Quality in primary care.* 2010;18(6):379–389.

6. Campbell JD, Ghushchyan V, Brett McQueen R, et al. Burden of multiple sclerosis on direct, indirect costs and quality of life: National US estimates. *Multiple sclerosis and related disorders.* 2014;3(2):227–236.

7. Janzen W, Turpin KV, Warren SA, Marrie RA, Warren KG. Change in the health-related quality of life of multiple sclerosis patients over 5 years. *Int J MS Care.* 2013;15(1):46–53.

8. Hadgkiss EJ, Jelinek GA, Weiland TJ, et al. Health-related quality of life outcomes at 1 and 5 years after a residential retreat promoting lifestyle modification for people with multiple sclerosis. *Neurol Sci.* 2013;34(2):187–195.

9. Weiland TJ, Jelinek GA, Hadgkiss EJ, et al. Clinically significant fatigue: prevalence and associated factors in an international sample of adults with multiple sclerosis. *PLOS One.* 2015;10(2):e0115541. doi: 10.1371/journal.pone.0115541.

10. Taylor KT, Hadgkiss EJ, Jelinek GA, et al. Lifestyle and demographic factors and medications associated with depression risk in an international sample of people with multiple sclerosis. *BMC Psychiatry.* 2014;14:327. doi: 10.1186/s12888-014-0327-3.

11. Ioannidis JP. Why most published research findings are false. *PLoS medicine.* 2005;2(8):e124.

12. Riccio P, Rossano R. Nutrition facts in multiple sclerosis. *ASN Neuro.* 2015;7(1). doi: 10.1177/1759091414568185.

13. Kern S, Ziemssen T. Review: brain–immune communication psychoneuroimmunology of multiple sclerosis. *Mult Scler.* 2007;14:6–21.

14. Marrie RA, Salter A, Tyry T, Fox RJ, Cutter GR. Health literacy association with health behaviors and health care utilization in multiple sclerosis: a cross-sectional study. *Interactive journal of medical research.* 2014;3(1):e3.

15. Sumowski JF, Wylie GR, DeLuca J, Chiaravalloti N. Intellectual enrichment is linked to cerebral efficiency in multiple sclerosis: functional magnetic resonance imaging evidence for cognitive reserve. *Brain* 2010;133:362–74.

16. Sumowski JF, Rocca MA, Leavitt VM, et al. Brain reserve and cognitive reserve in multiple sclerosis: what you've got and how you use it. *Neurology.* 2013;80(24):2186–2193.

17. Tan-Kristanto S, Kiropoulos LA. Resilience, self-efficacy, coping styles and depressive and anxiety symptoms in those newly diagnosed with multiple sclerosis. *Psychology, Health & Medicine.* 2015;20(6):635–645.

18. Baumhackl U. The search for a balance between short and long-term treatment outcomes in multiple sclerosis. *J Neurol.* 2008;255 Suppl 1:75–83.

19. Jelinek GA, Gawler RH. Thirty-year follow-up at pneumonectomy of a 58-year-old survivor of disseminated osteosarcoma. *Med J Aust.* 2008;189(11–12):663–665.

20. Ornish D, Magbanua MJ, Weidner G, et al. Changes in prostate gene expression in men undergoing an intensive nutrition and lifestyle intervention. *Proc Natl Acad Sci USA.* 2008;105(24):8369–8374.

21. Jelinek GA, Hassed CS. Managing multiple sclerosis in primary care: are we forgetting something? *Qual Prim Care.* 2009;17(1):55–61.

22. Brownson RC, Kreuter MW, Arrington BA, True WR. Translating scientific discoveries into public health action: how can schools of public health move us forward? *Public Health Rep.* 2006;121(1):97–103.

INDEX